# Skew-Normal Model Theories and Their Applications


**Rendao Ye**
College of Economics, Hangzhou Dianzi University
People's Republic of China

**Kun Luo**
Alibaba Business School, Hangzhou Normal University
People's Republic of China

**Wenyan Zhu**
College of Economics, Hangzhou Dianzi University
People's Republic of China

**Yue Qi**
College of Economics, Hangzhou Dianzi University
People's Republic of China

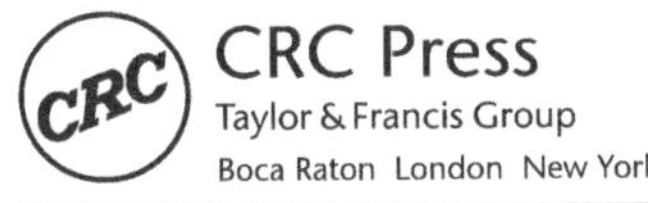


CRC Press
Taylor & Francis Group
Boca Raton  London  New York

CRC Press is an imprint of the
Taylor & Francis Group, an **informa** business

A SCIENCE PUBLISHERS BOOK

First edition published 2025
by CRC Press
2385 NW Executive Center Drive, Suite 320, Boca Raton FL 33431

and by CRC Press
4 Park Square, Milton Park, Abingdon, Oxon, OX14 4RN

© 2025 Rendao Ye, Kun Luo, Wenyan Zhu and Yue Qi

*CRC Press is an imprint of Taylor & Francis Group, LLC*



*Library of Congress Cataloging-in-Publication Data (applied for)*

ISBN: 978-1-032-69469-6 (hbk)
ISBN: 978-1-032-71149-2 (pbk)
ISBN: 978-1-032-71147-8 (ebk)

DOI: 10.1201/9781032711478

Typeset in Times New Roman
by Prime Publishing Services

# Preface

The mixed effects model is an important statistical model with broad application backgrounds. However, the classical theories and methods, mostly based on the assumption of normal distribution, can not be directly applied to statistical modeling with skew-normal data which are common in reality, and therefore are inadequate for practical data analysis and problem-solving. This book is aimed at the mixed effects model with skew-normal distribution, and discusses various statistical inference problems. This book is of academic value, since it helps to establish a series of statistical inference theories and methods for mixed effects models with skew-normal distribution. It will also provide efficient methods and tools for practical data analysis in various fields including economics, finance, biology and medical science, which features its application value.

Chapter 1 introduces various kinds of skew-normal mixed effects models, and their research status, methods, characteristics and content. Chapter 2 presents the preliminary knowledge including multivariate skew-normal and skew-normal matrix distributions. In Chapters 3 to 10 we employ matrix techniques, maximum likelihood estimation, the Bootstrap approach, the generalized approach and Monte Carlo simulation. Through these methods we set up a series of new and effective statistical inference methods for all kinds of skew-normal model. These include skew-normal population models, one-way classification models with skew-normal random effects, unbalanced one-way classification models with skew-normal random effects models, skew-normal unbalanced heteroscedastic one-way classification random effects model, skew-normal unbalanced panel models with one-way error components, two-way classification random effects models with skew-normal errors, and skew-normal mixed effects models.

This book owes much to many people. My Ph.D. supervisor, Professor Songgui Wang, provided extensive care, guidance and support during my time at the Beijing University of Technology. Next, I would like to express my gratitude to Professor Tonghui Wang from New Mexico State University, for his warm hospitality and guidance, which helped me delve into the field of skew-normal models. I am thankful to my master's graduate students from Hangzhou Dianzi University, including Zhongchi Wang, Lijun Xu, Jian Qi, Weixiao Du, Na An, Ya Lin, Ling Jiang, Bingni Fang and Yilan Zhang. Special appreciation goes to the editor Vijay at CRC press for her encouragement and assistance. Finally, I dedicate this book to my lovely daughter, Han Ye, and hope she grows up happily.

Dec. 2023                                                                     Rendao Ye

# Contents

# Chapter 1

# Introduction

The mixed effects model (MEM) has found broad applications in various fields such as economics, finance, business, biology, medical science, engineering technology and social science. The MEM proves effective in explaining many phenomena and problems in these areas. In comparison with the traditional statistical models, the MEM excels in describing correlated information among the data enhancing model precision by through the introduction of random effects. Consequently, this model serves as a valuable tool to analyze correlated data such as longitudinal data and panel data.

In practical applications, the skew data sets are by no means exceptions but facts of life in many diverse fields such as economics, finance, biomedicine, environment, demography, and pharmacokinetics. Usually for mathematical convenience, they are assumed to follow the normal distribution, despite their skewness. However, this restrictive may result in a lack of robustness against departures from normality, leading to invalid statistical inferences, especially when dealing with skewed data. Among numerous skew distributions, the skew-normal distribution is undoubtedly the most common one for fitting skewed data sets. However, existing classic theories and methods of the normal mixed effects model (MEM) may not sufficiently provide precise statistical inference for the practical skew data sets. Therefore, it is both theoretically and practically important to develop statistical models under the skew-normal assumption.

## 1.1 Model outline

The skew-normal MEM is given by

$$y = X\beta + Z\varepsilon + \varepsilon_0, \tag{1.1}$$

where $y$ is a $n \times 1$ random vector, $X$ and $Z$ are $n \times p$ and $n \times k$ design matrices, respectively, $\beta$ is a $p \times 1$ vector of fixed effects, $\varepsilon$ is a $k \times 1$ vector of random effects, and $\varepsilon_0$ a $n \times 1$ vector of random errors. Generally speaking, we assume that the random effect item or random error item is distributed as the skew-normal distribution. It is clear that the random part $Z\varepsilon + \varepsilon_0$ in model (1.1) could be decomposed as

$$Z\varepsilon + \varepsilon_0 = \sum_{i=1}^{k} Z_i \varepsilon_i + \varepsilon_0,$$

where $Z_i$ is a $n \times q_i$ known design matrix, $\varepsilon_i$ is a $q_i \times 1$ vector of random effects. Thus, model (1.1) could be further represented as

$$y = X\beta + \sum_{i=1}^{k} Z_i \varepsilon_i + \varepsilon_0, \tag{1.2}$$

In the literature, model (1.2) is called known as the variance component model. In model (1.2), when $X$ and $Z_i$ are the indicator matrices composed of 0 and 1, then it is named the mixed variance component model. When $X\beta = 1_n \mu$, then it is named the general random effects model, where $1_a$ is a $a \times 1$ vector with each component equals 1, and $\mu$ is the population mean. Note that model (1.2) encompasses many important statistical models, including the one-way classification model with random effects, the two-way classification random effects model with interaction, and the panel model with one-way error component.

**Example 1.1** This is an example of a one-way classification model with random effects In the exposure assessment, let $x_{ij}$ denote the $j$th shift-long exposure measurement for the $i$th worker, $i = 1, \cdots, k, j = 1, \cdots, b$. It is assumed that $y_{ij} = ln(x_{ij})$. The one-way classification model with random effects for $y_{ij}$'s is given by

$$y_{ij} = \mu + \alpha_i + e_{ij}, i = 1, \cdots, a, j = 1, \cdots, b, \tag{1.3}$$

where $\mu$ is the overall mean, $\alpha_i$ is the random effect due to the $i$th worker, and $e_{ij}$ is the random error. Using the matrix symbol, model (1.3) could be rewritten as the form of (1.1). Denote $y = (y_{11}, \cdots, y_{1b}, \cdots, y_{a1}, \cdots, y_{ab})', \varepsilon_0 = (e_{11}, \cdots, e_{1b}, \cdots, e_{a1}, \cdots, e_{ab})', Z = I_a \otimes 1_b, \varepsilon = (\alpha_1, \alpha_2, \cdots, \alpha_a)'$, where $\otimes$ denotes the Kronecker product and $I_m$ is an identity matrix of order $m$. Then model (1.3) is expressed as

$$y = 1_{ab}\mu + Z\varepsilon + \varepsilon_0. \tag{1.4}$$

**Example 1.2** Two-way classification random effects model with interaction. We consider a reliability study in which each of the $a$ subjects is independently measured by each of the $b$ raters with $k$ replicates. It is also assumed that both subjects and raters are randomly selected from their populations. The corresponding model is a two-way classification random effects model with interaction. Let $y_{ijk}$ be the $k$th measurement on the $i$th subject by the $j$th rater, which could be represented as

$$y_{ijk} = \mu + \alpha_i + \beta_j + \gamma_{ij} + e_{ijk}, i = 1, \cdots, a, j = 1, \cdots, b, k = 1, \cdots, c, \quad (1.5)$$

where $\mu$ is the overall mean, $\alpha_i$ is the random effect due to the $i$th subject, $\beta_j$ is the random effect due to the $j$th rater, $\gamma_{ij}$ is the effect of the interaction between the $i$th subject and the $j$th rater, and $e_{ijk}$ is the random error. Denote $y = (y_{111}, \cdots, y_{11c}, \cdots, y_{ab1}, \cdots, y_{abc})', \varepsilon_0 = (e_{111}, \cdots, e_{11c}, \cdots, e_{ab1}, \cdots, e_{abc})', Z_3 = I_a \otimes 1_a \otimes 1_c, Z_2 = I_a \otimes 1_a \otimes 1_c, Z_1 = I_a \otimes 1_a \otimes 1_c, \varepsilon_3 = (\alpha_1, \alpha_2, \cdots, \alpha_a)', \varepsilon_2 = (\beta_1, \beta_2, \cdots, \beta_b)', \varepsilon_1 = (\gamma_{11}, \cdots, \gamma_{1b}, \cdots, \gamma_{a1}, \cdots, \gamma_{ab})'$. Then model (1.5) is expressed as

$$y = 1_{abc}\mu + Z_3\varepsilon_3 + Z_2\varepsilon_2 + Z_1\varepsilon_1 + \varepsilon_0. \quad (1.6)$$

**Example 1.3** Panel model with one-way error component Panel model with one-way error component is one of the MEM with the widest applications in econometrics. Suppose that we observe $N$ individuals for $T$ time points. Let $y_{it}$ be some economic index of the $i$th individual at the $t$th time point, then we have

$$y_{it} = \alpha + x_{it}'\beta + \mu_i + e_{it}, i = 1, \cdots, N, t = 1, \cdots, T, \quad (1.7)$$

where $\alpha$ is a scalar, $x_{it}$ is a $k \times 1$ known vector, $\beta$ is a $k \times 1$ vector of regression coefficients, $\mu_i$ is the random effect of the $i$th individual, and $e_{it}$ is the random error. Denote $y = (y_{11}, \cdots, y_{1T}, \cdots, y_{N1}, \cdots, y_{NT})', X = (x_{11}, \cdots, x_{1T}, \cdots, x_{N1}, \cdots, x_{NT})', Z = I_N \otimes 1_T, \varepsilon = (\mu_1, \mu_2, \cdots, \mu_N)', \varepsilon_0 = (e_{11}, \cdots, e_{1T}, \cdots, e_{N1}, \cdots, e_{NT})', X^* = (1_{NT}, X), \beta^* = (\alpha, \beta')'$. Then model (1.7) is expressed as

$$y = X^*\beta^* + Z\varepsilon + \varepsilon_0. \quad (1.8)$$

## 1.2 Research status

### *1.2.1 Skew-normal distribution*

In recent years, the real data of economics, physics and epidemiology often show obvious skewed and asymmetric characteristics (Lin et al., 2007; Basso et al., 2010; Fruhwirth-Schnatter and Pyne, 2020). The routine use of the normality assumption has been questioned by many authors (Verbeke and Lesaffre, 1997; Zhang and Davidian, 2001; Pinheiro et al., 2001; Ghidey et al., 2004; Lin and Lee, 2008; Lachos et al., 2009; Ye et al., 2014). For this, Azzalini (1985) first proposed the skew-normal distribution by introducing the skewness parameter, whose alteration allows for a continuous variation from normality to skew-normality.

In view of the wide applications of the skew-normal distribution, many scholars further explored its statistical properties. Some recent studies include: characterizations of distributions (Arnold and Lin, 2004; Gupta et al., 2004), characteristic functions (Kim and Genton, 2011), sampling distributions (Su and Gupta, 2015), distribution of quadratic forms (Gupta and Huang, 2002; Wang et al., 2009; Ye et al., 2014), measures of skewness and divergence (Balakrishnan and Scarpa, 2012; Contreras-Reyes and Arellano-Valle, 2012), asymptotic expansions for moments of the extremes (Liao et al., 2013), rates of convergence of the extremes (Liao et al., 2014), exact density of the sum of independent random variables (Nadarajah and Li, 2017), identifiability of finite mixtures of the skew-normal distributions (Otiniano et al., 2015), and more. On this basis, we can use the skew-normal distribution as the fitted distribution of real data and establish a statistical model to solve the practical problem. Some recent applications include: modelling of air pollution data (Bartoletti and Loperfido, 2010), modelling of psychiatric measures (Counsell et al., 2011), modelling of bounded health scores (Hutton and Stanghellini, 2011), modelling of insurance claims (Eling, 2012), asset pricing (Carmichael and Coen, 2013), individual loss reserving (Pigeon et al., 2013), robust portfolio estimation (Taniguchi et al., 2015), growth estimates of cardinalfish (Contreras-Reyes et al., 2013), age-specific fertility rates (Mazzuco and Scarpa, 2015), reliability studies (Gupta and Brown, 2001), statistical process control (Figueiredo and Gomes, 2013), analysis of student satisfaction towards university courses (Montanari and Viroli, 2010), detecting differential expression to microRNA data (Hossain and Beyene, 2015), among others.

Due to the complex structure of the skew-normal distribution, the traditional parameter estimation method is difficult to be applied directly. To this end, Pewsey (2000a) studied the weaknesses of the direct parameterization in parameter estimation and proposed the centered parameterization method. Pewsey (2000b, 2006) applied this method to the wrapped skew-normal population and gave the methods of moment estimation and maximum likelihood (ML) estimation. Arellano-Valle and Azzalini (2008) extended the centered parameterization method to the multivariate skew-normal distribution and studied its information matrix. Furthermore, due to the wide application of the location parameter in econometrics, medicinal chemistry and life testing, the research on the location parameter of skew-normal distribution has attracted the attention of many scholars. For example, Wang et al. (2016) discussed the interval estimation of the location parameter when the coefficient of variation and skewness parameter are known. Thiuthad and Pal (2018) considered the hypothesis testing problem of the location parameter and constructed three test statistics when the scale parameter and skewness parameter are known. Ma et al. (2019) studied the interval estimation and hypothesis testing problems of the location parameter with known scale and skewness parameters. Based on the approximate likelihood equations, Gui and Guo (2018) derived the explicit estimators of the scale and location parameters.

On this basis, some inference problems of skew-normal statistical models are investigated. For example, within a Bayesian framework, Maleki and Wraith (2019) combined the skew-normal distribution with the factor analysis model to derive a mixture of the skew-normal factor analysis model and its parameter estimation. Based on the functional principal component analysis, Hu et al. (2020) discussed the ML estimation of the skew-normal partial functional linear model. Arellano-Valle et al. (2019) used the forward filtering and backward sampling method to study the Bayesian inference of the skew-normal dynamic linear model, and applied this methodology to the analysis of the condition factor index of male and female anchovies off northern Chile. Based on the penalized ML estimation and penalized EM-type algorithm, Jin et al. (2019) proposed the ML estimation of the skew-normal mixture model. Said et al. (2017) derived a detection procedure based on the likelihood ratio test for the change point problem of the skew-normal distribution, and applied it to the stock return problem.

### *1.2.2  Bootstrap approach*

Since it is difficult to directly apply the traditional test approaches to construct exact test statistics, Efron (1979) proposed the Bootstrap approach based on the computer numerical algorithm. This approach is very attractive as it performs satisfactorily in many cases, which has been widely used for statistical inference problems such as error estimation, hypothesis testing and interval estimation. For example, Krishnamoorthy et al. (2007) and Ma and Tian (2009) developed the Bootstrap test procedures for the equalities of several normal means and several inverse Gaussian means respectively. The given tests were compared with the generalized tests, and simulation results indicated that the Bootstrap tests tended to outperform the generalized tests in terms of size.

Furthermore, Yang et al. (2012) proposed the Bootstrap test of the variance component in the balanced one-way classification random effects model. Zhang et al. (2021) developed overall mean test procedures of heteroscedastic one-way analysis of variance problems based on parametric Bootstrap and objective Bayesian approaches. Xu et al. (2014, 2016) constructed the parametric Bootstrap tests for the main effects in unbalanced two-factor and three-factor nested designs under heteroscedasticity. Xu et al. (2015) studied the equivalence testing problem of factor effects in the two-way ANOVA model without interaction under heteroscedasticity, whose results showed that the Bootstrap approach is better than the generalized F approach. Yue et al. (2015) constructed the Bootstrap test statistics of regression coefficients for the two-way error component regression model. Sinha (2009), Ye and Jiang (2018) and Ye et al. (2022) applied the Bootstrap approach to the unbalanced two-way random effects model. Hypothesis testing problems for variance components in panel data models and generalized linear mixed models were studied by them.

## *1.2.3 Generalized approach*

For a complex statistical model, the unknown parameters could be divided into parameters of interest and nuisance parameters. Usually, the number of nuisance parameter is more than that of parameter of interest, making the study of the parameter of interest more complex. In such cases, conventional approaches may be difficult to apply or fail to provide effective inferences. However, it is productive to obtain test statistics and confidence intervals based on the generalized p-value and generalized confidence interval (Krishnamoorthy and Guo, 2005; Jose and Luke, 2012; Li and Li, 2005; Li, 2007; Ye et al., 2014; Ma and Wang, 2007; Zhao et al., 2014; Zhao et al., 2014). This approach proves valuable whenever standard test statistics and standard pivot quantities are either non-existent or difficult to obtain based on conventional methods.

Recently, the generalized approach has garnered significant attention from scholars, leading to important progress. For example, Tian (2006), Park (2010), Krishnamoorthy and Mathew (2003), Krishnamoorthy et al. (2011), and Gamage et al. (2004) studied the statistical inference problem of the overall mean in normal, lognormal and inverse Gaussian populations. Krishnamoorthy and Lu (2003), Lin and Lee (2005), and Ye et al. (2010) considered the inference problem of the common mean in normal and inverse Gaussian populations. Furthermore, Weerahandi (1991), Arendacka (2005), and Mathew and Webb (2005) discussed the hypothesis testing and confidence interval problems of variance components for various simple mixed effects models. Weerahandi and Berger (1999), Lin and Lee (2003), and Chi and Weerahandi (1998) explored the testing problem of fixed effects for various simple growth curve models.

Building on this, Tian (2005), Ye and Wang (2009), and Gilder et al. (2007) investigated inference problems of intraclass correlation coefficients for various random effects models. Weerahandi and Johnson (1992), Roy and Mathew (2005), and Krishnamoorthy and Lin (2010) researched interval estimation problems of reliability parameters in normal, exponential and Weibull populations. Mathew et al. (2007) and Hsu et al. (2008) considered the confidence interval of several process capability indexes in the normal population. Finally, Li et al. (2007) and Hannig et al. (2006) constructed the generalized p-value and generalized confidence interval by using fiducial inference theory. Xu and Liu (2008) studied the hypothesis testing and interval estimation problems of mixed ratio in the mixed model. Xiong et al. (2008) discussed the testing problems of location parameter and scale parameter in the heteroscedastic linear model. These results provide practical and reliable methods for real data analysis.

## 1.3  Research methods and ideas

This book focuses on the skew-normal population, one-way classification model with skew-normal random effects, unbalanced one-way classification model with skew-normal random effects, skew-normal unbalanced heteroscedastic one-way classification random effects model, skew-normal unbalanced panel model with one-way error component, skew-normal two-way classification random effects model with interaction, and skew-normal mixed effects model. At the same time, we comprehensively employ various research methods and tools, including matrix techniques, maximum likelihood estimation, EM algorithm, Bootstrap method, generalized method, and Monte Carlo method. The book addresses statistical inference problems such as excellent estimate and exact testing of unknown parameters. A series of novel and effective statistical inference methods are developed and applied to practical data analysis in fields such as economics, finance, biology, and medicine. The specific research methods are as follows.

(i) Fine matrix techniques: Matrix techniques play an indispensable role in thoroughly studying the statistical excellence of parameter estimation methods, particularly fine techniques involving vector operations and matrix derivatives. Cleverly integrating these matrix techniques with maximum likelihood estimation can significantly enhance efficiency in statistical analysis.

(ii) Maximum likelihood estimation and EM algorithm: Due to the complexity of the skew-normal density function, it is difficult to obtain explicit solutions for the parameters of interest based on maximum likelihood estimation. Therefore, the EM algorithm is employed to obtain maximum likelihood estimates for the parameters of interest.

(iii) Bootstrap approach and generalized approach: When considering hypothesis testing problem for parameters of interest, the Bootstrap approach and generalized approach are utilized to construct test statistics and pivotal quantities for parameters such as fixed effect, variance component function, and common location parameter.

(iv) Monte Carlo method: To validate the rationality and effectiveness of new methods, the Monte Carlo method is employed to calculate statistical indexes such as Type I error probability, power, coverage probability, and interval length.

Based the above various methods, the research framework of this book is as follows:

Firstly, when the scale parameter and skewness parameter are unknown, we focus on hypothesis testing and interval estimation problem for the location parameter and common location parameter in several skew-normal populations. This involves constructing moment and maximum likelihood estimates for unknown parameters and providing Bootstrap test statistics and Bootstrap confidence intervals for location and common location parameters.

Secondly, for various complex models such as one-way classification model with skew-normal random effects, unbalanced one-way classification model with skew-normal random effects, skew-normal unbalanced heteroscedastic one-way classification random effects model, skew-normal unbalanced panel model with one-way error components, skew-normal two-way classification random effects model with interaction. We investigate hypothesis testing and interval estimation problems for fixed effect and variance component functions. Using a combination of the Bootstrap approach, generalized approach, and fine matrix technique, we establish corresponding testing methods and confidence intervals. Furthermore, we explore theoretical properties, such as invariance and theoretical confidence levels.

Thirdly, for the skew-normal mixed effects model, we construct exact tests for regression coefficients and variance components based on the noncentral skew-F distribution, providing their statistical properties.

Fourthly, for the aforementioned research methods, we employ the Monte Carlo method to simulate evaluation indicators including Type I error probability, power, coverage probability, and interval length. This evaluation is conducted to assess the reasonability and effectiveness of these methods.

Finally, the methods established in this book are applied to practical data analysis in fields such as economics, finance, biology, and medicine. This provides a straightforward and effective approach to solve real-world problems.

## 1.4 Research characteristics and innovation points

This book delves into a theoretical exploration that deepens the existing understanding of parameter estimation and testing for skew-normal mixed effects models. Moreover, it aligns well with the skew-normal distribution, imbalance, and heteroscedasticity of actual longitudinal data, thereby enhancing the precision of statistical inferences and facilitating effective solutions to practical problems. Specifically, this book is characterized by the following innovations:

(i) Under the skew-normal distribution, fine matrix techniques are employed to construct excellent estimates for parameters of interest.

Under the assumption of skew-normal distribution, the existing traditional parameter estimation theories and methods which are based on the normal distribution are challenging to directly apply to mixed effects models. Therefore, this book ingeniously employs fine matrix techniques, such as vector operations and matrix derivatives, along with statistical methods like maximum likelihood estimation and EM algorithm. These techniques are used to construct excellent estimates for parameters of interest, including regression coefficients, variance component functions, skewness parameters, and common location parameters.

(ii) Under the skew-normal distribution, the Bootstrap approach and generalized approach are utilized to establish excellent tests for parameters of interest.

Due to the complexity of the density function under the skew-normal distribution assumption, traditional methods cannot be directly applied to construct test statistics for parameters of interest. Therefore, the study employs the Bootstrap approach and generalized approach to establish excellent tests for parameters of interest, such as regression coefficients, variance component functions, and common location parameters. This is a challenging task, but one that holds strong theoretical and practical significance, representing a key innovation in this research.

(iii) Based on the noncentral skew-F distribution, exact tests for parameters of interest are constructed, establishing hypothesis testing theories and methods for the skew-normal mixed effects model.

Previous studies have indicated that, under the assumption of skew-normal distribution, for parameters of interest such as regression coefficients and variance components, constructed based on the ratio of quadratic forms of two observed vectors do not follow a noncentral distribution in the usual sense. Consequently, corresponding testing methods cannot be established. In response to this, this book defines a new distribution, namely the noncentral skew-F distribution. This distribution is defined as the ratio of quadratic forms of two observed vectors under the assumption of a skew-normal distribution. Building upon this, exact tests for parameters of interest, including regression coefficients and variance components, are developed.

(iv) Applying the aforementioned statistical inference theories and methods, we analyze key and hot issues in the current economic and social fields. Our aim is to enhance the precision of statistical inference in practical economic and social problems, and improve the effectiveness of real data analysis.

Drawing upon the statistical inference theories and methods mentioned above, this book conducts statistical analyses on real-world issues such as regional GDP, birth rate, and gasoline consumption. The aim is to make more accurate and effective statistical inferences, contributing to the resolution of practical problems. The insights gained from this longitudinal data analysis in other fields also have relevance and applicability. These studies are instructive for longitudinal data analysis in other fields.

This work systematically investigates the fundamental theories, methods, and applications of several skew-normal mixed effects models, including skew-normal population, one-way classification model with skew-normal random effects, unbalanced one-way classification model with skew-normal random effects. The academic value and scientific significance are as follows.

(i) Constructing feasible estimation and testing for mixed effects models under conditions of skew-normal distribution, imbalance, and heteroscedasticity. The statistical excellence of these constructions is demonstrated, deepening and extending the existing statistical inference theories for such models.

(ii) The statistical inference theories and methods developed in this book can accurately capture the characteristics of real longitudinal data, such as asymmetry and multimodality. This enhances the precision of statistical inference, providing a new and effective statistical method.

(iii) The research outcomes of this work can, to a certain extent, reveal general patterns in statistical inference for skew-normal longitudinal data. These findings have informative implications for the analysis of other forms of skewed longitudinal data, such as skew-t and skew-elliptical distributions.

## 1.5 Research content and frame

This book focuses on the skew-normal population, one-way classification model with skew-normal random effects, unbalanced one-way classification model with skew-normal random effects, skew-normal unbalanced heteroscedastic one-way classification random effects model, skew-normal unbalanced panel model with one-way error component, skew-normal two-way classification random effects model with interaction, and skew-normal mixed effects model. This book systematically explores the statistical inference theories, methods, and applications of parameters of interest. The specific research content and framework are as follows:

Chapter 1 introduces various skew-normal mixed effects models through examples and provides an overview of the current state of domestic and international research, methods, characteristics, innovations, content, and framework. It aims to give readers some understanding of the rich practical background and related research of such models, facilitating comprehension of the content in the subsequent chapters.

Chapter 2 presents the preliminary knowledge to build statistical inference theories and methods for skew-normal mixed effects models, including multivariate skew-normal and skew-normal matrix distributions, Bootstrap approach, and generalized approach. Specific discussions contain statistical properties of skew-normal vectors and matrices, such as mean and covariance matrix, distributions of linear function and quadratic form. Additionally, it covers statistical methods like Bootstrap tests, Bootstrap confidence intervals, and fundamental concepts of generalized test variables, generalized p-values, generalized pivotal quantities, and generalized confidence intervals.

In Chapter 3, we research the problem of a homogeneous test of location parameters in several skew-normal populations when the scale parameters and skewness parameters are unknown. We construct the conditional test statistic and prove its approximate distribution. Furthermore, we estimate the unknown parameters based on the methods of moments and maximum likelihood estimation. Additionally, we construct Bootstrap test statistics, generalizing the results of Xu (2016) from the normal population to the skew-normal population.

In Chapter 4, we research the interval estimation and hypothesis testing problems for the common location parameter of several skew-normal populations when the scale parameters and skewness parameters are unknown. We construct Bootstrap confidence intervals and Bootstrap test statistics, which generalize the results given by Xu (2016) under several normal populations.

In Chapter 5, we present some statistical properties of one-way classification model with skew-normal random effects. Based on the EM algorithm, we provide the ML estimation of unknown parameters. Further, we discuss the hypothesis testing and interval estimation problems of fixed effects and variance component functions.

In Chapter 6, we consider the one-sided hypothesis testing and interval estimation problems for fixed effect and variance component functions in the unbalanced one-way classification model with skew-normal random effects. Based on the matrix decomposition technique, Bootstrap approach and generalized approach, we construct test statistics and confidence intervals for the fixed effect and variance component functions.

In Chapter 7, we consider the one-sided hypothesis testing and interval estimation problems for the fixed effect and variance component functions in the skew-normal unbalanced heteroscedastic one-way classification random effects model. The Bootstrap approach is used to establish the test statistic for the fixed effect. Further, we construct the test statistics and confidence intervals for variance component functions are constructed using the Bootstrap approach and generalized approach, and discuss their theoretical properties.

In Chapter 8, we discuss the hypothesis testing and interval estimation problems for the regression coefficients and variance component functions in the skew-normal unbalanced panel model with one-way error component. Based on the matrix decomposition technique, the exact test statistic for the regression coefficients is obtained. Further, the test statistics and confidence intervals for the single variance component and sum of variance components are constructed by the Bootstrap approach and generalized approach. Next, the exact test and approximate test for the ratio of variance components are established.

In Chapter 9, we discuss the statistical inference problems for the fixed effect and variance component functions in the two-way classification random effects model with skew-normal errors. We construct the exact test statistic for the fixed effect. Building upon this using the Bootstrap approach and generalized approach, we investigate the one-sided hypothesis testing and interval estimation problems for the single variance component, the sum and ratio of variance components are investigated respectively.

In Chapter 10, we focus on the skew-normal mixed effects model and systematically explores its statistical properties, including density function, moment generating function, mean vector, covariance matrix, and independence condition. Based on these properties, the chapter establishes the necessary and sufficient conditions under which the quadratic form of the observed vector in the skew-normal mixed effects model follows a noncentral skewed chi-square distribution and provides Cochran's theorem for this model. Finally, relying on the noncentral skew-F distribution, we construct exact tests for regression coefficient and variance component are constructed.

# Chapter 2

# Preliminary Knowledge

## 2.1 Multivariate skew-normal distribution

The multivariate skew-normal distribution is a distribution that combines the properties of the normal distribution with skewness characteristics. Widely applied in various fields such as environment, finance and biomedicine (Wang et al., 2009). It was first introduced by Azzalini and Dalla Valle (1996), who provided its probability density function. This chapter explores the properties of mean, covariance matrix, and distributions of linear function and quadratic forms for vectors with skew-normal distribution.

### 2.1.1 Skew-normal random vector

Let $M_{n \times k}$ be the set of all $n \times k$ matrices over the real field $\Re$ and $\Re^n = M_{n \times 1}$. For any $B \in M_{n \times k}$, use $B'$, $B^+$, $B^-$, and $rk(B)$ to denote the transpose, the Moore-Penrose inverse, the generalized inverse, and the rank of $B$, respectively. For any non-negative definite $T \in M_{n \times n}$ and $m > 0$, use $\rho(T)$ to denote the inverse of the largest eigenvalue of $T$, respectively, and use $T^m$ and $T^{-m}$ to denote the $m$th non-negative definite roots of $T$ and $T^+$, respectively. Also for $B \in M_{m \times n}$ and $C \in M_{p \times q}$, use $B \otimes C$ to denote the Kronecker product of $B$ and $C$.

**Definition 2.1.** *The random vector X follows a multivariate skew-normal distribution, denoted by $X \sim SN_n(\mu, \Sigma, \alpha)$, if its density function is*

$$f_X(x; \mu, \Sigma, \alpha) = 2\phi_n(x; \mu, \Sigma)\Phi(\alpha'\Sigma^{-1/2}(x - \mu)), \qquad x \in \Re^n, \qquad (2.1)$$

*where $\phi_n(x; \mu, \Sigma)$ is the n-dimensional normal density function with location parameter $\mu$, scale parameter $\Sigma$, skewness parameter $\alpha$, and $\Phi(\cdot)$ is the standard normal cumulative distribution function.*

From definition 2.1, we can see that the multivariate skew-normal distribution is completely determined by its location parameter $\mu$, scale parameter $\Sigma$, and skewness parameter $\alpha$. Specifically, when $\alpha=0$, the distribution of $X$ degenerates into a multivariate normal distribution $N_n(\mu,\Sigma)$. However, this definition is based on the probability density function to define the distribution, so $\Sigma>0$ is required.

**Lemma 2.1.** *Let* $U \sim N_n(\mu,\Sigma), c \in \Re, d \in \Re^n$, *then*

$$E(\Phi(c+d'U)) = \Phi\left(\frac{c}{(1+d'\Sigma d)^{1/2}}\right), \tag{2.2}$$

The proof of Lemma 2.1 can be found in Zacks (1981).

**Theorem 2.1.** *Suppose that the model* $X$ *is given in* (2.1). *Then the moment generating function (MGF) of* $X$ *is*

$$M_X(t) = 2\exp\left(t'\mu_x + \frac{t'\Sigma_x t}{2}\right)\Phi\left\{\frac{\alpha'\Sigma^{1/2}t}{(1+\alpha'\alpha)^{1/2}}\right\}, \qquad t \in \Re^n, \tag{2.3}$$

*Proof.* The MGF of X is

$$M_X(t) = \frac{2}{(2\pi)^{n/2}|\Sigma|^{1/2}}\int_{R_n}\exp(t'x - \frac{1}{2}(x-\mu)'\Sigma^{-1}(x-\mu))\Phi(\alpha'\Sigma^{-1/2}(x-\mu))dx$$

$$= 2\exp\left(t'\mu + \frac{t'\Sigma t}{2}\right)\int_{R_n}\frac{1}{(2\pi)^{n/2}|\Sigma|^{1/2}}\Phi(\alpha'\Sigma^{-1/2}(x-\mu))$$

$$\times \exp\left\{-\frac{1}{2}[x-(\mu+\Sigma t)]'\Sigma^{-1}(x-(\mu+\Sigma t))\right\}dx.$$

Let $U = x - (\mu + \Sigma t)$, from Lemma 2.1, we have

$$\int_{R^n}\frac{1}{(2\pi)^{n/2}|\Sigma|^{1/2}}\exp\left\{-\frac{1}{2}[x-(\mu+\Sigma t)]'\Sigma^{-1}(x-(\mu+\Sigma t))\right\}$$

$$\times\Phi\left(\alpha'\Sigma^{-1/2}(x-\mu)\right)dx$$

$$= E\left\{\Phi\left(\alpha'\Sigma^{-1/2}U+\alpha'\Sigma^{1/2}t\right)\right\} = \Phi\left(\frac{\alpha'\Sigma^{1/2}t}{(1+\alpha'\alpha)^{1/2}}\right).$$

Then,

$$M_X(t) = 2\exp\left(t'\mu + \frac{t'\Sigma t}{2}\right)\Phi\left(\frac{\alpha'\Sigma^{1/2}t}{(1+\alpha'\alpha)^{1/2}}\right).$$

Theorem 2.1 is proven. $\square$

**Corollary 2.1.** *The mean vector and covariance matrix of* $X$ *are*

$$E(X) = \mu + \sqrt{\frac{2}{\pi}}\frac{\Sigma^{1/2}\alpha}{(1+\alpha'\alpha)^{1/2}}, \qquad Cov(X) = \Sigma^{1/2}\left(I_n - \frac{2\alpha\alpha'}{\pi(1+\alpha'\alpha)}\right)\Sigma^{1/2}.$$

By calculating the first-order and second-order derivatives of Equation (2.3) with respect to $t$, it is easy to obtain the above expressions of the mean vector and covariance matrix of $X$.

**Theorem 2.2.** *Suppose* $X \sim SN_n(\mu, \Sigma, \alpha)$, $B$ *is the* $m \times n$ *matrix with full row rank, then* $Y = BX \sim SN_m(B\mu, B\Sigma B', \alpha_1)$, *where*
$$\alpha_1 = \frac{(B\Sigma B')^{-1/2} B\Sigma^{1/2}\alpha}{\left\{1 + \alpha'[I_n - \Sigma^{1/2}B'(B\Sigma B')^{-1}B\Sigma^{1/2}]\alpha\right\}^{1/2}}.$$

*Proof.* Suppose $Z \sim SN_m(B\mu, B\Sigma B', \alpha_1)$, where $\alpha_1$ is given in Theorem 2.2. From Theorem 2.1, the MGF of Z is

$$M_z(t) = 2\exp\left(t'B\mu + \frac{t'B\Sigma B't}{2}\right)\Phi\left(\frac{\alpha_1'(B\Sigma B')^{1/2}t}{(1+\alpha_1'\alpha_1)^{1/2}}\right). \qquad (2.4)$$

Substituting the expression for $\alpha_1$ into Equation (2.4), we get

$$M_z(t) = 2\exp\left(t'B\mu + \frac{t'B\Sigma B't}{2}\right)\Phi\left(\frac{\alpha'\Sigma^{1/2}B't}{(1+\alpha'\alpha)^{1/2}}\right). \qquad (2.5)$$

The MGF of Y is

$$M_Y(t) = E(\exp(t'Y)) = E(\exp(t'BX)) = M_X(B't).$$

Again using Theorem 2.1, we have

$$M_Y(t) = 2\exp\left(t'B\mu + \frac{t'B\Sigma B't}{2}\right)\Phi\left(\frac{\alpha'\Sigma^{1/2}B't}{(1+\alpha'\alpha)^{1/2}}\right). \qquad (2.6)$$

Compare Equation (2.5) with Equation (2.6), then $M_z(t) = M_Y(t)$. By the uniqueness of MGF, $Y \sim SN_m(B\mu, B\Sigma B', \alpha_1)$, Theorem 2.2 is proven.

$\square$

**Theorem 2.3.** *Suppose* $X \sim SN_n(\mu, \Sigma, \alpha)$, $B_i \in M_{m_i \times n}$, $Y_i = B_iX$, $i = 1, 2$, *where* $M_{m_i \times n}$ *denotes the set of all* $m_i \times n$ *matrices over the real field R. Then* $Y_1$ *and* $Y_2$ *are independent if and only if:*
*(i)* $B_1\Sigma B_2' = 0.$
*(ii)* $B_1\Sigma^{1/2}\alpha = 0$ *or* $B_2\Sigma^{1/2}\alpha = 0.$

*Proof.* Let $X = \mu + \Sigma^{1/2}V$, $V \sim SN_n(0, I_n, \alpha)$, $i = 1, 2$, then $Y_i = B_i\mu + B_i\Sigma^{1/2}V$. It can be seen from the conclusions of Theorem 2.2 in Wang et al. (2009), and the conclusions of Theorem 2.3 hold. $\square$

### 2.1.2 Quadratic form of a skew-normal random vector

According to Section 2.1.1, under certain conditions, the quadratic form of the normal random vector follows the $\chi^2$ distribution. Is there a similar conclusion for the quadratic form of the skew-normal random vector? Therefore, this section first defines a new distribution, namely the noncentral skew chi-square distribution (Ye and Wang, 2015), which is a direct extension of the noncentral $\chi^2$ distribution.

**Definition 2.2.** *Let* $U \sim SN_m(v, I_m, \alpha)$. *The distribution of* $T = U'U$ *is defined as the noncentral skew chi-square distribution with degrees of freedom m, noncentrality parameter* $\lambda = v'v$, *and skewness parameters* $\delta_1 = \alpha'v$ *and* $\delta_2 = \alpha'\alpha$, *denoted by* $T \sim S\chi_m^2(\lambda, \delta_1, \delta_2)$.

**Theorem 2.4.** *Let* $U \sim SN_m(v, I_m, \alpha)$ *and* $T = U'U \sim S\chi_m^2(\lambda, \delta_1, \delta_2)$ *with* $\lambda = v'v$, $\delta_1 = \alpha'v$ *and* $\delta_2 = \alpha'\alpha$. *Then the density function of* $T$ *is given by*

$$f_T(x; \lambda, \delta_1, \delta_2) = \frac{\exp\left\{-\frac{1}{2}(\lambda + x)\right\}}{\Gamma(\frac{1}{2})\Gamma(\frac{m-1}{2})2^{m/2-1}} h(x; \lambda, \delta_1, \delta_2), \qquad x > 0, \qquad (2.7)$$

*where* $\alpha_0 = \frac{\lambda^{-1/2}\delta_1}{(1+\delta_2-\delta_1^2/\lambda)^{1/2}}$ *and*

$$h(x; \lambda, \delta_1, \delta_2) = \int_{-\sqrt{x}}^{\sqrt{x}} \exp(\lambda^{1/2}s_1)(x - s_1^2)^{\frac{m-3}{2}} \Phi\left(\alpha_0(s_1 - \lambda^{1/2})\right) ds_1.$$

*For the case where* $\delta_1 = 0$, *the density function of* $T$ *can be degenerated into*

$$f_T(x; \lambda) = e^{-\lambda/2} \, _0F_1\left(\frac{1}{2}m; \frac{1}{4}\lambda x\right) \frac{1}{2^{m/2}\Gamma(\frac{m}{2})} e^{-x/2}x^{m/2-1}, \qquad x > 0, \qquad (2.8)$$

*which is free to* $\delta_2$ *and is denoted by* $T \sim \chi_m^2(\lambda)$, *where* $_0F_1(\kappa_1; \kappa_2)$ *denotes the Bessel function (Muirhead, 1982).*

*Proof.* Let $S = KU$ and $v = (v_1, \cdots, v_m)'$, where $K$ is a $m \times m$ orthogonal matrix whose elements in the first row are $v_i/\lambda^{1/2}$, $i = 1, \cdots, m$. Then $S \sim SN_m(Kv, I_m, K\alpha)$ with $Kv = (\lambda^{1/2}, 0, \cdots, 0)'$, so that

$$T = U'U = S'S = \sum_{i=1}^{m} S_i^2 = S_1^2 + W,$$

where, $W = \sum_{i=2}^{m} S_i^2 \sim \chi_{m-1}^2$ and $S_1 \sim SN(\lambda^{1/2}, 1, \alpha_0)$. Thus the conditional density function of $T$ given $S_1 = s_1$ is

$$f_{T|S_1=s_1}(x) = \frac{(x - s_1^2)^{\frac{m-3}{2}}}{\Gamma(\frac{m-1}{2})2^{\frac{m-1}{2}}} \exp\left(-\frac{x - s_1^2}{2}\right), \qquad x \geq s_1^2.$$

Let $f_{S_1}(s_1)$ denote the density function of $S_1$. Then the density function of $T$ is

$$
\begin{aligned}
f_T(x;\lambda,\delta_1,\delta_2) &= \int_{-\sqrt{x}}^{\sqrt{x}} f_{T|S_1=s_1}(x) f_{S_1}(s_1)\,ds_1 \\
&= \frac{1}{\Gamma(\frac{1}{2})\Gamma(\frac{m-1}{2})2^{m/2-1}} \int_{-\sqrt{x}}^{\sqrt{x}} \exp\left\{ -\frac{1}{2}(x-s_1^2) - \frac{1}{2}(s_1-\lambda^{1/2})^2 \right\} \\
&\quad \times (x-s_1^2)^{\frac{m-3}{2}} \Phi\{\alpha_0(s_1-\lambda^{1/2})\}\,ds_1 \\
&= \frac{\exp\left\{-\frac{1}{2}(\lambda+x)\right\}}{\Gamma(\frac{1}{2})\Gamma(\frac{m-1}{2})2^{m/2-1}} h(x;\lambda,\delta_1,\delta_2), \qquad x>0,
\end{aligned}
$$

where, $h(x;\lambda,\delta_1,\delta_2)$ is given in Equation (2.7). Note that when $\delta_1 = 0$, $f_T(x;\lambda,\delta_1,\delta_2)$ is reduced to

$$
f_T(x;\lambda) = \frac{\exp\left\{-\frac{1}{2}(\lambda+x)\right\}}{\Gamma(\frac{1}{2})\Gamma(\frac{m-1}{2})2^{m/2}} \int_{-\sqrt{x}}^{\sqrt{x}} \exp(\lambda^{1/2}s_1)(x-s_1^2)^{\frac{m-3}{2}}\,ds_1.
$$

Now make the change of variable $s_1 = x^{1/2}\cos\theta$ with $0 < \theta < \pi$. The Jacobian is easily calculated to be $-x^{1/2}\sin\theta$, so that

$$
\begin{aligned}
f_T(x;\lambda) &= \frac{\exp\left\{-\frac{1}{2}(\lambda+x)\right\}}{\Gamma(\frac{1}{2})\Gamma(\frac{m-1}{2})2^{m/2}} \int_0^\pi \exp(\lambda^{1/2}x^{1/2}\cos\theta)\sin^{m-2}\theta\, x^{m/2-1}\,d\theta \\
&= e^{-\lambda/2} \frac{\Gamma(\frac{m}{2})}{\Gamma(\frac{1}{2})\Gamma(\frac{m-1}{2})} \int_0^\pi \exp(\lambda^{1/2}x^{1/2}\cos\theta)\sin^{m-2}\theta\,d\theta \\
&\quad \times \frac{1}{2^{m/2}\Gamma(\frac{m}{2})} e^{-x/2} x^{m/2-1} \\
&= e^{-\lambda/2}\, {}_0F_1\left(\frac{1}{2}m;\frac{1}{4}\lambda x\right) \frac{1}{2^{m/2}\Gamma(\frac{m}{2})} e^{-x/2} x^{m/2-1}, \qquad x>0.
\end{aligned}
$$

$\qquad\qquad\qquad\qquad\qquad\qquad\qquad\qquad\qquad\qquad\qquad\qquad\qquad\qquad\square$

**Remark 2.1.** *From Theorem 2.4, we know that the density function of the noncentral skew chi-square distribution is uniquely decided by the parameters m, $\lambda$, $\delta_1$ and $\delta_2$. This noncentral skew chi-square distribution modifies the one given in Wang et al. (2009) to avoid the unidentifiability of $\alpha$.*

We graph density curves of noncentral skew chi-square distributions in Figures 2.1–2.3.

In Figure 2.1, the solid curve corresponds to the density of $S\chi_5^2(5,0,10)=\chi_5^2(5)$, the noncentral chi-square distribution with 5 degrees of freedom and noncentrality parameter 5. The dashed curve corresponds to the density of $S\chi_5^2(5,5,10)$. From Figure 2.1, we can see that skewness parameter $\delta_1$ plays an important

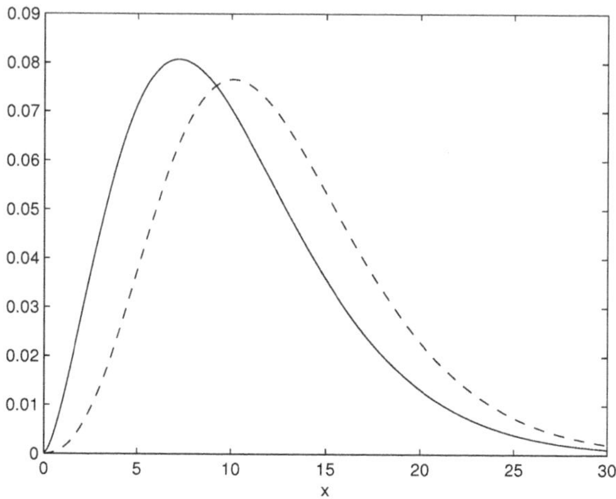

**Figure 2.1:** Density curves of $S\chi_5^2(5,0,10)$ (solid curve) and $S\chi_5^2(5,5,10)$ (dashed curve).

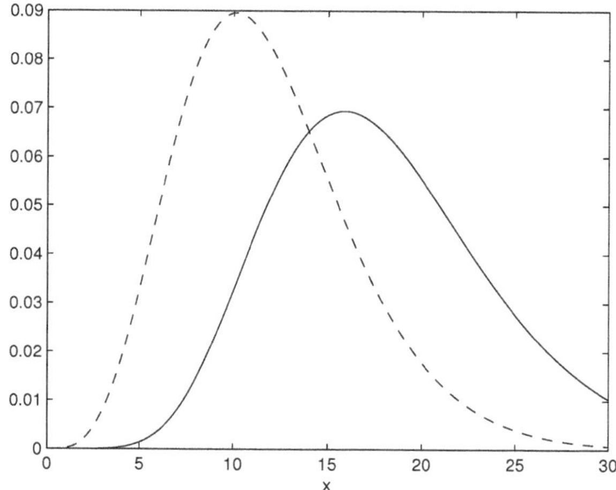

**Figure 2.2:** Density curves of $S\chi_{10}^2(5,10,25)$ (solid curve) and $S\chi_{10}^2(5,-10,25)$ (dashed curve).

role in the difference between the noncentral chi-square distribution and noncentral skew chi-square distribution. In Figure 2.2, the solid curve corresponds to the density of $S\chi_{10}^2(5,10,25)$ and the dashed curve corresponds to the density of $S\chi_{10}^2(5,-10,25)$. From Figure 2.2, we know that signs of $\delta_1$ can change the shapes of the densities. In Figure 2.3, the solid curve corresponds to the density of $S\chi_{25}^2(5,5,25)$ and the dashed curve corresponds to the density of $S\chi_{25}^2(2,-1,5)$. We know from Figure 2.3 that as the degrees of freedom $m$ increases, the shapes

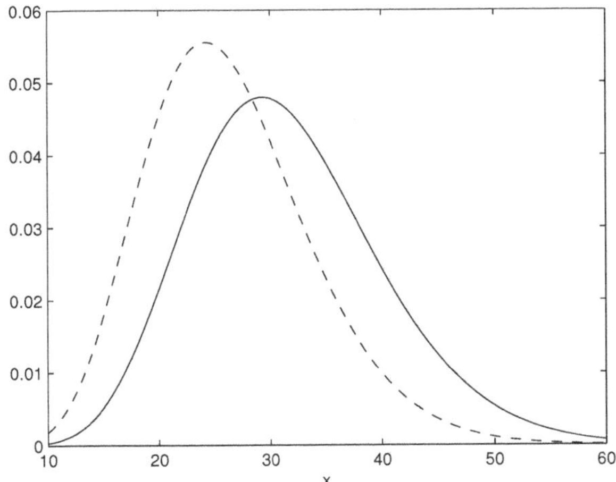

**Figure 2.3:** Density curves of $S\chi^2_{25}(5,5,25)$ (solid curve) and $S\chi^2_{25}(2,-1,5)$ (dashed curve).

of the densities are similar and the values of $\delta_1$ and $\delta_2$ have little impact to the densities.

**Theorem 2.5.** *Suppose that* $X \sim SN_n(\mu,\Sigma,\alpha)$ *and* $A$ *is a $n$-dimensional symmetric matrix, then the MGF of* $Q = X'AX$ *is*

$$
M_Q(t) = \frac{2\exp\left\{-\frac{1}{2}\mu'\Sigma^{-1}\mu + \frac{1}{2}\mu'\Sigma^{-1}(I_n - 2t\Sigma A)^{-1}\mu\right\}}{|I_n - 2t\Sigma A|^{1/2}}
$$
$$
\times \Phi\left\{\frac{\alpha'\Sigma^{-1/2}[(I_n - 2t\Sigma A)^{-1} - I_n]\mu}{[1 + \alpha'\Sigma^{-1/2}(I_n - 2t\Sigma A)^{-1}\Sigma^{1/2}\alpha]^{1/2}}\right\},
$$

*where* $t \in R$, $2|t| < \rho(\Sigma A)$ *and* $\rho(\Sigma A)$ *represents the inverse of the maximum eigenvalue of matrix* $\Sigma A$.

*Proof.* The MGF of Q is

$$
M_Q(t) = 2\int_{R_n} \exp(tx'Ax)\phi_n(x;\mu,\Sigma)\Phi(\alpha'\Sigma^{-1/2}(x-\mu))dx
$$
$$
= \frac{2\exp\left\{-\frac{1}{2}\mu'\Sigma^{-1}\mu\right\}}{(2\pi)^{n/2}|\Sigma|^{1/2}}\int_{R_n} \exp\left\{-\frac{1}{2}x'(\Sigma^{-1} - 2tA)x + \mu\Sigma^{-1}x\right\}
$$
$$
\times \Phi(\alpha'\Sigma^{-1/2}(x-\mu))dx
$$
$$
= \frac{2\exp\left\{-\frac{1}{2}\mu'\Sigma^{-1}\mu + \frac{1}{2}\mu'\Sigma^{-1}(I_n - 2t\Sigma A)^{-1}\mu\right\}}{(2\pi)^{n/2}|\Sigma|^{1/2}}
$$
$$
\times \int_{R_n} \exp\left\{-\frac{1}{2}H(t)'(\Sigma^{-1} - 2tA)H(t)\right\}\Phi(\alpha'\Sigma^{-1/2}(x-\mu))dx,
$$

where $H(t) = x - (I_n - 2t\Sigma A)^{-1}\mu$. Notice that

$$\alpha'\Sigma^{-1/2}(x - \mu) = \alpha'\Sigma^{-1/2}[(I_n - 2t\Sigma A)^{-1} - I_n]\mu + \alpha'\Sigma^{-1/2}H(t),$$

then by Lemma 2.1, we can get

$$
\begin{aligned}
M_Q(t) &= \frac{2exp\left\{-\frac{1}{2}\mu'\Sigma^{-1}\mu + \frac{1}{2}\mu'\Sigma^{-1}(I_n - 2t\Sigma A)^{-1}\mu\right\}}{|I_n - 2t\Sigma A|^{1/2}} \\
&\quad \times E\left\{\Phi\left\{\alpha'\Sigma^{-1/2}[(I_n - 2t\Sigma A)^{-1} - I_n]\mu + \alpha'\Sigma^{-1/2}H(t)\right\}\right\} \\
&= \frac{2exp\left\{-\frac{1}{2}\mu'\Sigma^{-1}\mu + \frac{1}{2}\mu'\Sigma^{-1}(I_n - 2t\Sigma A)^{-1}\mu\right\}}{|I_n - 2t\Sigma A|^{m/2}} \\
&\quad \times \Phi\left\{\frac{\alpha'\Sigma^{-1/2}[(I_n - 2t\Sigma A)^{-1} - I_n]\mu}{[1 + \alpha'\Sigma^{-1/2}(I_n - 2t\Sigma A)^{-1}\Sigma^{1/2}\alpha]^{1/2}}\right\}.
\end{aligned}
$$

Theorem 2.5 is proved. $\qquad\qquad\square$

**Corollary 2.2.** *Assume* $U \sim SN_m(v, I_m, \alpha)$, $T = U'U \sim S\chi_m^2(\lambda, \delta_1, \delta_2)$, *where* $\lambda = v'v, \delta_1 = \alpha'v, \delta_2 = \alpha'\alpha$. *Then the MGF of Y is*

$$M_T(t) = \frac{2\exp\left\{t(1 - 2t)^{-1}\lambda\right\}}{(1 - 2t)^{m/2}}\Phi\left\{\frac{2t(1 - 2t)^{-1}\delta_1}{[1 + (1 - 2t)^{-1}\delta_2]^{1/2}}\right\},$$

*where* $t \in R$, $|t| < \frac{1}{2}$.

From Theorem 2.5, it is easy to prove the conclusion of Corollary 2.2.

**Corollary 2.3.** *Let* $T \sim S\chi_m^2(\lambda, \delta_1, \delta_2)$, *then the mean and variance of T are respectively*

$$
\begin{aligned}
E(T) &= n + \lambda + \frac{4\delta_1}{\sqrt{2\pi(1 + \delta_2)}}, \\
Var(T) &= 2n + 4\lambda + \frac{4\delta_1[(2\pi)^{1/2}\delta_2 - 2\delta_1(1 + \delta_2)^1/2 + 2(2\pi)^1/2]}{\pi(1 + \delta_2)^{1/2}}.
\end{aligned}
$$

By calculating the first-order and second-order derivatives of $M_T(t)$ in Corollary 2.2, respectively, the above expressions of the mean and variance of $T$ can be obtained.

**Lemma 2.2.** *Let* $P(s,t), Q(s,t), R(s,t), S(s,t)$ *are polynomials of both s and t, and satisfy*

$$P(s,t)/Q(s,t) = \exp\left\{R(s,t)/S(s,t)\right\},$$

*where the range of values for s and t is around 0,* $P(0,0)/Q(0,0) = 1$ *and* $R(0,0)/S(0,0) = 0$, *then* $P(s,t)/Q(s,t) = 1$ *and* $R(s,t)/S(s,t) = 0$.

The process of proving this lemma can be found in Laha (1956) and Driscoll and Gundberg (1986).

**Lemma 2.3.** *Assume $\mu \in R_n$, $\lambda > 0$, m is a positive integer, $m \leq n$, $\Sigma$ is a positive definite matrix of order n, and A is a non-negative definite matrix of order n with $rk(A) = m$. If*

$$\frac{\exp\left\{-\frac{1}{2}\mu'\Sigma^{-1}\mu + \frac{1}{2}\mu'\Sigma^{-1}(I_n - 2t\Sigma A)^{-1}\mu\right\}}{|I_n - 2t\Sigma A|^{1/2}} = \frac{\exp\left\{t(1-2t)^{-1}\lambda\right\}}{(1-2t)^{m/2}},$$

*where $t \in R$, $2|t| < min\{1, \rho(\Sigma A)\}$, then*
*(i) $\Sigma A$ is an idempotent matrix of rank m,*
*(ii) $\lambda = \mu'A\mu$.*

*Proof.* Let

$$
\begin{aligned}
P(s,t)/Q(s,t) &= |I_n - 2t\Sigma A|^{1/2}/(1-2t)^{m/2}, \\
R(s,t)/S(s,t) &= -\frac{1}{2}\mu'\Sigma^{-1}\mu + \frac{1}{2}\mu'\Sigma^{-1}(I_n - 2t\Sigma A)^{-1}\mu - t(1-2t)^{-1}\lambda.
\end{aligned}
$$

Based on Lemma 2.2, we have

$$|I_n - 2t\Sigma A|^{1/2} = (1-2t)^{m/2}, \tag{2.9}$$

$$-\frac{1}{2}\mu'\Sigma^{-1}\mu + \frac{1}{2}\mu'\Sigma^{-1}(I_n - 2t\Sigma A)^{-1}\mu = t(1-2t)^{-1}\lambda. \tag{2.10}$$

Obviously, Equation (2.9) is equivalent to Conclusion (i), and based on Conclusion (i) and Taylor expansion, Equation (2.10) can be simplified to

$$(\mu'A\mu)\sum_{j=0}^{\infty}(2t)^j = \lambda\sum_{j=0}^{\infty}(2t)^j. \tag{2.11}$$

By comparing the coefficients of t on both sides in Equation (2.11), we can know $\lambda = \mu'A\mu$. Lemma 2.3 is proven. $\quad\square$

**Theorem 2.6.** *Let $X \sim SN_n(\mu, \Sigma, \alpha)$, A is a non-negative definite matrix of order n, $rk(A) = m$, then the necessary and sufficient conditions of $Q = X'AX \sim S\chi_m^2(\lambda, \delta_1, \delta_2)$ are*
*(i) $\Sigma A$ is an idempotent matrix with rank m,*
*(ii) $\lambda = \mu'A\mu$,*
*(iii) $\delta_1 = \alpha'\Sigma^{1/2}A\mu/d$,*
*(iv) $\delta_2 = \alpha'P_1P_1'\alpha/d^2$,*
*where $d = (1 + \alpha'P_2P_2'\alpha)^{1/2}$, $P = (P_1, P_2)$ is an orthogonal matrix, such that*

$$\Sigma^{1/2}A\Sigma^{1/2} = P\begin{pmatrix} I_m & 0 \\ 0 & 0 \end{pmatrix}P' = P_1P_1'. \tag{2.12}$$

*Proof.* First, we assume that (i)–(iv) hold. By (i), there exists an orthogonal matrix P such that Equation (2.12) holds. For any non-negative definite matrix A, we have

$$P_1 P_1' \Sigma^{1/2} A = \Sigma^{1/2} A. \tag{2.13}$$

Let $v = P_1' \Sigma^{1/2} A \mu$ and $U = v + P_1' V$, where $V \sim SN_n(0, I_n, \alpha)$. It is easy to show that $U \sim SN_m(v, I_m, \alpha_1)$, $\alpha_1 = P_1' \alpha / d$, $d = (1 + \alpha' P_2 P_2' \alpha)^{1/2}$. By Definition 2.2, $U'U \sim S\chi_m^2(\lambda, \delta_1, \delta_2)$, $\lambda = v'v$, $\delta_1 = \alpha_1' v$, $\delta_2 = \alpha_1' \alpha_1$. Notice that $\lambda$, $\delta_1$ and $\delta_2$ are equal to Condition (ii)–(iv), respectively. Thus it suffices to show that $Q \overset{d}{=} U'U$, that is, Q and $U'U$ have the same distribution.

By Equation (2.12) and Equation (2.13), we have

$$
\begin{aligned}
Q &= \left(\mu + \Sigma^{1/2} V\right)' A \left(\mu + \Sigma^{1/2} V\right) \\
&= \mu' A \mu + 2V' \Sigma^{1/2} A \mu + V' \Sigma^{1/2} A \Sigma^{1/2} V \\
&= v'v + 2V' P_1 P_1' \Sigma^{1/2} A \mu + V' P_1 P_1' V \\
&= v'v + 2V' P_1 v + V' P_1 P_1' V \\
&= (v + P_1' V)' (v + P_1' V) \overset{d}{=} U'U.
\end{aligned}
$$

Thus the desired result follows.

Next, assume that $Q \sim S\chi_m^2(\lambda, \delta_1, \delta_2)$. Let $U \sim SN_m(v, I_m, \alpha_1)$, $\lambda = v'v$, $\delta_1 = \alpha_1' v$, $\delta_2 = \alpha_1' \alpha_1$. By Definition 2.2, we know $Q \overset{d}{=} U'U$, so that $M_Q(t) = M_{U'U}(t)$, that is

$$
\frac{\exp\left\{-\frac{1}{2}\mu' \Sigma^{-1} \mu + \frac{1}{2}\mu' \Sigma^{-1}(I_n - 2t\Sigma A)^{-1} \mu\right\}}{|I_n - 2t\Sigma A|^{1/2}} \Phi\left\{\frac{\alpha' \Sigma^{-1/2}\left[(I_n - 2t\Sigma A)^{-1} - I_n\right]\mu}{\left[1 + \alpha' \Sigma^{-1/2}(I_n - 2t\Sigma A)^{-1} \Sigma^{1/2} \alpha\right]^{1/2}}\right\}
$$
$$
= \frac{\exp\left\{t(1-2t)^{-1}\lambda\right\}}{(1-2t)^{m/2}} \Phi\left\{\frac{2t(1-2t)^{-1}\delta_1}{[1+(1-2t)^{-1}\delta_2]^{1/2}}\right\}, t \in R, 2|t| < \min\{1, \rho(\Sigma A)\}.
$$

Note that when $\delta_1 = 0$, the distribution of Q is degenerated into a noncentral chi-square distribution, so the above equation is simplified to

$$
\frac{\exp\left\{-\frac{1}{2}\mu' \Sigma^{-1} \mu + \frac{1}{2}\mu' \Sigma^{-1}(I_n - 2t\Sigma A)^{-1} \mu\right\}}{|I_n - 2t\Sigma A|^{1/2}} = \frac{\exp\left\{t(1-2t)^{-1}\lambda\right\}}{(1-2t)^{m/2}}, \tag{2.14}
$$

$$
\Phi\left\{\frac{\alpha' \Sigma^{-1/2}\left[(I_n - 2t\Sigma A)^{-1} - I_n\right]\mu}{\left[1 + \alpha' \Sigma^{-1/2}(I_n - 2t\Sigma A)^{-1} \Sigma^{1/2} \alpha\right]^{1/2}}\right\} = \Phi\left\{\frac{2t(1-2t)^{-1}\delta_1}{\left[1+(1-2t)^{-1}\delta_2\right]^{1/2}}\right\}. \tag{2.15}
$$

According to Lemma 2.3, Equation (2.14) implies (i) and (ii) with $P = (P_1, P_2)$ is an orthogonal matrix satisfying (2.12). As $\Phi(x)$ is a strictly monotonically increasing function of $x$, so based on (2.15), we can get

$$\frac{\alpha'\Sigma^{-1/2}\left[(I_n - 2t\Sigma A)^{-1} - I_n\right]\mu}{\left[1 + \alpha'\Sigma^{-1/2}(I_n - 2t\Sigma A)^{-1}\Sigma^{1/2}\alpha\right]^{1/2}} = \frac{2t(1-2t)^{-1}\delta_1}{\left[1 + (1-2t)^{-1}\delta_2\right]^{1/2}},$$

where $t \in R$ and $|t| < \frac{1}{2}$. By Taylor expansion, we have

$$\alpha'\Sigma^{1/2}A\mu\,(1 + \delta_2)^{1/2} = \delta_1\,(1 + \alpha'\alpha)^{1/2}, \tag{2.16}$$

$$\alpha'\Sigma^{1/2}A\mu\,\delta_2^{1/2} = \delta_1\left(\alpha'\Sigma^{1/2}A\Sigma^{1/2}\alpha\right)^{1/2}. \tag{2.17}$$

Further, their ratio is

$$\frac{1 + \delta_2}{\delta_2} = \frac{1 + \alpha'\alpha}{\alpha'\Sigma^{1/2}A\Sigma^{1/2}\alpha}. \tag{2.18}$$

From (2.12) and (2.18), we get,

$$\delta_2 = \frac{\alpha'P_1P_1'\alpha}{1 + \alpha'P_2P_2'\alpha} = \frac{\alpha'P_1P_1'\alpha}{d^2}.$$

So (iv) holds. In addition, substituting $\delta_2$ back to (2.17), it is easy to get (iii). The necessity is proved. $\qquad\square$

## 2.2 Distribution of a skew-normal matrix quadratic form

With the rise of big data and high-dimensional data, statistical inference methods on random matrices have found widespread applications various fields such as economics, finance, biology, psychology, and physics (Adhikari, 2007; Gupta and Nagar, 2000; Gupta et al., 2013). Therefore, under the assumption of a skew-normal distribution, this book systematically investigates the statistical properties of random matrices, encompassing density functions, moment generating functions (MGF), independence conditions, and distributions of quadratic forms, among others. Some findings in this work are generalizations of the conclusions on the skew-normal random matrix in Gupta et al. (2013).

### 2.2.1  Skew-normal random matrix

For any non-negative definite matrix $T \in M_{n \times n}$ and $m > 0$, use $\mathrm{etr}(T)$ to denote the exponential trace. Suppose $A = (a_1, \cdots, a_n)' \in M_{n \times m}$, $B \in M_{m \times p}$, $C \in M_{p \times q}$, Define $\mathrm{Vec}^*(A) = (a_1', \cdots, a_n')'$, $\mathrm{Vec}^*(ABC) = (A \otimes C')\mathrm{Vec}^*(B)$ and $(A \otimes C')(B) = ABC$. Use $E$ and $F$ to denote certain $p$- and $k$-dimensional inner product spaces over the real field $\Re$, use $\mathcal{L}(E, F)$ to denote the vector space of all linear maps of $E$ into $F$, and $\mathcal{L}(E, F)$ will be equipped with the trace inner product: $\langle A, B \rangle = tr(A'B)$ for all $A, B \in \mathcal{L}(E, F)$.

**Definition 2.3.** *Suppose $Y$ is a $n \times p$ random matrix, and $y = \mathrm{Vec}^*(Y) \sim SN_{np}(\mu^*, V \otimes \Sigma, \gamma \otimes \alpha)$, where $\mu^* = \mathrm{Vec}^*(\mu)$, $\mu \in M_{n \times p}, V \in M_{n \times n}, \Sigma \in M_{p \times p}$, $\gamma \in \Re^n$, $\alpha \in \Re^p$, and $V$ is known. Then $Y$ is said to have a skew-normal matrix distribution with location matrix $\mu$, scale matrix $V \otimes \Sigma$, and skewness parameter matrix $\gamma \otimes \alpha'$, denoted by $Y \sim SN_{n \times p}(\mu, V \otimes \Sigma, \gamma \otimes \alpha')$.*

**Theorem 2.7.** *Let $Z \sim SN_{k \times p}(0, I_{kp}, 1_k \otimes \alpha')$ with $1_k = (1, \cdots, 1)' \in \Re^k$. Then*

*(i) The density function of $Z$ is*

$$f(Z) = 2\phi_{k \times p}(Z)\Phi(1_k' Z\alpha), \quad Z \in M_{k \times p}, \tag{2.19}$$

*where $\phi_{k \times p}(Z) = (2\pi)^{-kp/2}\mathrm{etr}(-Z'Z/2)$ and $\Phi(\cdot)$ is the standard normal cumulative distribution function.*

*(ii) The MGF of $Z$ is*

$$M_Z(T) = 2\mathrm{etr}(T'T/2)\Phi\left\{ \frac{1_k' T\alpha}{(1 + k\alpha'\alpha)^{1/2}} \right\}, \quad T \in M_{k \times p}. \tag{2.20}$$

*Proof.* We know that $Z \sim SN_{k \times p}(0, I_{kp}, 1_k \otimes \alpha')$ is equivalent to $z = \mathrm{Vec}^*(Z) \sim SN_{kp}(0, I_{kp}, 1_k \otimes \alpha)$. Then the density function of $z$ is

$$f(z) = \frac{2}{(2\pi)^{kp/2}} \exp(-z'z/2)\Phi((1_k \otimes \alpha)'z). \tag{2.21}$$

Replacing $z$ with $\mathrm{Vec}^*(Z)$ in Equation (2.21), we obtain

$$\begin{aligned} f(z) &= \frac{2}{(2\pi)^{kp/2}} \exp(-\mathrm{Vec}^*(Z)'\mathrm{Vec}^*(Z)/2)\Phi((1_k \otimes \alpha)'\mathrm{Vec}^*(Z)) \\ &= \frac{2}{(2\pi)^{kp/2}} \mathrm{etr}(-Z'Z/2)\Phi(1_k' Z\alpha). \end{aligned}$$

Further, the MGF of $z$ is

$$M_z(t) = E(\exp(t'z)) = 2\exp(t't/2)\Phi\left\{ \frac{(1_k \otimes \alpha)'t}{(1 + k\alpha'\alpha)^{1/2}} \right\} \quad t \in \Re^{kp}. \tag{2.22}$$

Let $t = \text{Vec}^*(T)$ in Equation (2.22), we have

$$
\begin{aligned}
M_z(t) &= 2\exp(\text{Vec}^*(T)'\text{Vec}^*(T)/2)\Phi\left\{\frac{(1_k \otimes \alpha)'\text{Vec}^*(T)}{(1+k\alpha'\alpha)^{1/2}}\right\} \\
&= 2\text{etr}(T'T/2)\Phi\left\{\frac{1_k'T\alpha}{(1+k\alpha'\alpha)^{1/2}}\right\}.
\end{aligned}
$$

The desired result is obtained. $\qquad\qquad\qquad\qquad\qquad\qquad\square$

**Remark 2.2.** *Let $Z = (Z_1,\cdots,Z_k)' \sim SN_{k\times p}(0,I_{kp},1_k \otimes \alpha')$ with $Z_i \in \Re^p$. From Theorem 2.7, it is easy to see that $Z_1,\cdots,Z_k$, the components of $Z$, are identically distributed as $SN_p(0,I_p,\alpha_*)$ with $\alpha_* = \alpha/[1+(k-1)\alpha'\alpha]^{1/2}$. Also for distinct $i,j \in \{1,\cdots,k\}$, $Z_i$ and $Z_j$ are not independent as $Cov(Z_i,Z_j) = -2\alpha\alpha'/[\pi(1+k\alpha'\alpha)]$.*

*Let $\mu \in M_{n\times p}$, $A \in M_{k\times n}$, and $\Sigma$ be non-singular with $\Sigma \in M_{p\times p}$. Consider the random matrix $Y = \mu + A'Z\Sigma^{1/2}$ with $Z \sim SN_{k\times p}(0,I_{kp},1_k \otimes \alpha')$. We know that the density function of $Y$ may not exist. The following results list the properties of the distribution of $Y$.*

**Theorem 2.8.** *Let $Z \sim SN_{k\times p}(0,I_{kp},1_k \otimes \alpha')$ and $Y = \mu + A'Z\Sigma^{1/2}$. Then*

*(i) The MGF of $Y$ is*

$$
M_Y(T) = 2\text{etr}\left(T'\mu + \frac{\Sigma T'VT}{2}\right)\Phi\left\{\frac{1_k'AT\Sigma^{1/2}\alpha}{(1+k\alpha'\alpha)^{1/2}}\right\} \qquad T \in M_{n\times p}, \quad (2.23)
$$

*where $V = A'A$.*

*(ii) The mean and covariance matrix of $Y$ are*

$$
E(Y) = \mu + \sqrt{\frac{2}{\pi}}\frac{A'1_k\alpha'\Sigma^{1/2}}{(1+k\alpha'\alpha)^{1/2}}, Cov(y) = (A' \otimes \Sigma^{1/2})\left(I_{kp} - \frac{2(J_k \otimes \alpha\alpha')}{\pi(1+k\alpha'\alpha)}\right)(A \otimes \Sigma^{1/2}),
$$
$$
(2.24)
$$

*where $y = \text{Vec}^*(Y)$ and $J_k = 1_k 1_k'$.*

*(iii) The density function of $Y$, if it exists, is*

$$
f(Y;\mu,A,\Sigma,\alpha) = 2\phi_{n\times p}(Y;\mu,V,\Sigma)\Phi\left\{\frac{1_k'AV^{-1}(Y-\mu)\Sigma^{-1/2}\alpha}{[1+(k-1_k'P_A1_k)\alpha'\alpha]^{1/2}}\right\}, \quad (2.25)
$$

*where $\phi_{n\times p}(Y;\mu,V,\Sigma) = (2\pi)^{-np/2}|V|^{-p/2}|\Sigma|^{-n/2}\text{etr}[-\Sigma^{-1}(Y-\mu)'V^{-1}(Y-\mu)/2]$.*

*Proof.* For (i), by (ii) of Theorem 2.7, we have

$$
\begin{aligned}
M_Y(T) &= E(\operatorname{etr}(T'Y)) = \operatorname{etr}(T'\mu)E\{\operatorname{etr}[(AT\Sigma^{1/2})'Z]\} \\
&= 2\operatorname{etr}(T'\mu)\operatorname{etr}[(AT\Sigma^{1/2})'(AT\Sigma^{1/2})/2]\Phi\left\{\frac{1'_k AT\Sigma^{1/2}\alpha}{(1+k\alpha'\alpha)^{1/2}}\right\} \\
&= 2\operatorname{etr}\left(T'\mu+\frac{\Sigma T'VT}{2}\right)\Phi\left\{\frac{1'_k AT\Sigma^{1/2}\alpha}{(1+k\alpha'\alpha)^{1/2}}\right\}.
\end{aligned}
$$

Conclusion (i) holds. For (ii), by calculating the first-order and second-order derivatives of Equation (2.23) with respect to $t = \operatorname{Vec}*(T)$, the mean vector and covariance matrix of $y = \operatorname{Vec}*(Y)$ are obtained as follows.

$$
E(y) = \operatorname{Vec}*(\mu) + \sqrt{\frac{2}{\pi}}\frac{(A'1_k)\otimes(\Sigma^{1/2}\alpha)}{(1+k\alpha'\alpha)^{1/2}},
$$

$$
\operatorname{Cov}(y) = (A'\otimes\Sigma^{1/2})\left(I_{kp} - \frac{2(J_k\otimes\alpha\alpha')}{\pi(1+k\alpha'\alpha)}\right)(A\otimes\Sigma^{1/2}),
$$

where $J_k$ is given in Equation (2.24). Replacing $y$ with $\operatorname{Vec}*(Y)$ in the first equation, we obtain

$$
E(Y) = \mu + \sqrt{\frac{2}{\pi}}\frac{A'1_k\alpha'\Sigma^{1/2}}{(1+k\alpha'\alpha)^{1/2}}.
$$

Conclusion (ii) holds.

For (iii), suppose that $A$ is of the full column rank. Let $Y_1 = \mu + V^{1/2}Z_1\Sigma^{1/2}$ and $Z_1 \sim SN_{n\times p}(0, I_{np}, \gamma\otimes\alpha')$, where $V = A'A$ and

$$
\gamma = \frac{V^{-1/2}A'1_k}{[1+(k-1'_k P_A 1_k)\alpha'\alpha]^{1/2}}.
$$

By (i), the MGF of $Y_1$ is

$$
M_{Y_1}(T) = 2\operatorname{etr}\left(T'\mu+\frac{\Sigma T'VT}{2}\right)\Phi\left\{\frac{\gamma'V^{1/2}T\Sigma^{1/2}\alpha}{(1+\gamma'\gamma\alpha'\alpha)^{1/2}}\right\}. \tag{2.26}
$$

Substituting $\gamma$ back in Equation (2.26), it is obvious that Equation (2.23) and Equation (2.26) are equivalent, i.e., $M_Y(T) = M_{Y_1}(T)$. Thus by the uniqueness of MGF, $Y$ and $Y_1$ have the same density function. By (i) of Theorem 2.7, the density function of $Y_1$ is

$$
f(Y_1;\mu,A,\Sigma,\alpha) = \frac{2\operatorname{etr}[-\Sigma^{-1}(Y_1-\mu)'V^{-1}(Y_1-\mu)/2]}{(2\pi)^{np/2}|V|^{p/2}|\Sigma|^{n/2}}\Phi\left\{\frac{1'_k AV^{-1}(Y_1-\mu)\Sigma^{-1/2}\alpha}{[1+(k-1'_k P_A 1_k)\alpha'\alpha]^{1/2}}\right\}.
$$

Conclusion (iii) holds. $\qquad\square$

**Theorem 2.9.** *Suppose that $Z \sim SN_{k \times p}(0, I_{kp}, 1_k \otimes \alpha')$. For $i = 1, 2$, let $Y_i = \mu_i + A_i' Z \Sigma_i^{1/2}$ with $A_i \in M_{k \times n_i}$ and $\Sigma_i \in M_{p \times p}$. Then $Y_1$ and $Y_2$ are independent if and only if*

*(i) $A_1' A_2 = 0$,*

*(ii) $(A_1' 1_k) \otimes \alpha = 0$ or $(A_2' 1_k) \otimes \alpha = 0$.*

*Proof.* It suffices to show that $\text{Vec}^*(Y_1)$ and $\text{Vec}^*(Y_2)$ are independent if and only if (i) and (ii) hold. For $i = 1, 2$, $\text{Vec}^*(Y_i) = \text{Vec}^*(\mu_i) + (A_i' \otimes \Sigma_i^{1/2}) \text{Vec}^*(Z)$. By Theorem 2.2 of Wang et al. (2009), the desired result is obtained. $\qquad\square$

### 2.2.2 Distribution of a quadratic form

For the distribution of the quadratic form of $Y = \mu + A' Z \Sigma^{1/2}$, we have the following definition of the noncentral skew Wishart distribution.

**Definition 2.4.** *Let $X \sim SN_{k \times p}(v, I_k \otimes \Sigma, 1_k \otimes \alpha')$. The distribution of $X'X$ is defined as the noncentral skew Wishart distribution with $k$ degrees of freedom, the scale matrix $\Sigma$, the noncentral parameter matrix $\lambda = v'v$, and skewness parameter matrices $\delta_1 = \alpha 1_k' v$ and $\delta_2 = k \alpha \alpha'$, denoted by $X'X \sim SW_p(k, \Sigma, \lambda, \delta_1, \delta_2)$.*

**Theorem 2.10.** *Let $Z \sim SN_{k \times p}(0, I_{kp}, 1_k \otimes \alpha')$, $Y = \mu + A' Z \Sigma^{1/2}$, and $Q = Y' W Y$ with symmetric $W \in M_{n \times n}$. Then the MGF of $Q$ is*

$$
M_Q(T) = \frac{2 \exp\{\langle T, \mu' W \mu \rangle + 2 \langle \mu, [(WA' \otimes T \Sigma^{1/2})(I_{kp} - 2\Psi)^{-1}(AW \otimes \Sigma^{1/2} T)](\mu) \rangle\}}{|I_{kp} - 2\Psi|^{1/2}}
$$
$$
\times \Phi \left\{ \frac{\langle 1_k \otimes \alpha', [(I_{kp} - 2\Psi)^{-1}(A \otimes \Sigma^{1/2})](L) \rangle}{[1 + (1_k \otimes \alpha)'(I_{kp} - 2\Psi)^{-1}(1_k \otimes \alpha)]^{1/2}} \right\}, \tag{2.27}
$$

*for symmetric $T \in M_{p \times p}$ such that $\rho(\Psi) < 1/2$, where $\Psi = (AWA') \otimes (\Sigma^{1/2} T \Sigma^{1/2})$ and $L = 2W\mu T$.*

*Proof.* Note that $Y = \mu + A' Z \Sigma^{1/2} = \mu + (A' \otimes \Sigma^{1/2})(Z)$, then we have

$$
\begin{aligned}
Q &= Y'WY = [\mu + (A' \otimes \Sigma^{1/2})(Z)]' W [\mu + (A' \otimes \Sigma^{1/2})(Z)] \\
&= \mu' W \mu + \mu' W [(A' \otimes \Sigma^{1/2})(Z)] + [(A' \otimes \Sigma^{1/2})(Z)]' W \mu \\
&\quad + [(A' \otimes \Sigma^{1/2})(Z)]' W [(A' \otimes \Sigma^{1/2})(Z)],
\end{aligned}
$$

and

$$
\begin{aligned}
\langle T, Q \rangle &= \langle T, \mu' W \mu \rangle + \langle T, \mu' W [(A' \otimes \Sigma^{1/2})(Z)] + [(A' \otimes \Sigma^{1/2})(Z)]' W \mu \rangle \\
&\quad + \langle T, [(A' \otimes \Sigma^{1/2})(Z)]' W [(A' \otimes \Sigma^{1/2})(Z)] \rangle \\
&= \langle T, \mu' W \mu \rangle + \langle Z, (A \otimes \Sigma^{1/2})(L) \rangle + \langle Z, \Psi(Z) \rangle,
\end{aligned}
$$

where $L$ and $\Psi$ are given in Equation (2.27). By (i) of Theorem 2.7, the MGF of $Q$ is given by

$$
\begin{aligned}
M_Q(T) &= \int_{\mathcal{L}(E,F)} \exp\{\langle T,\mu'W\mu\rangle + \langle Z,(A\otimes\Sigma^{1/2})(L)\rangle + \langle Z,\Psi(Z)\rangle\}f(Z)dZ \\
&= \frac{2\exp\{\langle T,\mu'W\mu\rangle\}}{(2\pi)^{kp/2}}\int_{\mathcal{L}(E,F)}\exp\Big\{-\frac{1}{2}\mathrm{Vec}^*(Z)'(I_{kp}-2\Psi)\mathrm{Vec}^*(Z) \\
&\qquad +\mathrm{Vec}^*(Z)'\mathrm{Vec}^*((A\otimes\Sigma^{1/2})(L))\Big\}\Phi\{(1_k\otimes\alpha)'\mathrm{Vec}^*(Z)\}dZ \\
&= \frac{2\exp\{\langle T,\mu'W\mu\rangle + 2\langle\mu,[(WA'\otimes T\Sigma^{1/2})(I_{kp}-2\Psi)^{-1}(AW\otimes\Sigma^{1/2}T)](\mu)\rangle\}}{(2\pi)^{kp/2}} \\
&\qquad \times\int_{\mathcal{L}(E,F)}\exp\Big\{-\frac{1}{2}H'(I_{kp}-2\Psi)H\Big\}\Phi\{(1_k\otimes\alpha)'\mathrm{Vec}^*(Z)\}dZ,
\end{aligned}
$$

where $H = \mathrm{Vec}^*(Z) - (I_{kp}-2\Psi)^{-1}\mathrm{Vec}^*((A\otimes\Sigma^{1/2})(L))$. Note that

$$
(1_k\otimes\alpha)'\mathrm{Vec}^*(Z) = (1_k\otimes\alpha)'H + \langle 1_k\otimes\alpha',[(I_{kp}-2\Psi)^{-1}(A\otimes\Sigma^{1/2})](L)\rangle.
$$

By Lemma 2.1, we obtain

$$
\begin{aligned}
M_Q(T) &= \frac{2\exp\{\langle T,\mu'W\mu\rangle + 2\langle\mu,[(WA'\otimes T\Sigma^{1/2})(I_{kp}-2\Psi)^{-1}(AW\otimes\Sigma^{1/2}T)](\mu)\rangle\}}{|I_{kp}-2\Psi|^{1/2}} \\
&\qquad \times E\Big\{\Phi\{(1_k\otimes\alpha)'H + \langle 1_k\otimes\alpha',[(I_{kp}-2\Psi)^{-1}(A\otimes\Sigma^{1/2})](L)\rangle\}\Big\} \\
&= \frac{2\exp\{\langle T,\mu'W\mu\rangle + 2\langle\mu,[(WA'\otimes T\Sigma^{1/2})(I_{kp}-2\Psi)^{-1}(AW\otimes\Sigma^{1/2}T)](\mu)\rangle\}}{|I_{kp}-2\Psi|^{1/2}} \\
&\qquad \times\Phi\left\{\frac{\langle 1_k\otimes\alpha',[(I_{kp}-2\Psi)^{-1}(A\otimes\Sigma^{1/2})](L)\rangle}{[1+(1_k\otimes\alpha)'(I_{kp}-2\Psi)^{-1}(1_k\otimes\alpha)]^{1/2}}\right\}.
\end{aligned}
$$

$\square$

From Theorem 2.10, it is easy to obtain the MGF of $X'X \sim SW_p(k,\Sigma,\lambda,\delta_1,\delta_2)$, where $X = v + Z\Sigma^{1/2}$.

**Corollary 2.4.** *Let $X = v + Z\Sigma^{1/2}$ and $Z \sim SN_{k\times p}(0,I_{kp},1_k\otimes\alpha')$. Then the MGF of $K = X'X \sim SW_p(k,\Sigma,\lambda,\delta_1,\delta_2)$ is given by*

$$
\begin{aligned}
M_K(T) &= \frac{2\exp\{\langle T,\lambda\rangle + 2\langle\lambda,T\Sigma^{1/2}(I_p-2\Sigma^{1/2}T\Sigma^{1/2})^{-1}\Sigma^{1/2}T\rangle\}}{|I_p-2\Sigma^{1/2}T\Sigma^{1/2}|^{k/2}} \\
&\qquad \times\Phi\left\{\frac{2\langle T,\Sigma^{1/2}(I_p-2\Sigma^{1/2}T\Sigma^{1/2})^{-1}\delta_1\rangle}{[1+\langle\bar{J}_k\otimes\delta_2,I_k\otimes(I_p-2\Sigma^{1/2}T\Sigma^{1/2})^{-1}\rangle]^{1/2}}\right\}, \quad (2.28)
\end{aligned}
$$

*for symmetric $T \in M_{p\times p}$ such that $\rho(T\Sigma) < 1/2$, where $\bar{J}_k = 1_k 1_k'/k$.*

**Remark 2.3.** *Note that when the skewness parameter matrix* $\delta_1 = 0$, *then the MGF of* $K = X'X$ *is reduced to*

$$M_K(T) = \frac{\exp\{\langle T,\lambda\rangle + 2\langle\lambda, T\Sigma^{1/2}(I_p - 2\Sigma^{1/2}T\Sigma^{1/2})^{-1}\Sigma^{1/2}T\rangle\}}{|I_p - 2\Sigma^{1/2}T\Sigma^{1/2}|^{k/2}},$$

*which is free to* $\delta_2$, *denoted by* $K \sim W_p(k,\Sigma,\lambda)$.

**Lemma 2.4.** *Let* $A \in M_{k\times n}$, $\mu \in M_{n\times p}$, $\lambda \in M_{p\times p}$, $m \le k$ *be a positive integer,* $\Sigma \in M_{p\times p}$ *be positive definite, and* $W \in M_{n\times n}$ *be non-negative definite with rank* $m$. *If*

$$\frac{\exp\{\langle T,\mu'W\mu\rangle + 2\langle\mu, [(WA'\otimes T\Sigma^{1/2})(I_{kp} - 2\Psi)^{-1}(AW\otimes\Sigma^{1/2}T)](\mu)\rangle\}}{|I_{kp} - 2\Psi|^{1/2}}$$

$$= \frac{\exp\{\langle T,\lambda\rangle + 2\langle\lambda, T\Sigma^{1/2}(I_p - 2\Sigma^{1/2}T\Sigma^{1/2})^{-1}\Sigma^{1/2}T\rangle\}}{|I_p - 2\Sigma^{1/2}T\Sigma^{1/2}|^{m/2}},$$

*where* $T \in M_{p\times p}$; $\min\{\rho(\Psi),\rho(T\Sigma)\} > 2$; $\Psi = (AWA')\otimes(\Sigma^{1/2}T\Sigma^{1/2})$, *then*

*(i)* $AWA'$ *is idempotent of rank* $m$ *and*

*(ii)* $\lambda = \mu'W\mu = \mu'WVW\mu = \mu'WVWVW\mu$ *with* $V = A'A$.

The proof of Lemma 2.4 is similar to that of Corollary 2.3.2 given in Wong et al. (1991).

**Theorem 2.11.** *Let* $Z \sim SN_{k\times p}(0,I_{kp},1_k\otimes\alpha')$, $Y = \mu + A'Z\Sigma^{1/2}$, *and* $Q = Y'WY$ *with non-negative definite* $W \in M_{n\times n}$. *Then the necessary and sufficient conditions under which* $Q \sim SW_p(m,\Sigma,\lambda,\delta_1,\delta_2)$, *for some* $\delta_1 \in M_{p\times p}$ *including* $\delta_1 = 0$, *are:*

*(i)* $AWA'$ *is idempotent of rank* $m$,

*(ii)* $\lambda = \mu'W\mu = \mu'WVW\mu = \mu'WVWVW\mu$,

*(iii)* $\delta_1 = \alpha 1'_k AW\mu/d$, *and*

*(iv)* $\delta_2 = 1'_k P_1 P'_1 1_k \alpha\alpha'/d^2$,
*where* $V = A'A$, $d = \sqrt{1 + 1'_k P_2 P'_2 1_k \alpha'\alpha}$ *and* $P = (P_1,P_2)$ *is an orthogonal matrix in* $M_{k\times k}$ *such that*

$$AWA' = P\begin{pmatrix} I_m & 0 \\ 0 & 0 \end{pmatrix}P' = P_1 P'_1. \tag{2.29}$$

*Proof.* First, we assume that (i)-(iv) hold. By (i), there exists an orthogonal matrix $P \in M_{k\times k}$ such that Equation (2.29) holds. Then for non-negative definite $W$, we get

$$P_1 P'_1 AW = AW. \tag{2.30}$$

Let $v = P_1'AW\mu$ and $X = v + P_1'Z\Sigma^{1/2}$, where $Z \sim SN_{kp \times p}(0, I_{kp}, 1_k \otimes \alpha')$. It is easy to show that $X \sim SN_{m \times p}(v, I_m \otimes \Sigma, \gamma_* \otimes \alpha')$, where $\gamma_* = P_1'1_k/d$ and $d = \sqrt{1 + 1_k'P_2P_2'1_k\alpha'\alpha}$. By Definition 2.4, $X'X \sim SW_p(m, \Sigma, \lambda, \delta_1, \delta_2)$ with $\lambda = v'v$, $\delta_1 = \alpha\gamma_*'v$ and $\delta_2 = \gamma_*'\gamma_*\alpha\alpha'$. Note that $\lambda$, $\delta_1$ and $\delta_2$ chosen here are equivalent to (ii), (iii) and (iv), respectively. Thus it suffices to show that $Q \overset{d}{=} X'X$, which means that $Q$ and $X'X$ have the same distribution.

By Equation (2.29) and Equation (2.30), we have

$$
\begin{aligned}
Q &= (\mu + A'Z\Sigma^{1/2})'W(\mu + A'Z\Sigma^{1/2}) \\
&= \mu'W\mu + \Sigma^{1/2}Z'AW\mu + \mu'WA'Z\Sigma^{1/2} + \Sigma^{1/2}Z'AWA'Z\Sigma^{1/2} \\
&= v'v + \Sigma^{1/2}Z'P_1v + v'P_1'Z\Sigma^{1/2} + \Sigma^{1/2}Z'P_1P_1'Z\Sigma^{1/2} \\
&= (v + P_1'Z\Sigma^{1/2})'(v + P_1'Z\Sigma^{1/2}) \overset{d}{=} X'X. 
\end{aligned}
\tag{2.31}
$$

Thus the desired result follows.

Next, assume that $Q \sim SW_p(m, \Sigma, \lambda, \delta_1, \delta_2)$. Let $X \sim SN_{m \times p}(v, I_m \otimes \Sigma, \gamma_* \otimes \alpha')$, $\lambda = v'v$, $\delta_1 = \alpha\gamma_*'v$ and $\delta_2 = \gamma_*'\gamma_*\alpha\alpha'$. By Definition 2.4, we know that $Q \overset{d}{=} X'X$ so that $M_Q(T) = M_{X'X}(T)$. Note that for the case where the skewness parameter matrix $\delta_1 = 0$, the distribution of $Q$ is the noncentral Wishart distribution. By Theorem 2.10 and Corollary 2.4, we obtain

$$
\frac{\exp\{\langle T, \mu'W\mu\rangle + 2\langle \mu, [(WA' \otimes T\Sigma^{1/2})(I_{kp} - 2\Psi)^{-1}(AW \otimes \Sigma^{1/2}T)](\mu)\rangle\}}{|I_{kp} - 2\Psi|^{1/2}}
$$
$$
= \frac{\exp\{\langle T, \lambda\rangle + 2\langle \lambda, T\Sigma^{1/2}(I_p - 2\Sigma^{1/2}T\Sigma^{1/2})^{-1}\Sigma^{1/2}T\rangle\}}{|I_p - 2\Sigma^{1/2}T\Sigma^{1/2}|^{m/2}}
\tag{2.32}
$$

and

$$
\Phi\left\{\frac{\langle 1_k \otimes \alpha', [(I_{kp} - 2\Psi)^{-1}(A \otimes \Sigma^{1/2})](L)\rangle}{[1 + (1_k \otimes \alpha)'(I_{kp} - 2\Psi)^{-1}(1_k \otimes \alpha)]^{1/2}}\right\}
$$
$$
= \Phi\left\{\frac{2\langle T, \Sigma^{1/2}(I_p - 2\Sigma^{1/2}T\Sigma^{1/2})^{-1}\delta_1\rangle}{[1 + \langle \bar{J}_k \otimes \delta_2, I_k \otimes (I_p - 2\Sigma^{1/2}T\Sigma^{1/2})^{-1}\rangle]^{1/2}}\right\},
\tag{2.33}
$$

for symmetric $T \in M_{p \times p}$ such that $\max\{\rho(\Psi), \rho(T\Sigma)\} < 1/2$, where $L = 2W\mu T$ and $\Psi = (AWA') \otimes (\Sigma^{1/2}T\Sigma^{1/2})$. By Lemma 2.4, Equation (2.32) implies (i) and (ii) with $P = (P_1, P_2)$ is an orthogonal matrix in $M_{k \times k}$ satisfying Equation (2.29).

Since $\Phi(x)$ is a strictly increasing function of $x$, Equation (2.33) is reduced to

$$
\frac{\langle 1_k \otimes \alpha', [(I_{kp} - 2\Psi)^{-1}(A \otimes \Sigma^{1/2})](L)\rangle}{[1 + (1_k \otimes \alpha)'(I_{kp} - 2\Psi)^{-1}(1_k \otimes \alpha)]^{1/2}} = \frac{2\langle T, \Sigma^{1/2}(I_p - 2\Sigma^{1/2}T\Sigma^{1/2})^{-1}\delta_1\rangle}{[1 + \langle \bar{J}_k \otimes \delta_2, I_k \otimes (I_p - 2\Sigma^{1/2}T\Sigma^{1/2})^{-1}\rangle]^{1/2}}.
\tag{2.34}
$$

Let $\Gamma = I_p - 2\Sigma^{1/2}T\Sigma^{1/2}$, then $(I_{kp} - 2\Psi)^{-1} = (I_k - AWA') \otimes I_p + (AWA') \otimes \Gamma^{-1}$ and Equation (2.34) is reduced to

$$\frac{\langle 1_k \otimes \alpha', AW\mu T\Sigma^{1/2}\Gamma^{-1}\rangle}{[d^2 + 1_k'P_1P_1'\alpha\Gamma^{-1}\alpha]^{1/2}} = \frac{\langle T, \Sigma^{1/2}\Gamma^{-1}\delta_1\rangle}{[1 + \langle \delta_2, \Gamma^{-1}\rangle]^{1/2}}. \tag{2.35}$$

Note that $\Gamma^{-1} = \sum_{i=0}^{\infty}(2\Sigma^{1/2}T\Sigma^{1/2})^i$. Let $\Gamma^{-1} = I_p$ in Equation (2.35), then we have

$$\langle \Sigma^{1/2}T, \delta_1\rangle = \sqrt{\frac{1 + \langle \delta_2, I_p\rangle}{1 + k\alpha'\alpha}}\langle \Sigma^{1/2}T, \alpha 1_k'AW\mu\rangle,$$

so that

$$\delta_1 = \sqrt{\frac{1 + \langle \delta_2, I_p\rangle}{1 + k\alpha'\alpha}}\alpha 1_k'AW\mu. \tag{2.36}$$

Let $\Gamma^{-1} = 2\Sigma^{1/2}T\Sigma^{1/2}$ and substitute $\delta_1$ back to (2.35), then we obtain

$$\frac{1 + \langle \delta_2, I_p\rangle}{1 + \langle \delta_2, 2\Sigma^{1/2}T\Sigma^{1/2}\rangle} = \frac{1 + k\alpha'\alpha}{d^2 + 21_k'P_1P_1'1_k\alpha'\Sigma^{1/2}T\Sigma^{1/2}\alpha}. \tag{2.37}$$

Further, let $T = 0$ in Equation (2.37), we get

$$1 + \langle \delta_2, I_p\rangle = (1 + k\alpha'\alpha)/d^2. \tag{2.38}$$

By Equations (2.36)-(2.38), we have

$$\delta_1 = \alpha 1_k'AW\mu/d \quad \text{and} \quad \delta_2 = 1_k'P_1P_1'1_k\alpha\alpha'/d^2.$$

$\square$

**Corollary 2.5.** *Let* $Z \sim SN_{k \times p}(0, I_{kp}, 1_k \otimes \alpha')$, $Y = \mu + A'Z\Sigma^{1/2}$ *and* $W$ *be nonnegative definite in* $M_{n \times n}$ *with rank m. Then* $Q = Y'WY \sim SW_p(m, \Sigma, \lambda, \delta_1, \delta_2)$ *if and only if for some* $\delta_1 \in M_{p \times p}$ *including* $\delta_1 = 0$:

*(i)* $W = WVW$,

*(ii)* $\lambda = \mu'W\mu$,

*(iii)* $\delta_1 = \alpha 1_k'AW\mu/d$, and

*(iv)* $\delta_2 = 1_k'P_1P_1'1_k\alpha\alpha'/d^2$,
*where* $V = A'A$, $d = \sqrt{1 + 1_k'P_2P_2'1_k\alpha'\alpha}$ *and* $P = (P_1, P_2)$ *is an orthogonal matrix in* $M_{k \times k}$ *such that*

$$AWA' = P\begin{pmatrix} I_m & 0 \\ 0 & 0 \end{pmatrix}P' = P_1P_1'.$$

**Remark 2.4.** *On the basis of Theorem 2.11, let $Q_i = Y'W_iY$, where $W_i$ is non-negative definite in $M_{n \times n}$, $rk(W_i) = m_i$, $i = 1, \cdots, \ell$. The necessary and sufficient conditions of the quadratic vector $Q = (Q_1, \cdots, Q_\ell)'$ distribution can be further studied, that is, Cohcran's theorem under the skew-normal random matrix, which can be obtained in Ye et al. (2014). This theorem generalizes Cochran theorem (Wong et al., 1991; Gupta and Huang, 2002; Genton et al., 2001; Khatri, 1980; Mathew and Nordstrom, 1997; Wang, 1997; Wang et al., 2009) for normal matrix and skew-normal random vector.*

## 2.3   Bootstrap approach

Suppose that $F(x; \beta)$ is a known cumulative distribution function, where $\beta$ is an unknown parameter or parameter vector. Let $X_1, \ldots, X_n$ be samples from the population $F(x; \beta)$. Firstly, based on the ML equation, we get the ML estimate $\hat{\beta}$ of $\beta$. Then, replacing $\beta$ with $\hat{\beta}$ in the $F(x; \beta)$, we obtain the estimation function $F(x; \hat{\beta})$. Next, generate the samples with sample capacity $n$ from $F(x; \hat{\beta})$, namely,

$$X_{B1}, \cdots, X_{Bn} \sim F(x; \hat{\beta}),$$

which are called the Bootstrap samples. Using the above Bootstrap samples, we can construct the statistical inference method for $\beta$, which is defined as the parameter Bootstrap approach. Next, we apply the Bootstrap approach to discuss the hypothesis testing and interval estimation problems of the mean in the two normal populations.

### 2.3.1   Bootstrap test

Suppose we let $X_1, \ldots, X_n$ and $Y_1, \ldots, Y_n$ be samples from $N(\mu_1, \sigma_1^2)$ and $N(\mu_2, \sigma_2^2)$, respectively, and all the samples are mutually independent. The sample means and sample variances are given by

$$\overline{X} = \frac{1}{n} \sum_{i=1}^{n} X_i, S_1^2 = \frac{1}{n-1} \sum_{i=1}^{n} (X_i - \bar{X})^2,$$

$$\overline{Y} = \frac{1}{m} \sum_{i=1}^{m} Y_i, S_2^2 = \frac{1}{m-1} \sum_{i=1}^{m} (Y_i - \bar{Y})^2.$$

The hypothesis testing problem is considered as

$$H_0 : \mu_1 = \mu_2 \quad versus \quad H_1 : \mu_1 \neq \mu_2. \tag{2.39}$$

If $\sigma_1^2$ and $\sigma_2^2$ are known, then a natural test statistic is defined as

$$T(\overline{X}, \overline{Y}; \sigma_1^2, \sigma_2^2) = \frac{\overline{X} - \overline{Y}}{\sqrt{\sigma_1^2/n + \sigma_2^2/m}}. \tag{2.40}$$

When the null hypothesis $H_0$ is true, $T(\overline{X},\overline{Y};\sigma_1^2,\sigma_2^2) \sim N(0,1)$. Therefore, we can establish the testing method based on $T(\overline{X},\overline{Y};\sigma_1^2,\sigma_2^2)$.

However, generally speaking, $\sigma_1^2$ and $\sigma_2^2$ are unknown. Then replacing $\sigma_i^2$ with $S_i^2$ $(i=1,2)$ in (2.40), the new test statistic is represented as

$$T(\overline{X},\overline{Y};S_1^2,S_2^2) = \frac{\overline{X}-\overline{Y}}{\sqrt{S_1^2/n+S_2^2/m}}. \tag{2.41}$$

It is obvious that the exact distribution for $T(\overline{X},\overline{Y};S_1^2,S_2^2)$ is not obtained under the null hypothesis $H_0$, so we can not get the exact test for the hypothesis testing problem (2.39). Then, we can set up the testing method by using the Bootstrap approach.

Let $(\bar{x},\bar{y},s_1^2,s_2^2)$ be the observed values of $(\overline{X},\overline{Y},S_1^2,S_2^2)$. Let

$$\overline{X}_B \sim N(0,s_1^2/n), S_{B1}^2 \sim s_1^2\chi_{n-1}^2/(n-1),$$

$$\overline{Y}_B \sim N(0,s_2^2/m), S_{B2}^2 \sim s_2^2\chi_{m-1}^2/(m-1).$$

By (2.41), the Bootstrap test statistic given by Xu (2016) is expressed as

$$T_B = \frac{\overline{X}_B-\overline{Y}_B}{\sqrt{S_{B1}^2/n+S_{B2}^2/m}}. \tag{2.42}$$

The Bootstrap p-value is computed as

$$p = 2\min\{P(T_B>t),P(T_B<t)\},$$

where $t = T(\bar{x},\bar{y};s_1^2,s_2^2)$ is the observed value of $T(\overline{X},\overline{Y};S_1^2,S_2^2)$. The null hypothesis $H_0$ in (2.39) is rejected whenever the above Bootstrap p-value is less than the nominal significance level of $\gamma$.

### 2.3.2  Bootstrap confidence interval

In this subsection, using the Bootstrap approach, the confidence interval of $\mu_1-\mu_2$ is constructed based on the sufficient statistics $(\overline{X},\overline{Y},S_1^2,S_2^2)$. If $\sigma_1^2$ and $\sigma_2^2$ are known, then a natural pivot quantity is defined as

$$T^*(\overline{X},\overline{Y};\sigma_1^2,\sigma_2^2) = \frac{\overline{X}-\overline{Y}-(\mu_1-\mu_2)}{\sqrt{\sigma_1^2/n+\sigma_2^2/m}}. \tag{2.43}$$

Clearly, $T^*(\overline{X},\overline{Y};\sigma_1^2,\sigma_2^2) \sim N(0,1)$. Let $z_\gamma$ denote the $100\gamma$ percentile of the standard normal distribution. Then the $100(1-\gamma)\%$ confidence interval for $\mu_1-\mu_2$ is given by

$$\left[\bar{x}-\bar{y}-z_{\gamma/2}\sqrt{\sigma_1^2/n+\sigma_2^2/m},\bar{x}-\bar{y}+z_{\gamma/2}\sqrt{\sigma_1^2/n+\sigma_2^2/m}\right].$$

In practice, $\sigma_1^2$ and $\sigma_2^2$ are often unknown. Replacing $\sigma_i^2$ with $S_i^2$ ($i = 1, 2$) in (2.43), the new pivot quantity is represented as

$$T^*(\overline{X}, \overline{Y}; S_1^2, S_2^2) = \frac{\overline{X} - \overline{Y} - (\mu_1 - \mu_2)}{\sqrt{S_1^2/n + S_2^2/m}}. \tag{2.44}$$

Obviously, the exact distribution of $T^*(\overline{X}, \overline{Y}; S_1^2, S_2^2)$ is not obtained, so we can not get the exact confidence interval for $\mu_1 - \mu_2$. Then, the Bootstrap pivot quantity proposed by Xu (2016) is given by

$$T_B^* = \frac{(\overline{X}_B - \overline{Y}_B) - (\overline{x} - \overline{y})}{\sqrt{S_{B1}^2/n + S_{B2}^2/m}}. \tag{2.45}$$

where $\overline{X}_B, \overline{Y}_B, S_{B1}^2, S_{B2}^2$ are from (2.42). Let $T_B^*(\gamma)$ be the $100\gamma$ empirical percentile of $T_B^*$. The $100(1 - \gamma)\%$ Bootstrap confidence interval for $\mu_1 - \mu_2$ is expressed as

$$\left[ \overline{x} - \overline{y} - T_B^*(1 - \gamma/2)\sqrt{s_1^2/n + s_2^2/m}, \ \overline{x} - \overline{y} + T_B^*(\gamma/2)\sqrt{s_1^2/n + s_2^2/m} \right].$$

## 2.4 Generalized p-value and generalized confidence interval

The concept of the generalized p-value and generalized confidence interval was initially introduced by Tsui and Weerahandi (1989) and Weerahandi (1993), respectively. This approach finds wide application in hypothesis testing problems where the number of nuisance parameters exceeds that of the parameters of interest. Building on references (Abdel-Karim, 2005; Weerahandi, 1995; Weerahandi, 2004), we present the notions of generalized test variables, generalized p-values, generalized pivot quantities, and generalized confidence intervals.

Let $X$ be a random variable relying on $\zeta = (\theta, \eta)$, where $\theta$ is the parameter of interest, $\eta$ is the nuisance parameter, and $\eta$ may be a vector of parameters. Let $\mathscr{X}$ be the sample space of $X$, $\Theta$ be the parameter space of $\theta$, and $x$ be the observed value of $X$. Consider the hypothesis testing problem.

$$H_0 : \theta \in \Theta_0 \quad versus \quad H_1 : \theta \in \Theta_1, \tag{2.46}$$

where $\Theta_0$ and $\Theta_1$ are two disjoint subsets of $\Theta$.

**Definition 2.5.** *Given a value $\theta_0$ and an observed value $x$, if there exists a real-valued function $T(X;\theta_0)$ satisfying the following conditions:*

*(i) The distribution of $T(X;\theta_0)$ is free of the nuisance parameter $\eta$,*

*(ii) $T(X;\theta_0)$ is stochastically monotonic with respect to $\theta$, i.e., $P(T(X;\theta_0) \geq t)$ is a monotonic function of $\theta$, where $t$ is the observed value of $T(X;\theta_0)$.*

*Then $T(X;\theta_0)$ is called the test statistic for $\theta$.*

**Definition 2.6.** *Let $C(X;x)$ be a subset of the sample space $\mathscr{X}$. If $C(X;x)$ satisfies the following conditions:*

*(i) The observed value $x$ of $X$ lies on the boundary of $C(X;x)$,*

*(ii) $C(X;z)$ is free of the nuisance parameter $\eta$,*

*(iii) The probability of $C(X;x)$ is free of $\zeta$, where $\theta = \theta_0$ and $P(C(X;x)|\theta \in \Theta_0) \leq P(C(X;x)|\theta \in \Theta_1)$.*

*Then $C(X;x)$ is called the extreme region.*

**Definition 2.7.** *Let $C(X;x)$ be the extreme region, and the p-value based on this extreme region can be computed as*

$$p = \sup\{P(C(X;x)|\theta \in \Theta_0)\}. \tag{2.47}$$

**Definition 2.8.** *Let $R(X;\theta)$ be a real-valued function of $X$ and $\theta$. If the distribution of $R(X;\theta)$ is free of $\theta$, then $R(X;\theta)$ is called a pivot quantity.*

**Definition 2.9.** *Let $L(X)$ and $U(X)$ be functions of $X$ satisfying $P(L(X) \leq \theta \leq U(X)) = 1 - \gamma$. Then $[L(X),U(X)]$ is called a confidence interval for $\theta$ with a confidence level of $100(1 - \gamma)\%$, where $\gamma$ is the nominal significance level.*

**Definition 2.10.** *For an observed value $x$ and a parameter $\zeta$, if there exists a real-valued function $T(X;x,\zeta)$ satisfying the following conditions:*

*(i) The distribution of $T(X;x,\zeta)$ is free of the nuisance parameter $\eta$,*

*(ii) The observed value $t$ of $T(X;x,\zeta)$ is free of any unknown parameters,*

*(iii) Given $x$ and $\eta$, $T(X;x,\zeta)$ is stochastically monotonic with respect to $\theta$, i.e., $P(T(X;x,\zeta) \geq t)$ is a monotonic function of $\theta$.*

*Then $T$ is called a generalized test variable.*

**Remark 2.5.** *Condition (ii) in Definition 2.10 can be omitted because if $T(X;x,\zeta)$ does not satisfy this condition, $\widetilde{T}(X;x,\zeta) = T(X;x,\zeta) - T(x;x,\zeta)$ can be redefined. It is evident that $\widetilde{T}(X;x,\zeta)$ satisfies Condition (ii) in Definition 2.10. Additionally, Condition (i) ensures that the p-value based on the generalized test variable is computable, and Condition (iii) makes this testing method unbiased.*

**Definition 2.11.** *Let $C(X;x,\zeta)$ be a subset of the sample space $\mathscr{X}$. If $C(X;x,\zeta)$ satisfies the following conditions:*

*(i) The observed value $x$ of $X$ lies on the boundary of $C(X;x,\zeta)$,*

*(ii) The probability of $C(X;x,\zeta)$ is free of the nuisance parameter $\eta$ and satisfies $P(C(X;x,\zeta)|\theta \in \Theta_0) \leqslant P(C(X;x,\zeta)|\theta \in \Theta_1)$.*

*Then $C(X;x,\zeta)$ is called a generalized extreme region.*

**Definition 2.12.** *Let $C(X;x,\zeta)$ be a generalized extreme region. The generalized p-value based on this extreme region can be computed as*

$$p = \sup\{P(C(X;x,\zeta)|\theta \in \Theta_0)\}, \tag{2.48}$$

**Remark 2.6.** *Considering the hypothesis testing problem:*

$$H_0 : \theta \leqslant \theta_0 \quad versus \quad H_1 : \theta > \theta_0,$$
$$H_0 : \theta \geqslant \theta_0 \quad versus \quad H_1 : \theta < \theta_0.$$

*Assuming the generalized test variable $T(X;x,\zeta)$ is stochastically monotonic increasing with respect to $\theta$, then the generalized p-values for the above-mentioned hypothesis testing problems can be respectively computed as*

$$p = P(T(X;x,\zeta) \geqslant t|\theta = \theta_0),$$
$$p = P(T(X;x,\zeta) \leqslant t|\theta = \theta_0),$$

*where $t = T(x;x,\zeta)$.*

**Definition 2.13.** *The hypothesis testing problem (2.46) is invariant under a transformation $G$ in the sample space $\chi$. For any given $x \in \mathscr{X}, \theta \in \Theta, g \in G$, and the power $\pi(x;\theta) = P(X \in C(X;x,\zeta)|\theta)$, if $\pi(g(x);\theta) = \pi(x;\theta)$, then the test based on the generalized extreme region $C(X;x,\zeta)$ is called a p-invariant test.*

**Definition 2.14.** *Let $R(X;x,\zeta)$ be a real-valued function of $X,x$ and $\zeta$. If $R(X;x,\zeta)$ satisfies the following conditions:*

*(i) The distribution of $R(X;x,\zeta)$ is free of any unknown parameters,*

*(ii) The observed value $r$ of $R(X;x,\zeta)$ is free of the nuisance parameter $\eta$.*

*Then $R(X;x,\zeta)$ is called a generalized pivot quantity.*

**Definition 2.15.** *Let $C_\gamma$ be a subset of the sample space $\mathscr{R}$ of $R(X;x,\zeta)$, which satisfies*

$$P(R(X;x,\zeta) \in C_\gamma) = 1 - \gamma.$$

*Then the subset $\Theta_c(x) = \{\theta \in \Theta | R(x;x,\zeta) \in C_\gamma\}$ of parameter space $\Theta$ is called a generalized confidence interval for $\theta$ with the confidence level of $100(1-\gamma)\%$.*

**Remark 2.7.** *If $R(x;x,\zeta) = \theta$, then $[R(\gamma/2), R(1-\gamma/2)]$ is a generalized confidence interval for $\theta$ with a confidence level of $100(1-\gamma)\%$, where $R = R(X;x,\zeta)$ and $R(k)$ represents the $100k$ empirical percentile of $R$.*

**Definition 2.16.** *The distribution family $F(X|\theta)$ of $X$ is invariant under a transformation $G$ in the sample space $\mathscr{X}$, and the induced transformation on the parameter space is $\theta \to \theta$ (i.e., uneffected by $\theta$). For any given $x \in \mathscr{X}, g \in G$, if the generalized confidence interval $\Theta_c(x)$ satisfies $\Theta_c(g(x)) = \Theta_c(x)$, then the generalized confidence interval $\Theta_c(x)$ is invariant.*

# Chapter 3

# Location Parameter of Skew-Normal Population

Consider the skew-normal population density function

$$f(y;\xi,\eta^2,\alpha) = 2\phi(y;\xi,\eta^2)\Phi[\alpha\eta^{-1}(y-\xi)], \tag{3.1}$$

where $\xi \in R$ denotes the location parameter, $\eta^2 \in R^+$ denotes the scale parameter, $\alpha \in R$ denotes the skewness parameter, $\phi(y;\xi,\eta^2)$ is the normal density function with mean $\xi$ and variance $\eta^2$, and $\Phi(\cdot)$ is the standard normal cumulative distribution function. Denote $Y \sim SN(\xi,\eta^2,\alpha)$. When $\xi = 0$ and $\eta^2 = 1$, (3.1) is degenerated into the standard skew-normal distribution $SN(\alpha)$. When $\alpha = 0$, (3.1) is degenerated into the normal distribution $N(\xi,\eta^2)$. In short, the alteration of the skewness parameter allows for a continuous variation from normality to skew-normality.

For (3.1), in this section we address the issue of homogeneous testing of location parameters in several skew-normal populations. Initially, we construct the conditional test statistic and establish its approximate distribution. Subsequently, we estimate the unknown parameters using the methods of moments and maximum likelihood estimation. We the proceed to construct the Bootstrap test statistics. Finally, we present Monte Carlo results from both methods and illustrate the aforementioned approaches with two real examples involving gross domestic product and turbine bearing performance.

## 3.1 Conditional test statistic

For convenience, let $\overset{asy}{\sim}$ denote the approximate distribution, and $D(X)$ denote the variance of random variable $X$. In this section, the conditional test statistic for homogeneous testing of location parameters in $k$ skew-normal populations is constructed, and then the relevant properties of the skew-normal distributions are given.

**Lemma 3.1.** *Suppose* $X_j \overset{asy}{\sim} N(0,1)$, $j = 1,...,k$, *and* $X_1,...,X_k$ *are mutually independent of each other, then* $\sum\limits_{j=1}^{k} X_j^2 \overset{asy}{\sim} \chi^2(k)$.

*Proof.* Suppose the distribution function of $X_j$ is $F_j(x)$, $j = 1,...,k$. Additionally, let $F(x)$ denote the standard normal cumulative distribution function. From the weak convergence Theorem (Hu, 2009), we get

$$\int e^{itx^2} dF_j(x) \to \int e^{itx^2} dF(x), \ j = 1,...,k,$$

namely

$$E(e^{itx_j^2}) \to E(e^{itx^2}), \ j = 1,...,k.$$

By the continuity Theorem (Wu et al., 1979), we obtain

$$X_j^2 \overset{asy}{\sim} \chi^2(1), \ j = 1,...,k.$$

Since $X_1,...,X_k$ are mutually independent of each other, according to Zhong (2010)

$$\sum_{j=1}^{k} X_j^2 \overset{asy}{\sim} \chi^2(k).$$

Therefore, the proof of Lemma 3.1 is completed. $\qquad\qquad\square$

Suppose $Y_{i1},...,Y_{in_i}$ is a group of random samples from the skew-normal distribution $SN(\xi_i, \eta_i^2, \alpha_i)$, $i = 1,...,k$. The sample mean, the second-order and third-order central moments can be expressed as

$$\bar{Y}_i = \frac{1}{n_i} \sum_{j=1}^{n_i} Y_{ij}, \ S_{2i} = \frac{1}{n_i} \sum_{j=1}^{n_i} (Y_{ij} - \bar{Y}_i)^2, \ S_{3i} = \frac{1}{n_i} \sum_{j=1}^{n_i} (Y_{ij} - \bar{Y}_i)^3, \ i = 1,...,k. \quad (3.2)$$

Obviously, the moment generating function of $Y_i$ is

$$M_{Y_i}(t) = 2\exp\left(t\xi_i + \frac{t^2 \eta_i^2}{2}\right) \Phi(t\eta_i \delta_i), \ i = 1,...,k. \quad (3.3)$$

From (3.3), we get,

$$
\begin{aligned}
E(Y_i) &= M'_{Y_i}(t)|_{t=0} = \xi_i + b\eta_i\delta_i, \\
E(Y_i^2) &= M''_{Y_i}(t)|_{t=0} = \xi_i^2 + 2b\xi_i\eta_i\delta_i + \eta_i^2, \\
E(Y_i^3) &= M'''_{Y_i}(t)|_{t=0} = \xi_i^3 + 3b\xi_i^2\eta_i\delta_i + 3\xi_i\eta_i^2 + 3b\eta_i^3\delta_i - b\eta_i^3\delta_i^3,
\end{aligned}
\tag{3.4}
$$

where $\delta_i = \alpha_i/(1+\alpha_i^2)^{1/2}$, and $b = (2/\pi)^{1/2}$, $i = 1,...,k$. For a given $(\eta_i, \delta_i)$, the estimator of $\xi_i$ and its variance can be expressed as

$$
\hat{\xi}_i|_{(\eta_i,\delta_i)} = \bar{Y}_i - b\eta_i\delta_i, \quad D(\hat{\xi}_i|_{(\eta_i,\delta_i)}) = \frac{\eta_i^2(1-b^2\delta_i^2)}{n_i}, \quad i = 1,...,k.
\tag{3.5}
$$

For $i = 1,...,k$, let $\xi_i = \xi + \Delta\xi_i$, where $\Delta\xi_i$ denotes the difference between the $i$th population location parameter $\xi_i$ and common location parameter $\xi$. Then the homogeneous test of location parameters is equal to

$$
H_0 : \Delta\xi_1 = \Delta\xi_2 = ... = \Delta\xi_k = 0 \qquad versus \qquad H_1 : \exists\, i,\ \Delta\xi_i \neq 0.
\tag{3.6}
$$

When the null hypothesis $H_0$ is true and $(\eta_i, \delta_i)$ is known, using the idea of Graybill-Deal estimation (Graybill and Deal, 1959), the estimator of the common location parameter $\xi$ is

$$
\hat{\xi} = \frac{\displaystyle\sum_{i=1}^{k} \frac{1}{D(\hat{\xi}_i|_{(\eta_i,\delta_i)})} \hat{\xi}_i|_{(\eta_i,\delta_i)}}{\displaystyle\sum_{i=1}^{k} \frac{1}{D(\hat{\xi}_i|_{(\eta_i,\delta_i)})}} = \frac{\displaystyle\sum_{i=1}^{k} \frac{n_i}{\eta_i^2(1-b^2\delta_i^2)} \hat{\xi}_i|_{(\eta_i,\delta_i)}}{\displaystyle\sum_{i=1}^{k} \frac{n_i}{\eta_i^2(1-b^2\delta_i^2)}} = \sum_{i=1}^{k} \omega_i \hat{\xi}_i|_{(\eta_i,\delta_i)},
\tag{3.7}
$$

where $\omega_i = \dfrac{\frac{n_i}{\eta_i^2(1-b^2\delta_i^2)}}{\sum_{i=1}^{k} \frac{n_i}{\eta_i^2(1-b^2\delta_i^2)}}, i = 1,...,k.$

Then, define a statistic

$$
Z_i = \frac{n_i}{\eta_i^2(1-b^2\delta_i^2)}\left(\hat{\xi}_i|_{(\eta_i,\delta_i)} - \sum_{i=1}^{k} \omega_i \hat{\xi}_i|_{(\eta_i,\delta_i)}\right), \quad i = 1,...,k.
\tag{3.8}
$$

Under $H_0$ in (3.6), the expectation and variance of $Z_i$ are

$$E(Z_i) = \frac{n_i}{\eta_i^2(1-b^2\delta_i^2)} \left( E(\hat{\xi}_i|_{(\eta_i,\delta_i)}) - \sum_{i=1}^{k} \omega_i E(\hat{\xi}_i|_{(\eta_i,\delta_i)}) \right) = 0,$$

$$D(Z_i) = \left( \frac{n_i}{\eta_i^2(1-b^2\delta_i^2)} \right)^2 D\left( (1-\omega_i)\hat{\xi}_i|_{(\eta_i,\delta_i)} + \sum_{j\neq i}^{k} \omega_j \hat{\xi}_j|_{(\eta_j,\delta_j)} \right)$$

$$= \left( \frac{n_i}{\eta_i^2(1-b^2\delta_i^2)} \right)^2 \left[ (1-\omega_i)^2 \frac{\eta_i^2(1-b^2\delta_i^2)}{n_i} + \sum_{j\neq i}^{k} \omega_j^2 \frac{\eta_j^2(1-b^2\delta_j^2)}{n_j} \right]$$

$$= \left( \frac{n_i}{\eta_i^2(1-b^2\delta_i^2)} \right)^2 \left( \frac{\eta_i^2(1-b^2\delta_i^2)}{n_i} - \frac{1}{\sum\limits_{i=1}^{k} \frac{n_i}{\eta_i^2(1-b^2\delta_i^2)}} \right), \ i = 1,...,k.$$

By the central limit theorem, we have

$$\frac{Z_i - E(Z_i)}{\sqrt{D(Z_i)}} = \frac{\xi_i|_{(\eta_i,\delta_i)} - \sum\limits_{i=1}^{k} \omega_i \hat{\xi}_i|_{(\eta_i,\delta_i)}}{\sqrt{\frac{\eta_i^2(1-b^2\delta_i^2)}{n_i}}\, (1-\omega_i)}, \ i = 1,...,k. \tag{3.9}$$

When $n_i \to \infty$, the approximate distribution of $\frac{Z_i - E(Z_i)}{\sqrt{D(Z_i)}}$ is a standard normal distribution $N(0,1)$, $i = 1,...,k$. Under $H_0$ in (3.6), define the conditional test statistic as

$$T = \sum_{i=1}^{k} \left( \frac{\xi_i|_{(\eta_i,\delta_i)} - \sum\limits_{i=1}^{k} \omega_i \hat{\xi}_i|_{(\eta_i,\delta_i)}}{\sqrt{\frac{\eta_i^2(1-b^2\delta_i^2)}{n_i}}\, (1-\omega_i)} \right)^2$$

$$= \sum_{i=1}^{k} \frac{n_i}{\eta_i^2(1-b^2\delta_i^2)} \frac{\left( (\bar{Y}_i - b\eta_i\delta_i) - \sum\limits_{i=1}^{k} \omega_i(\bar{Y}_i - b\eta_i\delta_i) \right)^2}{1-\omega_i}. \tag{3.10}$$

Due to Lemma 3.1, we get $T \overset{asy}{\sim} \chi^2(k)$.

Denote

$$\bar{Y} = (\bar{Y}_1 - b\eta_1\delta_1, \bar{Y}_2 - b\eta_2\delta_2, ..., \bar{Y}_k - b\eta_k\delta_k)',$$

$$\Delta = diag\left( \frac{\eta_1^2(1-b^2\delta_1^2)}{n_1}, \frac{\eta_2^2(1-b^2\delta_2^2)}{n_2}, ..., \frac{\eta_k^2(1-b^2\delta_k^2)}{n_k} \right).$$

Obviously, the conditional test statistic $T$ can be expressed as

$$T = \left( \Delta^{-1/2}\bar{Y} \right)' AB^{-1}A \left( \Delta^{-1/2}\bar{Y} \right), \tag{3.11}$$

where $A = I_k - \left( \Delta^{-1/2}11'\Delta^{-1/2} \right)/(1'\Delta^{-1}1)$ is an idempotent matrix with rank $k-1$, $B = I_k - \Delta^{-1}/(1'\Delta^{-1}1)$, and $I_k$ is an identity matrix of order $k$. By the properties of an identity matrix and orthogonal decomposition, we have $A = P \begin{pmatrix} I_{k-1} & 0 \\ 0 & 0 \end{pmatrix} P^{-1}$, where $P$ is an orthogonal matrix. Accordingly, we obtain

$$AB^{-1}A = P \begin{pmatrix} I_{k-1} & 0 \\ 0 & 0 \end{pmatrix} P^{-1} B^{-1} P \begin{pmatrix} I_{k-1} & 0 \\ 0 & 0 \end{pmatrix} P^{-1}. \tag{3.12}$$

Let $Z = \begin{pmatrix} I_{k-1} & 0 \\ 0 & 0 \end{pmatrix} P^{-1} B^{-1} P \begin{pmatrix} I_{k-1} & 0 \\ 0 & 0 \end{pmatrix}$. Based on the orthogonal decomposition, we have $Z = Q\Lambda Q^{-1}$, where $\Lambda = diag(\lambda_1, ..., \lambda_k)$, and $Q$ is the eigenvector matrix corresponding to $\Lambda$. Thus, Equation (3.11) can be expressed as

$$T = \left( \Delta^{-1/2}\bar{Y} \right)' PQ\Lambda Q^{-1} P^{-1} \left( \Delta^{-1/2}\bar{Y} \right). \tag{3.13}$$

**Theorem 3.1.** *Let $\tau = \zeta' \Delta^{-1} \zeta$, where $\zeta = (\xi_1, ..., \xi_k)'$. If $\alpha_1 = \alpha_2 = ... = \alpha_k = 0$, then $T \sim \sum_{i=1}^{k} \lambda_i \chi_i^2(1, \tau)$, where $\chi_i^2(1, \tau)$ represents the noncentral $\chi^2$ distribution with degree of freedom 1 and noncentrality parameter $\tau$, $i = 1, ..., k$. And $\chi_1^2(1, \tau), ..., \chi_k^2(1, \tau)$ are mutually independent of each other.*

*Proof.* If $\alpha_1 = \alpha_2 = ... = \alpha_k = 0$, then

$$\Delta^{-1/2}\bar{Y} \sim N_k(\Delta^{-1/2}\zeta, I_k),$$
$$\left( \Delta^{-1/2}\bar{Y} \right)' PQQ^{-1} P^{-1} \left( \Delta^{-1/2}\bar{Y} \right) \sim \chi_k^2(\zeta' \Delta^{-1}\zeta).$$

Further,

$$T = \left( \Delta^{-1/2}\bar{Y} \right)' PQ\Lambda Q^{-1} P^{-1} \left( \Delta^{-1/2}\bar{Y} \right) \sim \sum_{i=1}^{k} \lambda_i \chi_i^2(1, \tau).$$

Therefore, the proof of Theorem 3.1 is complete. $\qquad\square$

**Remark 3.1.** *If $\alpha_1 = \alpha_2 = ... = \alpha_k = 0$ in (3.10), then $T$ can be expressed as*

$$T = \sum_{i=1}^{k} \frac{n_i}{\eta_i^2} \frac{\left( \bar{Y}_i - \sum_{i=1}^{k} \omega_{1i}\bar{Y}_i \right)^2}{1 - \omega_{1i}},$$

*where $\omega_{1i} = \left( \frac{n_i}{\eta_i^2} \right) / \left( \sum_{i=1}^{k} \frac{n_i}{\eta_i^2} \right)$, $i = 1, ..., k$. By Theorem 3.1, $T$ can be used as the conditional test statistic of the homogeneous test of means in several normal populations. Hence, $T$ is an extension of the result given by Xu (2016).*

## 3.2 Parameter estimation

For $i = 1,...,k$, it is well-known that $(\eta_i^2, \delta_i)$ is often unknown in practical issues. Then we consider the parameter estimation problem of $(\eta_i^2, \delta_i)$.

**Theorem 3.2.** *If $Y_i \sim SN(\xi_i, \eta_i^2, \alpha_i)$, then the moment estimators of $(\xi_i, \eta_i^2, \alpha_i)$ satisfy*

$$\hat{\xi}_i = \bar{Y}_i - cS_{3i}^{1/3}, \quad \hat{\eta}_i^2 = S_{2i} + c^2 S_{3i}^{2/3}, \quad \hat{\alpha}_i = \hat{\delta}_i / \left(1 - \hat{\delta}_i^2\right)^{1/2}, i = 1,...,k, \qquad (3.14)$$

*where* $c = [2/(4 - \pi)]^{1/3}$ *and* $\hat{\delta}_i = \dfrac{cS_{3i}^{1/3}}{b(S_{2i} + c^2 S_{3i}^{2/3})^{1/2}}.$

*Proof.* Let $(\bar{y}_i, s_{2i}, s_{3i})$ be the observed value of $(\bar{Y}_i, S_{2i}, S_{3i})$. Standardizing $Y_{ij}$, namely

$$X_{ij} = (Y_{ij} - \bar{y}_i)/\sqrt{s_{2i}}, i = 1,...,k, j = 1,...,n_i, \qquad (3.15)$$

then $X_{i1},...,X_{in_i}$ are the standardized samples from $X_i \sim SN(\xi_{si}, \eta_{si}^2, \alpha_i)$, where

$$\xi_{si} = (\xi_i - \bar{y}_i)/\sqrt{s_{2i}}, \quad \eta_{si} = \eta_i/\sqrt{s_{2i}}, \quad i = 1,...,k. \qquad (3.16)$$

Obviously, the moment generating function of $X_i$ is

$$M_{X_i}(t) = 2\exp\left(t\xi_{si} + \frac{t^2\eta_{si}^2}{2}\right)\Phi\left(t\eta_{si}\delta_i\right), i = 1,...,k. \qquad (3.17)$$

From (3.17), we can obtain

$$\begin{aligned}
M'_{X_i}(t)|_{t=0} &= \xi_{si} + b\eta_{si}\delta_i = 0, \\
M''_{X_i}(t)|_{t=0} &= \xi_{si}^2 + 2b\xi_{si}\eta_{si}\delta_i + \eta_{si}^2 = 1, \\
M'''_{X_i}(t)|_{t=0} &= \xi_{si}^3 + 3b\xi_{si}^2\eta_{si}\delta_i + 3\xi_{si}\eta_{si}^2 + 3b\eta_{si}^3\delta_i - b\eta_{si}^3\delta_i^3 = s_{2i}^{-3/2}s_{3i}.
\end{aligned} \qquad (3.18)$$

By (3.16) and (3.18), we get the moment estimates of $(\xi_i, \eta_i^2, \alpha_i)$ as follows.

$$\hat{\xi}_i^* = \bar{y}_i - cs_{3i}^{1/3}, \quad \hat{\eta}_i^{*2} = s_{2i} + c^2 s_{3i}^{2/3}, \quad \hat{\alpha}_i^* = \frac{\hat{\delta}_i^*}{\sqrt{1 - \hat{\delta}_i^{*2}}}, \qquad (3.19)$$

where $\hat{\delta}_i^* = \dfrac{cs_{3i}^{1/3}}{b(s_{2i} + c^2 s_{3i}^{2/3})^{1/2}}$, $i = 1,...,k$. Then the proof of Theorem 3.2 is completed. $\qquad\qquad\square$

As the results of using numerical techniques to maximize the log-likelihood for direct parameters $(\xi_i, \eta_i^2, \alpha_i)$ may be highly misleading as for this case no unique solution exists. For this, we derive the ML estimators of the unknown parameters based on the method of centred parametrization by Azzalini (1985), Azzalini and Capitanio (2014) and Pewsey (2000a). Denoting

$$W_i = \frac{Y_i - \xi_i}{\eta_i} \sim SN(\alpha_i), \ Y_{Ci} = \mu_i + \sigma_i \left( \frac{W_i - E(W_i)}{\sqrt{D(W_i)}} \right) \sim SN_C(\mu_i, \sigma_i^2, \gamma_i), \quad (3.20)$$

where $SN_C(\mu_i, \sigma_i^2, \gamma_i)$ represents the skew-normal distribution with mean $\mu_i \in R$, variance $\sigma_i^2 \in R^+$, and skewness coefficient $\gamma_i$, $i = 1, ..., k$. Pewsey (2006) introduced the following relationship between the direct parameter $(\xi_i, \eta_i^2, \alpha_i)$ and the centered one $(\mu_i, \sigma_i^2, \gamma_i)$

$$\xi_i = \mu_i - c\gamma_i^{1/3}\sigma_i, \ \eta_i^2 = \sigma_i^2(1 + c_i^2\gamma_i^{2/3}), \ \alpha_i = \frac{c\gamma_i^{1/3}}{\sqrt{b^2 + c^2(b^2 - 1)\gamma_i^{2/3}}}, \ i = 1, ..., k.$$

$$(3.21)$$

**Theorem 3.3.** *Suppose* $Y_i \sim SN(\xi_i, \eta_i^2, \alpha_i)$. *Let*

$$W_i = \frac{Y_i - \xi_i}{\eta_i} \ \ and \ \ Y_{Ci} = \mu_i + \sigma_i \left( \frac{W_i - E(W_i)}{\sqrt{D(W_i)}} \right),$$

*then* $Y_{Ci} = Y_i$, $i = 1, ..., k$.

*Proof.* By (3.3), we can derive the skewness coefficient $\gamma_i$ as follows.

$$\gamma_i = \frac{E\left[(Y_i - EY_i)^3\right]}{\left[E(Y_i - EY_i)^2\right]^{3/2}} = \frac{b^3\delta_i^3}{c^3(1 - b^2\delta_i^2)^{3/2}}. \quad (3.22)$$

From (3.21) and (3.22), we have

$$\sigma_i = \eta_i\sqrt{1 - b^2\delta_i^2}, \ \mu_i = \xi_i + b\eta_i\delta_i, \ i = 1, ..., k. \quad (3.23)$$

For $W_i \sim SN(\alpha_i)$, it is easy to see that

$$E(W_i) = b\delta_i, \ D(W_i) = 1 - b^2\delta_i^2, \ i = 1, ..., k.$$

Then,

$$Y_{Ci} = \xi_i + b\eta_i\delta_i + \eta_i\sqrt{1 - b^2\delta_i^2} \left( \frac{\frac{Y_i - \xi_i}{\eta_i} - b\delta_i}{\sqrt{1 - b^2\delta_i^2}} \right) = Y_i.$$

Therefore, the proof of Theorem 3.3 is complete. $\qquad\qquad\square$

**Remark 3.2.** *If* $|\alpha_i| \to \infty$, *then* $|\delta_i| \to 1$. *By* (3.22), *we have* $\gamma_i \in (-0.99527, 0.99527)$, $i = 1, ..., k$.

Now consider the ML estimators of the centered parameter $(\mu_i, \sigma_i^2, \gamma_i)$, $i = 1, ..., k$. Denote the observed value of $(\bar{Y}_{Ci}, S_{C2i}, S_{C3i})$ by $(\bar{y}_{Ci}, s_{C2i}, s_{C3i})$. Similarly, let $Y_{sij} = (Y_{Cij} - \bar{y}_{Ci})/\sqrt{s_{C2i}}$, where $Y_{si1}, ..., Y_{sin_i}$ is a group of samples from $Y_{si} \sim SN_C(\mu_{si}, \sigma_{si}^2, \gamma_i)$ with $\mu_{si} = (\mu_i - \bar{y}_{Ci})/\sqrt{s_{C2i}}$ and $\sigma_{si} = \sigma_i/\sqrt{s_{C2i}}$, $i = 1, ..., k, \ j = 1, ..., n_i$. The density function of $Y_{si}$ is obtained as follows.

$$f\left(y_{si}; \mu_{si}, \sigma_{si}^2, \gamma_i\right) = \frac{2}{\sigma_{si}\sqrt{s_{C2i}\left(1+c^2\gamma_i^{2/3}\right)}} \phi\left[\left(\frac{y_{si}-\mu_{si}}{\sigma_{si}} + c\gamma_i^{1/3}\right)\frac{1}{\sqrt{1+c^2\gamma_i^{2/3}}}\right]$$

$$\times \Phi\left\{\left(\frac{y_{si}-\mu_{si}}{\sigma_{si}} + c\gamma_i^{1/3}\right)\frac{c\gamma_i^{1/3}}{\sqrt{\left(1+c^2\gamma_i^{2/3}\right)\left[b^2+c^2\gamma_i^{2/3}(b^2-1)\right]}}\right\}. \tag{3.24}$$

By (3.24), we derive the logarithmic likelihood function (without constant terms)

$$l\left(y_{si1}, ..., y_{sin_i}; \mu_{si}, \sigma_{si}^2, \gamma_i\right) = -n_i\log\sigma_{si} - \frac{n_i}{2}\log\left(1+c^2\gamma_i^{2/3}\right)$$

$$+ \sum_{i=1}^{n_i}\log\phi\left[\left(\frac{y_{sij}-\mu_{si}}{\sigma_{si}} + c\gamma_i^{1/3}\right)\frac{1}{\left(1+c^2\gamma_i^{2/3}\right)^{1/2}}\right]$$

$$+ \sum_{i=1}^{n_i}\log\Phi\left\{\frac{\frac{(y_{sij}-\mu_{si})c\gamma_i^{1/3}}{\sigma_{si}}+c^2\gamma_i^{2/3}}{\left(1+c^2\gamma_i^{2/3}\right)^{1/2}\left[b^2+c^2\gamma_i^{2/3}(b^2-1)\right]^{1/2}}\right\}, \ i = 1, ..., k. \tag{3.25}$$

Therefore, let $(\tilde{\mu}_{si}^*, \tilde{\sigma}_{si}^{*2}, \tilde{\gamma}_i^*)$ denote the ML estimate of $(\mu_{si}, \sigma_{si}^2, \gamma_i)$ in (3.25) with the default starting value given by the moment estimates of $(\mu_{si}, \sigma_{si}^2, \gamma_i)$. Namely

$$\hat{\mu}_{si} = -cS_{C2i}^{-1/2}S_{C3i}^{1/3}, \quad \hat{\sigma}_{si}^2 = 1 + cS_{C2i}^{-1}S_{C3i}^{2/3}, \quad \hat{\gamma}_i = \frac{b\hat{\delta}_i^3\left(2b^2-1\right)}{\left(1-b^2\hat{\delta}_i^2\right)^{3/2}}, \ i = 1, ..., k. \tag{3.26}$$

Further, the ML estimates of $(\mu_i, \sigma_i^2)$ are available, namely

$$\tilde{\mu}_i^* = \bar{y}_{Ci} + s_{C2i}^{1/2}\tilde{\mu}_{si}^*, \quad \tilde{\sigma}_i^{*2} = s_{C2i}\tilde{\sigma}_{si}^{*2}, \ i = 1, ..., k. \tag{3.27}$$

From (3.21), we obtain the ML estimates of the direct parameter $(\xi_i, \eta_i^2, \alpha_i)$ as follows

$$\tilde{\xi}_i^* = \tilde{\mu}_i^* - c\tilde{\gamma}_i^{*1/3}\tilde{\sigma}_i^*, \quad \tilde{\eta}_i^{*2} = \tilde{\sigma}_i^{*2}(1+c^2\tilde{\gamma}_i^{*2/3}), \quad \tilde{\alpha}_i^* = \frac{c\tilde{\gamma}_i^{*1/3}}{\sqrt{b^2+c^2(b^2-1)\tilde{\gamma}_i^{*2/3}}}. \tag{3.28}$$

Then the ML estimate of $\delta_i$ is $\tilde{\delta}_i^* = \tilde{\alpha}_i^*/\left(1+\tilde{\alpha}_i^{*2}\right)^{1/2}$, $i = 1, ..., k$. Accordingly, we have the following results.

**Theorem 3.4.** *Suppose* $(\tilde{\mu}_{si}, \tilde{\sigma}_{si}^2, \tilde{\gamma}_i)$ *be the ML estimator corresponding to* $(\tilde{\mu}_{si}^*, \tilde{\sigma}_{si}^{*2}, \tilde{\gamma}_i^*)$, *then we get the ML estimators of the direct parameter* $(\xi_i, \eta_i^2, \alpha_i)$

$$\tilde{\xi}_i = \tilde{\mu}_i - c\tilde{\gamma}_i^{1/3}\tilde{\sigma}_i, \quad \tilde{\eta}_i^2 = \tilde{\sigma}_i^2(1 + c^2\tilde{\gamma}_i^{2/3}), \quad \tilde{\alpha}_i = \frac{c\tilde{\gamma}_i^{1/3}}{\sqrt{b^2 + c^2(b^2 - 1)\tilde{\gamma}_i^{2/3}}}, \quad (3.29)$$

*where* $(\tilde{\mu}_i, \tilde{\sigma}_i^2)$ *denotes the ML estimator corresponding to* $(\tilde{\mu}_i^*, \tilde{\sigma}_i^{*2})$. *Further, the ML estimator of* $\delta_i$ *is* $\tilde{\delta}_i = \tilde{\alpha}_i/(1 + \tilde{\alpha}_i^2)^{1/2}$, $i = 1, ..., k$.

## 3.3  Bootstrap test

For hypothesis testing problem (3.6), we can establish the Bootstrap test statistics. Firstly, by replacing $(\eta_i^2, \delta_i)$ with its moment estimators and ML estimators in (3.10), we construct the following test statistics

$$T_1 = \sum_{i=1}^{k} \frac{n_i}{\hat{\eta}_i^2(1 - b^2\hat{\delta}_i^2)} \frac{\left(\left(\bar{Y}_i - b\hat{\eta}_i\hat{\delta}_i\right) - \sum_{i=1}^{k} \hat{\omega}_i\left(\bar{Y}_i - b\hat{\eta}_i\hat{\delta}_i\right)\right)^2}{1 - \hat{\omega}_i}, \quad (3.30)$$

$$T_2 = \sum_{i=1}^{k} \frac{n_i}{\tilde{\eta}_i^2(1 - b^2\tilde{\delta}_i^2)} \frac{\left(\left(\bar{Y}_i - b\tilde{\eta}_i\tilde{\delta}_i\right) - \sum_{i=1}^{k} \tilde{\omega}_i\left(\bar{Y}_i - b\tilde{\eta}_i\tilde{\delta}_i\right)\right)^2}{1 - \tilde{\omega}_i}, \quad (3.31)$$

where $\hat{\omega}_i = \dfrac{\frac{n_i}{\hat{\eta}_i^2(1 - b^2\hat{\delta}_i^2)}}{\sum_{i=1}^{k} \frac{n_i}{\hat{\eta}_i^2(1 - b^2\hat{\delta}_i^2)}}$, and the definition of $\tilde{\omega}_i$ is similar to $\hat{\omega}_i$.

Under $H_0$ in (3.6), denote $Y_{BMij} \sim SN(\hat{\xi}^*, \hat{\eta}_i^{*2}, \hat{\alpha}_i^*)$, $i = 1, ..., k$, $j = 1, ..., n_i$, where

$$\hat{\xi}^* = \sum_{i=1}^{k} \hat{\omega}_i^* \hat{\xi}_i^*\big|_{(\hat{\eta}_i^*, \hat{\delta}_i^*)}, \quad \hat{\omega}_i^* = \frac{\frac{n_i}{\hat{\eta}_i^{*2}(1 - b^2\hat{\delta}_i^{*2})}}{\sum_{i=1}^{k} \frac{n_i}{\hat{\eta}_i^{*2}(1 - b^2\hat{\delta}_i^{*2})}}, \quad \hat{\xi}_i^*\big|_{(\hat{\eta}_i^*, \hat{\delta}_i^*)} = \bar{y}_i - b\hat{\eta}_i^*\hat{\delta}_i^*. \quad (3.32)$$

The sample mean, the second-order and third-order central moments can be expressed as $(\bar{Y}_{BMi}, S_{BM2i}, S_{BM3i})$, $i = 1, ..., k$. By Theorem 3.2, we obtain the moment estimators of $(\eta_i^2, \delta_i)$ as

$$\hat{\eta}_{BMi}^2 = S_{BM2i} + c^2 S_{BM3i}^{2/3}, \quad \hat{\delta}_{BMi} = \frac{c S_{BM3i}^{1/3}}{b\sqrt{S_{BM2i} + c^2 S_{BM3i}^{2/3}}}, \quad i = 1, ..., k. \quad (3.33)$$

Similarly, suppose $Y_{BLij} \sim SN(\tilde{\xi}^*, \tilde{\eta}_i^{*2}, \tilde{\alpha}_i^*), i = 1, ..., k, \ j = 1, ..., n_i$, where the definition of $\tilde{\xi}^*$ is analogous to $\hat{\xi}^*$ in (3.32), and its sample mean is $\bar{Y}_{BLi}$. By Theorem 3.4, $(\tilde{\eta}_{BLi}^2, \tilde{\delta}_{BLi})$ denotes the ML estimator of $(\eta_i^2, \delta_i)$, $i = 1, ..., k$. Furthermore, similar to (3.30) and (3.31), construct the Bootstrap test statistics

$$T_{B1} = \sum_{i=1}^{k} \frac{n_i}{\hat{\eta}_{BMi}^2(1 - b^2\hat{\delta}_{BMi}^2)} \frac{\left( \left( \bar{Y}_{BMi} - b\hat{\eta}_{BMi}\hat{\delta}_{BMi} \right) - \sum_{i=1}^{k} \hat{\omega}_{BMi} \left( \bar{Y}_{BMi} - b\hat{\eta}_{BMi}\hat{\delta}_{BMi} \right) \right)^2}{1 - \hat{\omega}_{BMi}},$$

(3.34)

$$T_{B2} = \sum_{i=1}^{k} \frac{n_i}{\tilde{\eta}_{BLi}^2(1 - b^2\tilde{\delta}_{BLi}^2)} \frac{\left( \left( \bar{Y}_{BLi} - b\tilde{\eta}_{BLi}\tilde{\delta}_{BLi} \right) - \sum_{i=1}^{k} \tilde{\omega}_{BLi} \left( \bar{Y}_{BLi} - b\tilde{\eta}_{BLi}\tilde{\delta}_{BLi} \right) \right)^2}{1 - \tilde{\omega}_{BLi}},$$

(3.35)

where $\hat{\omega}_{BMi} = \frac{\frac{n_i}{\hat{\eta}_{BMi}^{*2}(1-b^2\hat{\delta}_{BMi}^{*2})}}{\sum_{i=1}^{k} \frac{n_i}{\hat{\eta}_{BMi}^{*2}(1-b^2\hat{\delta}_{BMi}^{*2})}}$, and the definition of $\tilde{\omega}_{BLi}$ is similar to $\hat{\omega}_{BMi}$. Then, based on $T_{B1}$ and $T_{B2}$, we have

$$p_i = 2\min\{P(T_{Bi} > t_i), P(T_{Bi} < t_i)\}, \ i = 1, 2,$$

(3.36)

where $t_1$ and $t_2$ denote the observed values of $T_1$ and $T_2$ respectively. The null hypothesis $H_0$ in (3.6) is rejected whenever the above p-values are less than the nominal significance level of $\beta$, which means that there are at least two location parameters are unequal.

**Remark 3.3.** *If* $\alpha_1 = \alpha_2 = \cdots = \alpha_k = 0$, *then* $T_{B1}$ *can be expressed as*

$$T_{B1} = \sum_{i=1}^{k} \frac{n_i}{\hat{\eta}_{BMi}^2} \frac{\left( \bar{Y}_{BMi} - \sum_{i=1}^{k} \hat{\omega}_{1BMi}\bar{Y}_{BMi} \right)^2}{1 - \hat{\omega}_{1BMi}},$$

*where* $\hat{\omega}_{1BMi} = \left( \frac{n_i}{\hat{\eta}_{BMi}^2} \right) / \left( \sum_{i=1}^{k} \frac{n_i}{\hat{\eta}_{BMi}^2} \right)$, $i = 1, ..., k$. *Thus,* $T_{B1}$ *can be used as the Bootstrap test statistic for the homogeneous test of means in several normal populations, namely the result of Xu (2016).*

## 3.4 Monte Carlo simulation

In this section, the Monte Carlo simulation is adopted to study numerically the Type I error probability and power of the above test approaches. For the hypothesis testing problem (3.6), we only provide the steps of the Bootstrap approach based on the moment estimator in $k$ skew-normal populations as follows.

**Step 1**: For a given $(n_i, \xi_i, \eta_i^2, \alpha_i)$, generate a group of random samples $Y_{ij} \sim SN(\xi_i, \eta_i^2, \alpha_i)$, and $(\bar{Y}_i, S_{2i}, S_{3i})$ is computed by (3.2), $i = 1, \ldots, k$, $j = 1, \ldots, n_i$.

**Step 2**: Using (3.19) and (3.32), $(\hat{\bar{\xi}}^*, \hat{\xi}_i^*, \hat{\eta}_i^{*2}, \hat{\alpha}_i^*)$, the feasible estimate of $(\xi, \xi_i, \eta_i^2, \alpha_i)$ is computed, $i = 1, \ldots, k$. Further, $T_1$ is computed by (3.30).

**Step 3**: Under $H_0$, generate the Bootstrap samples $Y_{BMij} \sim SN(\hat{\bar{\xi}}^*, \hat{\eta}_i^{*2}, \hat{\alpha}_i^*)$, and compute $(\bar{Y}_{BMi}, S_{2BMi}, S_{3BMi})$ for $i = 1, \ldots, k$, $j = 1, \ldots, n_i$.

**Step 4**: From (3.19), $(\hat{\eta}_{BMi}^{*2}, \hat{\alpha}_{BMi}^*)$, the moment estimate of $(\eta^2, \alpha)$ from Bootstrap samples is computed, $i = 1, \ldots, k$. Then $T_{B1}$ is obtained by (3.34).

**Step 5**: Repeat Steps 3–4 $n_1$ times and compute $p_1$ by (3.36). If $p_1 < 0.05$, then $Q = 1$; otherwise, $Q = 0$.

**Step 6**: Repeat Steps 1–5 $n_2$ times and we get $Q_1, \cdots, Q_{n_2}$. Then the Type I error probability is $\frac{1}{n_2} \sum_{i=1}^{n_2} Q_i$.

Based on the above steps, the power of the hypothesis testing problem (3.6) under $H_1$ can be obtained similarly.

In the simulation, the parameters and sample sizes are set as follows. Initially, let the nominal significance level be 5%, the number of inner loops $n_1$ and number of outer loops $n_2$, let both be 2500, and $\xi = 2$. Subsequently, for the two populations, we set $\eta_1^2 = (0.2^2, 0.6^2), \eta_2^2 = (0.3^2, 0.9^2), \eta_3^2 = (0.5^2, 0.7^2), \eta_4^2 = (0.9^2, 1.2^2), \eta_5^2 = (1.5^2, 2^2), (\alpha_1, \alpha_2) = (3, 4), (6, 7),$ and $(n_1, n_2) = (30, 40), (40, 60), (50, 80), (80, 120), (180, 240)$.

For three populations, we set $\eta_1^2 = (0.2^2, 0.4^2, 0.6^2), \eta_2^2 = (0.3^2, 0.5^2, 0.7^2), \eta_3^2 = (0.5^2, 0.7^2, 0.9^2), \eta_4^2 = (0.9^2, 1.2^2, 1.5^2), \eta_5^2 = (1.5^2, 2^2, 2.5^2),$ $(\alpha_1, \alpha_2, \alpha_3) = (2, 3, 4), (5, 5, 6),$ and $(n_1, n_2, n_3) = (30, 40, 40), (60, 60, 80), (80, 100, 120), (120, 150, 150), (180, 240, 300)$.

For five populations, we set $\eta_1^2 = (0.1^2, 0.3^2, 0.5^2, 0.7^2, 0.9^2), \eta_2^2 = (0.2^2, 0.4^2, 0.6^2, 0.8^2, 1^2), \eta_3^2 = (0.3^2, 0.5^2, 0.7^2, 0.9^2, 0.9^2), \eta_4^2 = (0.4^2, 0.6^2, 0.8^2, 1^2, 1.2^2), \eta_5^2 = (0.5^2, 0.7^2, 0.9^2, 1.1^2, 1.3^2), (\alpha_1, \alpha_2, \alpha_3, \alpha_4, \alpha_5) = (3, 4, 4, 5, 6), (5, 5, 6, 7, 8),$ and $(n_1, n_2, n_3, n_4, n_5) = (30, 30, 40, 40, 50), (40, 50, 60, 60, 70), (60, 70, 80, 80, 90), (80, 90, 90, 100, 120), (90, 100, 100, 120, 150)$.

For hypothesis testing problem (3.6), Tables 3.1–3.3 present the simulated Type I error probabilities of the proposed two approaches $p_1$ and $p_2$. No matter in two populations, three populations or five populations, the actual levels of $p_1$ are all strictly less than the nominal significance level of 5%, which can effectively control the Type I error probabilities under certain parameter settings. The performance of $p_2$ is liberal relatively when sample sizes and skewness parameters are small. With the increase of skewness parameters, $p_2$ appears conservative individually. However, in the case of five populations, the actual levels of $p_2$ are controlled around the nominal significance level of 5%, and perform well generally.

Tables 3.4–3.6 present the simulated powers of the proposed approaches. As $\xi_i$ departs from the null hypothesis, the powers of the proposed approaches are significantly improved even in two populations, three populations or five populations. However, the power of the Bootstrap test statistic based on the moment estimator performs significantly better than that based on the ML estimator. In terms of the Bootstrap test statistic based on the ML estimator, the power rises more slowly as $\xi_i$ departs from the null hypothesis when scale parameters are small. With the increase of scale parameters and sample sizes, the power is improved significantly.

Tables 3.7 and 3.8 respectively present the simulated powers under the condition of $\xi_1 \neq \xi_2 \neq \cdots \neq \xi_k$ in three and five populations. The simulated results from Tables 3.7 and 3.8 are respectively similar to those of Tables 3.5 and 3.6. However, the powers of the proposed approach based on the ML estimator decrease slightly as $\xi_i$ departs from the null hypothesis with k=5.

**Table 3.1:** Simulation results on Type I error probability at nominal significance level of 5% ($k = 2$).

| | \multicolumn{10}{c}{$(\alpha_1,\alpha_2)=(3,4)$} | | | | | | | | | |
|---|---|---|---|---|---|---|---|---|---|---|
| | N1 | | N2 | | N3 | | N4 | | N5 | |
| | p1 | p2 | p1 | p2 | p1 | p2 | p1 | p2 | p1 | p2 |
| $\eta_1^2$ | 0.0416 | 0.0644 | 0.0364 | 0.0668 | 0.0300 | 0.0588 | 0.0240 | 0.0396 | 0.0328 | 0.0248 |
| $\eta_2^2$ | 0.0416 | 0.0644 | 0.0364 | 0.0668 | 0.0300 | 0.0588 | 0.0240 | 0.0396 | 0.0328 | 0.0248 |
| $\eta_3^2$ | 0.0476 | 0.0888 | 0.0472 | 0.0748 | 0.0476 | 0.0672 | 0.0328 | 0.0404 | 0.0340 | 0.0228 |
| $\eta_4^2$ | 0.0532 | 0.0892 | 0.0452 | 0.0748 | 0.0476 | 0.0652 | 0.0336 | 0.0436 | 0.0304 | 0.0240 |
| $\eta_5^2$ | 0.0532 | 0.0892 | 0.0452 | 0.0748 | 0.0476 | 0.0652 | 0.0336 | 0.0436 | 0.0304 | 0.0240 |
| | \multicolumn{10}{c}{$(\alpha_1,\alpha_2)=(6,7)$} | | | | | | | | | |
| | N1 | | N2 | | N3 | | N4 | | N5 | |
| | p1 | p2 | p1 | p2 | p1 | p2 | p1 | p2 | p1 | p2 |
| $\eta_1^2$ | 0.0356 | 0.0420 | 0.0304 | 0.0412 | 0.0304 | 0.0412 | 0.0304 | 0.0412 | 0.0304 | 0.0412 |
| $\eta_2^2$ | 0.0356 | 0.0420 | 0.0304 | 0.0412 | 0.0304 | 0.0412 | 0.0304 | 0.0412 | 0.0304 | 0.0412 |
| $\eta_3^2$ | 0.0336 | 0.0644 | 0.0304 | 0.0520 | 0.0304 | 0.0520 | 0.0304 | 0.0520 | 0.0304 | 0.0520 |
| $\eta_4^2$ | 0.0356 | 0.0640 | 0.0340 | 0.0420 | 0.0340 | 0.0420 | 0.0340 | 0.0420 | 0.0340 | 0.0420 |
| $\eta_5^2$ | 0.0356 | 0.0640 | 0.0340 | 0.0420 | 0.0340 | 0.0420 | 0.0340 | 0.0420 | 0.0340 | 0.0420 |

*Note:* $\eta_1^2=(0.2^2,0.6^2)$, $\eta_2^2=(0.3^2,0.9^2)$, $\eta_3^2=(0.5^2,0.7^2)$, $\eta_4^2=(0.9^2,1.2^2)$, $\eta_5^2=(1.5^2,2^2)$; $N1 = (30,40)$, $N2 = (40,60)$, $N3 = (50,80)$, $N4 = (80,120)$, $N5 = (180,240)$.

**Table 3.2:** Simulation results on Type I error probability at nominal significance level of 5% ($k = 3$).

| | $(\alpha_1,\alpha_2,\alpha_3)$=(2,3,4) | | | | | | | | | |
| | N1 | | N2 | | N3 | | N4 | | N5 | |
| | p1 | p2 | p1 | p2 | p1 | p2 | p1 | p2 | p1 | p2 |
|---|---|---|---|---|---|---|---|---|---|---|
| $\eta_1^2$ | 0.0372 | 0.0784 | 0.0308 | 0.0632 | 0.0312 | 0.0548 | 0.0260 | 0.0404 | 0.0252 | 0.0180 |
| $\eta_2^2$ | 0.0320 | 0.0756 | 0.0324 | 0.0648 | 0.0408 | 0.0592 | 0.0392 | 0.0420 | 0.0280 | 0.0184 |
| $\eta_3^2$ | 0.0388 | 0.0748 | 0.0408 | 0.0652 | 0.0504 | 0.0636 | 0.0420 | 0.0472 | 0.0264 | 0.0364 |
| $\eta_4^2$ | 0.0404 | 0.0704 | 0.0432 | 0.0660 | 0.0500 | 0.0624 | 0.0396 | 0.0464 | 0.0272 | 0.0400 |
| $\eta_5^2$ | 0.0404 | 0.0704 | 0.0432 | 0.0660 | 0.0500 | 0.0624 | 0.0396 | 0.0464 | 0.0272 | 0.0400 |

| | $(\alpha_1,\alpha_2,\alpha_3)$=(5,5,6) | | | | | | | | | |
| | N1 | | N2 | | N3 | | N4 | | N5 | |
| | p1 | p2 | p1 | p2 | p1 | p2 | p1 | p2 | p1 | p2 |
|---|---|---|---|---|---|---|---|---|---|---|
| $\eta_1^2$ | 0.0376 | 0.0612 | 0.0304 | 0.0312 | 0.0268 | 0.0236 | 0.0172 | 0.0120 | 0.0208 | 0.0102 |
| $\eta_2^2$ | 0.0380 | 0.0576 | 0.0240 | 0.0352 | 0.0228 | 0.0224 | 0.0148 | 0.0128 | 0.0260 | 0.0104 |
| $\eta_3^2$ | 0.0344 | 0.0544 | 0.0264 | 0.0364 | 0.0268 | 0.0248 | 0.0232 | 0.0328 | 0.0252 | 0.0500 |
| $\eta_4^2$ | 0.0352 | 0.0588 | 0.0292 | 0.0344 | 0.0244 | 0.0260 | 0.0244 | 0.0340 | 0.0252 | 0.0568 |
| $\eta_5^2$ | 0.0352 | 0.0588 | 0.0292 | 0.0344 | 0.0244 | 0.0260 | 0.0244 | 0.0340 | 0.0252 | 0.0568 |

*Note:* $\eta_1^2$=(0.2^2, 0.4^2, 0.6^2)$, $\eta_2^2$=(0.3^2, 0.5^2, 0.7^2)$, $\eta_3^2$=(0.5^2, 0.7^2, 0.9^2)$, $\eta_4^2$=(0.9^2, 1.2^2, 1.5^2)$, $\eta_5^2$=(1.5^2, 2^2, 2.5^2)$; $N1 = (30, 40, 40), N2 = (60, 60, 80), N3 = (80, 100, 120), N4 = (120, 150, 150), N5 = (180, 240, 300)$.

## 3.5 Illustrative examples

To verify the reasonableness and effectiveness of the proposed approaches in this section, two real examples of the regional GDP of China and performance data of high-speed turbine bearings are presented.

**Example 3.1** The above approaches are applied to the GDP data of Tianjin and Chongqing Municipalities from 1996 to 2018. As in Figures 3.1 and 3.2, the distributions of the GDPs of Tianjin and Chongqing don't follow the normal distribution but show asymmetric and right-skewed characteristics. To confirm the conclusion, we first conduct the normality test for these data. It turns out that the p-values of the Shapiro-Wilk test and Kolmogorov-Smirnov test for Tianjin's GDP are 0.001 and 0.016, and for Chongqing's GDP are 0.001 and 0.005. Hence, the GDPs of Tianjin and Chongqing are not normally distributed at the nominal significance level of 5%. In addition, we should prove whether the distributions of the GDPs of Tianjin and Chongqing are skew-normal by the chi-square goodness-of-fit test. By calculation, the fitted value of Tianjin is $\chi_t^2 = 5.9149 < \chi_2^2(0.95) = 5.99$ with p-value 0.0520, and the one of Chongqing is $\chi_c^2 = 4.2243 < \chi_2^2(0.95) = 5.99$ with p-value 0.1210. Therefore, the GDPs of

**Table 3.3:** Simulation results on Type I error probability at nominal significance level of 5% ($k = 5$).

| | $(\alpha_1,\alpha_2,\alpha_3,\alpha_4,\alpha_5)=(3,4,4,5,6)$ | | | | | | | | | |
|---|---|---|---|---|---|---|---|---|---|---|
| | N1 | | N2 | | N3 | | N4 | | N5 | |
| | p1 | p2 | p1 | p2 | p1 | p2 | p1 | p2 | p1 | p2 |
| $\eta_1^2$ | 0.0408 | 0.0444 | 0.0364 | 0.0544 | 0.0224 | 0.0464 | 0.0220 | 0.0548 | 0.0220 | 0.0600 |
| $\eta_2^2$ | 0.0384 | 0.0456 | 0.0320 | 0.0468 | 0.0248 | 0.0408 | 0.0268 | 0.0360 | 0.0240 | 0.0356 |
| $\eta_3^2$ | 0.0392 | 0.0516 | 0.0328 | 0.0500 | 0.0244 | 0.0444 | 0.0312 | 0.0332 | 0.0280 | 0.0308 |
| $\eta_4^2$ | 0.0400 | 0.0560 | 0.0368 | 0.0548 | 0.0252 | 0.0464 | 0.0332 | 0.0308 | 0.0308 | 0.0324 |
| $\eta_5^2$ | 0.0424 | 0.0560 | 0.0364 | 0.0588 | 0.0276 | 0.0536 | 0.0324 | 0.0392 | 0.0284 | 0.0364 |
| | $(\alpha_1,\alpha_2,\alpha_3,\alpha_4,\alpha_5)=(5,5,6,7,8)$ | | | | | | | | | |
| | N1 | | N2 | | N3 | | N4 | | N5 | |
| | p1 | p2 | p1 | p2 | p1 | p2 | p1 | p2 | p1 | p2 |
| $\eta_1^2$ | 0.0396 | 0.0440 | 0.0332 | 0.0560 | 0.0204 | 0.0476 | 0.0220 | 0.0560 | 0.0220 | 0.0616 |
| $\eta_2^2$ | 0.0380 | 0.0436 | 0.0308 | 0.0468 | 0.0220 | 0.0300 | 0.0252 | 0.0296 | 0.0220 | 0.0284 |
| $\eta_3^2$ | 0.0372 | 0.0492 | 0.0300 | 0.0420 | 0.0232 | 0.0316 | 0.0288 | 0.0284 | 0.0252 | 0.0236 |
| $\eta_4^2$ | 0.0428 | 0.0516 | 0.0352 | 0.0476 | 0.0232 | 0.0336 | 0.0300 | 0.0256 | 0.0248 | 0.0268 |
| $\eta_5^2$ | 0.0448 | 0.0540 | 0.0348 | 0.0552 | 0.0220 | 0.0396 | 0.0316 | 0.0340 | 0.0284 | 0.0328 |

*Note:* $\eta_1^2 = (0.1^2, 0.3^2, 0.5^2, 0.7^2, 0.9^2)$, $\eta_2^2=(0.2^2, 0.4^2, 0.6^2, 0.8^2, 1^2)$, $\eta_3^2=(0.3^2, 0.5^2, 0.7^2, 0.9^2, 0.9^2)$, $\eta_4^2=(0.4^2, 0.6^2, 0.8^2, 1^2, 1.2^2)$, $\eta_5^2=(0.5^2, 0.7^2, 0.9^2, 1.1^2, 1.3^2)$; $N1 = (30, 30, 40, 40, 50)$, $N2 = (40, 50, 60, 60, 70)$, $N3 = (60, 70, 80, 80, 90)$, $N4 = (80, 90, 90, 100, 120)$, $N5 = (90, 100, 100, 120, 150)$.

Tianjin and Chongqing from 1996 to 2018 follow the skew-normal distributions $SN(\xi_t, \eta_t^2, \alpha_t)$ and $SN(\xi_c, \eta_c^2, \alpha_c)$ respectively at the nominal significance level of 5%.

Consider the hypothesis testing problem

$$H_0 : \xi_t = \xi_c \qquad versus \qquad H_1 : \xi_t \neq \xi_c \, .$$

The p-values of the Bootstrap test statistics based on the moment estimator and ML estimator are 0.5666 and 0.6694 respectively. Thus, the null hypothesis $H_0$ can not be rejected at the nominal significance level of 5%, which means that there is no significant difference between the location parameters of the GDPs of Tianjin and Chongqing from 1996 to 2018.

**Example 3.2** Consider comparing the performance of high-speed turbine bearings made of two different compounds. In this study, 10 bearings of each type were tested, and the failure times of each bearing were recorded in units of millions of cycles. Similar to Example 3.1, we conduct the normality test for the bearings made of two different compounds, named $X$ and $Y$. It turns out that the p-values of Shapiro-Wilk test and Kolmogorov-Smirnov test for $X$ are

**Table 3.4:** Simulated powers of hypothesis testing problem (3.6) as $k = 2$ and $\xi_1 = 2$.

| | $(\eta_1^2,\eta_2^2)=(0.3,0.8)$ | | | | | | | | | | | |
| | $(\alpha_1,\alpha_2)=(3,4)$ | | | | | | $(\alpha_1,\alpha_2)=(6,7)$ | | | | | |
| | N1 | | N2 | | N3 | | N1 | | N2 | | N3 | |
| $\xi_2$ | p1 | p2 | p1 | p2 | p1 | p2 | p1 | p2 | p1 | p2 | p1 | p2 |
|---|---|---|---|---|---|---|---|---|---|---|---|---|
| 2.5 | 0.1928 | 0.1072 | 0.3592 | 0.0780 | 0.6292 | 0.0620 | 0.2388 | 0.0704 | 0.5096 | 0.0624 | 0.8096 | 0.0536 |
| 2.6 | 0.3464 | 0.1220 | 0.5532 | 0.0992 | 0.7696 | 0.0820 | 0.4428 | 0.0884 | 0.7076 | 0.0720 | 0.9208 | 0.1256 |
| 2.7 | 0.5044 | 0.1520 | 0.7356 | 0.1340 | 0.9128 | 0.1812 | 0.6328 | 0.1168 | 0.8748 | 0.1396 | 0.9892 | 0.2944 |
| 2.8 | 0.6880 | 0.2032 | 0.8844 | 0.2224 | 0.9832 | 0.3656 | 0.8124 | 0.1932 | 0.9684 | 0.2768 | 0.9992 | 0.5236 |
| 2.9 | 0.8268 | 0.2792 | 0.9624 | 0.3624 | 0.9968 | 0.5768 | 0.9184 | 0.2948 | 0.9956 | 0.4560 | 0.9996 | 0.7308 |

| | $(\eta_1^2,\eta_2^2)=(0.5,0.7)$ | | | | | | | | | | | |
| | $(\alpha_1,\alpha_2)=(3,4)$ | | | | | | $(\alpha_1,\alpha_2)=(6,7)$ | | | | | |
| | N1 | | N2 | | N3 | | N1 | | N2 | | N3 | |
| $\xi_2$ | p1 | p2 | p1 | p2 | p1 | p2 | p1 | p2 | p1 | p2 | p1 | p2 |
|---|---|---|---|---|---|---|---|---|---|---|---|---|
| 2.5 | 0.3344 | 0.1292 | 0.5364 | 0.1048 | 0.7684 | 0.1480 | 0.4344 | 0.0972 | 0.6976 | 0.0964 | 0.7684 | 0.1480 |
| 2.6 | 0.5092 | 0.1700 | 0.7196 | 0.1784 | 0.9144 | 0.3092 | 0.6560 | 0.1540 | 0.8760 | 0.2348 | 0.9144 | 0.3092 |
| 2.7 | 0.6808 | 0.2440 | 0.8632 | 0.3228 | 0.9776 | 0.5460 | 0.8216 | 0.2656 | 0.9692 | 0.4360 | 0.9776 | 0.5460 |
| 2.8 | 0.8092 | 0.3524 | 0.9408 | 0.5052 | 0.9908 | 0.7552 | 0.9236 | 0.4148 | 0.9928 | 0.6480 | 0.9908 | 0.7552 |
| 2.9 | 0.8980 | 0.4944 | 0.9732 | 0.6792 | 0.9972 | 0.8896 | 0.9732 | 0.5812 | 0.9980 | 0.8100 | 0.9972 | 0.8896 |

| | $(\eta_1^2,\eta_2^2)=(0.6,0.6)$ | | | | | | | | | | | |
| | $(\alpha_1,\alpha_2)=(3,4)$ | | | | | | $(\alpha_1,\alpha_2)=(6,7)$ | | | | | |
| | N1 | | N2 | | N3 | | N1 | | N2 | | N3 | |
| $\xi_2$ | p1 | p2 | p1 | p2 | p1 | p2 | p1 | p2 | p1 | p2 | p1 | p2 |
|---|---|---|---|---|---|---|---|---|---|---|---|---|
| 2.5 | 0.3944 | 0.1168 | 0.5640 | 0.2092 | 0.8384 | 0.3516 | 0.5500 | 0.1148 | 0.7492 | 0.2908 | 0.9548 | 0.5532 |
| 2.6 | 0.6416 | 0.1940 | 0.7952 | 0.3112 | 0.9572 | 0.4800 | 0.7892 | 0.2180 | 0.9260 | 0.4232 | 0.9972 | 0.7028 |
| 2.7 | 0.7984 | 0.3156 | 0.8944 | 0.4596 | 0.9724 | 0.6820 | 0.9148 | 0.3796 | 0.9756 | 0.6048 | 0.9992 | 0.8660 |
| 2.8 | 0.8612 | 0.4968 | 0.9248 | 0.6428 | 0.9764 | 0.8736 | 0.9488 | 0.6016 | 0.9880 | 0.7884 | 0.9996 | 0.9628 |
| 2.9 | 0.8860 | 0.6548 | 0.9424 | 0.8200 | 0.9876 | 0.9604 | 0.9612 | 0.7792 | 0.9924 | 0.9212 | 1.0000 | 0.9952 |

*Note:* $N1 = (20,30), N2 = (30,40), N3 = (50,60)$.

0.014 and 0.026 and for $Y$ are 0.001 and 0.011. Hence, the failure times of each type are not normally distributed at the nominal significance level of 5%. Furthermore, to verify the skew-normality of the failure times of each type, we intend to test the null hypothesis $H_0$ : the failure times of $X$ and $Y$ are skew-normally distributed. It can be obtained by calculation that the fitted values of $X$ is $\chi_x^2 = 1.5498 < \chi_1^2(0.95) = 3.84$ with p-value 0.2132, and the one of $Y$ is $\chi_y^2 = 3.5732 < \chi_2^2(0.95) = 5.99$ with p-value 0.1675. Therefore, the fail-

**Table 3.5:** Simulated powers of hypothesis testing problem (3.6) as $k = 3$ and $\xi_1 = \xi_2 = 2$.

$(\eta_1^2,\eta_2^2,\eta_3^2)=(0.1,0.4,0.7)$

| | $(\alpha_1,\alpha_2,\alpha_3)=(2,3,4)$ | | | | | | $(\alpha_1,\alpha_2,\alpha_3)=(5,5,6)$ | | | | | |
| | N1 | | N2 | | N3 | | N1 | | N2 | | N3 | |
| $\xi_3$ | p1 | p2 | p1 | p2 | p1 | p2 | p1 | p2 | p1 | p2 | p1 | p2 |
|---|---|---|---|---|---|---|---|---|---|---|---|---|
| 2.6 | 0.3616 | 0.1112 | 0.6604 | 0.1152 | 0.8800 | 0.1960 | 0.5028 | 0.0780 | 0.8344 | 0.1636 | 0.9736 | 0.2516 |
| 2.7 | 0.5408 | 0.1556 | 0.8512 | 0.2416 | 0.9628 | 0.3920 | 0.6752 | 0.1296 | 0.9312 | 0.3376 | 0.9904 | 0.4692 |
| 2.8 | 0.6956 | 0.2320 | 0.9524 | 0.3880 | 0.9924 | 0.5576 | 0.7996 | 0.2376 | 0.9776 | 0.5012 | 0.9980 | 0.6976 |
| 2.9 | 0.8272 | 0.3260 | 0.9856 | 0.5092 | 0.9992 | 0.6924 | 0.8924 | 0.3708 | 0.9936 | 0.6388 | 0.9996 | 0.8356 |
| 3.0 | 0.9124 | 0.4356 | 0.9968 | 0.6140 | 1.0000 | 0.7860 | 0.9484 | 0.4960 | 0.9976 | 0.7368 | 1.0000 | 0.9144 |

$(\eta_1^2,\eta_2^2,\eta_3^2)=(0.4,0.8,0.8)$

| | $(\alpha_1,\alpha_2,\alpha_3)=(2,3,4)$ | | | | | | $(\alpha_1,\alpha_2,\alpha_3)=(5,5,6)$ | | | | | |
| | N1 | | N2 | | N3 | | N1 | | N2 | | N3 | |
| $\xi_3$ | p1 | p2 | p1 | p2 | p1 | p2 | p1 | p2 | p1 | p2 | p1 | p2 |
|---|---|---|---|---|---|---|---|---|---|---|---|---|
| 2.6 | 0.1500 | 0.0812 | 0.4984 | 0.0516 | 0.8056 | 0.0584 | 0.2012 | 0.0548 | 0.7524 | 0.0540 | 0.9572 | 0.1048 |
| 2.7 | 0.2504 | 0.0928 | 0.7112 | 0.0640 | 0.9140 | 0.1132 | 0.3668 | 0.0596 | 0.8860 | 0.1180 | 0.9780 | 0.2100 |
| 2.8 | 0.4052 | 0.1112 | 0.8636 | 0.1408 | 0.9588 | 0.2580 | 0.5628 | 0.0924 | 0.9472 | 0.2480 | 0.9908 | 0.3796 |
| 2.9 | 0.5556 | 0.1436 | 0.9416 | 0.2644 | 0.9872 | 0.4256 | 0.7332 | 0.1356 | 0.9784 | 0.3992 | 0.9960 | 0.5708 |
| 3.0 | 0.7132 | 0.1972 | 0.9720 | 0.4140 | 0.9960 | 0.5896 | 0.8548 | 0.2116 | 0.9892 | 0.5628 | 0.9988 | 0.7260 |

$(\eta_1^2,\eta_2^2,\eta_3^2)=(0.6,0.7,0.8)$

| | $(\alpha_1,\alpha_2,\alpha_3)=(2,3,4)$ | | | | | | $(\alpha_1,\alpha_2,\alpha_3)=(5,5,6)$ | | | | | |
| | N1 | | N2 | | N3 | | N1 | | N2 | | N3 | |
| $\xi_3$ | p1 | p2 | p1 | p2 | p1 | p2 | p1 | p2 | p1 | p2 | p1 | p2 |
|---|---|---|---|---|---|---|---|---|---|---|---|---|
| 2.6 | 0.1544 | 0.0768 | 0.4596 | 0.0540 | 0.7412 | 0.0912 | 0.2504 | 0.0596 | 0.7228 | 0.0964 | 0.9384 | 0.2436 |
| 2.7 | 0.2884 | 0.0924 | 0.6552 | 0.0788 | 0.8704 | 0.1480 | 0.4280 | 0.0676 | 0.8580 | 0.1832 | 0.9704 | 0.3856 |
| 2.8 | 0.4284 | 0.1108 | 0.8112 | 0.1264 | 0.9420 | 0.2308 | 0.6136 | 0.0984 | 0.9316 | 0.2880 | 0.9892 | 0.5572 |
| 2.9 | 0.5632 | 0.1484 | 0.8952 | 0.2156 | 0.9752 | 0.3696 | 0.7552 | 0.1508 | 0.9712 | 0.4200 | 0.9960 | 0.6892 |
| 3.0 | 0.6884 | 0.2028 | 0.9416 | 0.3316 | 0.9904 | 0.5068 | 0.8520 | 0.2292 | 0.9904 | 0.5536 | 0.9988 | 0.7852 |

*Note:* $N1 = (30, 40, 40), N2 = (60, 60, 80), N3 = (80, 100, 120)$.

ure times of $X$ and $Y$ follow the skew-normal distributions $SN(\xi_x, \eta_x^2, \alpha_x)$ and $SN(\xi_y, \eta_y^2, \alpha_y)$ respectively at the nominal significance level of 5%.

Consider the hypothesis testing problem

$$H_0 : \xi_x = \xi_y \qquad versus \qquad H_1 : \xi_x \neq \xi_y .$$

The p-values of the Bootstrap test statistics based on the moment estimator and ML estimator are 0.8480 and 0.8432 respectively. Thus, the null hypothesis $H_0$ can not be rejected at the nominal significance level of 5%, which means that

**Table 3.6:** Simulated powers of hypothesis testing problem (3.6) as $k = 5$ and $\xi_1 = \xi_2 = \xi_3 = \xi_4 = 2$.

$(\eta_1^2,\eta_2^2,\eta_3^2,\eta_4^2,\eta_5^2)$=(0.1,0.3,0.5,0.7,0.9)

| | $(\alpha_1,\alpha_2,\alpha_3,\alpha_4,\alpha_5)$=(3,4,4,5,6) | | | | | | $(\alpha_1,\alpha_2,\alpha_3,\alpha_4,\alpha_5)$=(5,5,6,7,8) | | | | | |
| | N1 | | N2 | | N3 | | N1 | | N2 | | N3 | |
| $\xi_5$ | p1 | p2 | p1 | p2 | p1 | p2 | p1 | p2 | p1 | p2 | p1 | p2 |
|---|---|---|---|---|---|---|---|---|---|---|---|---|
| 3.1 | 0.4940 | 0.0996 | 0.7552 | 0.1296 | 0.8148 | 0.1840 | 0.5544 | 0.0932 | 0.8200 | 0.1572 | 0.8628 | 0.2368 |
| 3.2 | 0.6448 | 0.1344 | 0.8500 | 0.1796 | 0.8848 | 0.2464 | 0.6952 | 0.1288 | 0.8948 | 0.2180 | 0.9232 | 0.3192 |
| 3.3 | 0.7700 | 0.1736 | 0.9180 | 0.2420 | 0.9444 | 0.3160 | 0.8080 | 0.1676 | 0.9452 | 0.2928 | 0.9612 | 0.4020 |
| 3.4 | 0.8620 | 0.2152 | 0.9580 | 0.3144 | 0.9768 | 0.3936 | 0.8916 | 0.2160 | 0.9740 | 0.3692 | 0.9860 | 0.4808 |
| 3.5 | 0.9240 | 0.2688 | 0.9824 | 0.3864 | 0.9896 | 0.4680 | 0.9412 | 0.2712 | 0.9900 | 0.4388 | 0.9936 | 0.5476 |

$(\eta_1^2,\eta_2^2,\eta_3^2,\eta_4^2,\eta_5^2)$=(0.2,0.4,0.6,0.8,1)

| | $(\alpha_1,\alpha_2,\alpha_3,\alpha_4,\alpha_5)$=(3,4,4,5,6) | | | | | | $(\alpha_1,\alpha_2,\alpha_3,\alpha_4,\alpha_5)$=(5,5,6,7,8) | | | | | |
| | N1 | | N2 | | N3 | | N1 | | N2 | | N3 | |
| $\xi_5$ | p1 | p2 | p1 | p2 | p1 | p2 | p1 | p2 | p1 | p2 | p1 | p2 |
|---|---|---|---|---|---|---|---|---|---|---|---|---|
| 3.1 | 0.2096 | 0.0652 | 0.4368 | 0.0592 | 0.5716 | 0.0568 | 0.2348 | 0.0552 | 0.5476 | 0.0612 | 0.6812 | 0.0652 |
| 3.2 | 0.3064 | 0.0716 | 0.5692 | 0.0760 | 0.6808 | 0.0784 | 0.3416 | 0.0636 | 0.6712 | 0.0824 | 0.7696 | 0.0972 |
| 3.3 | 0.4172 | 0.0852 | 0.6976 | 0.1004 | 0.7704 | 0.1252 | 0.4780 | 0.0768 | 0.7828 | 0.1112 | 0.8364 | 0.1572 |
| 3.4 | 0.5372 | 0.1040 | 0.7952 | 0.1376 | 0.8492 | 0.1752 | 0.5960 | 0.0972 | 0.8480 | 0.1500 | 0.8924 | 0.2232 |
| 3.5 | 0.6508 | 0.1332 | 0.8636 | 0.1736 | 0.9012 | 0.2288 | 0.7112 | 0.1312 | 0.9072 | 0.2012 | 0.9332 | 0.2892 |

$(\eta_1^2,\eta_2^2,\eta_3^2,\eta_4^2,\eta_5^2)$=(0.3,0.5,0.7,0.9,0.9)

| | $(\alpha_1,\alpha_2,\alpha_3,\alpha_4,\alpha_5)$=(3,4,4,5,6) | | | | | | $(\alpha_1,\alpha_2,\alpha_3,\alpha_4,\alpha_5)$=(5,5,6,7,8) | | | | | |
| | N1 | | N2 | | N3 | | N1 | | N2 | | N3 | |
| $\xi_5$ | p1 | p2 | p1 | p2 | p1 | p2 | p1 | p2 | p1 | p2 | p1 | p2 |
|---|---|---|---|---|---|---|---|---|---|---|---|---|
| 3.1 | 0.5048 | 0.0944 | 0.7792 | 0.1128 | 0.8408 | 0.1328 | 0.5628 | 0.0876 | 0.8348 | 0.1204 | 0.8892 | 0.1648 |
| 3.2 | 0.6396 | 0.1252 | 0.8636 | 0.1640 | 0.9068 | 0.2016 | 0.7020 | 0.1212 | 0.9108 | 0.1880 | 0.9420 | 0.2520 |
| 3.3 | 0.7636 | 0.1704 | 0.9260 | 0.2276 | 0.9568 | 0.2788 | 0.8188 | 0.1680 | 0.9508 | 0.2616 | 0.9732 | 0.3376 |
| 3.4 | 0.8612 | 0.2192 | 0.9652 | 0.3132 | 0.9820 | 0.3576 | 0.8940 | 0.2248 | 0.9800 | 0.3444 | 0.9912 | 0.4408 |
| 3.5 | 0.9224 | 0.2732 | 0.9860 | 0.3872 | 0.9940 | 0.4572 | 0.9464 | 0.2772 | 0.9912 | 0.4380 | 0.9964 | 0.5220 |

*Note:* $N1 = (30,30,40,40,50), N2 = (40,50,60,60,70), N3 = (60,70,80,80,90)$.

there is no significant difference between high-speed turbine bearings made of these two different compounds.

**Table 3.7:** Simulated powers of hypothesis testing problem (3.6) as $k = 3$, $\xi_1 = 1$ and $\xi_2 = 1.1$.

$(\eta_1^2,\eta_2^2,\eta_3^2)=(0.4,0.4,0.8)$

| | $(\alpha_1,\alpha_2,\alpha_3)=(2,3,4)$ | | | | | | $(\alpha_1,\alpha_2,\alpha_3)=(5,5,6)$ | | | | | |
| | N1 | | N2 | | N3 | | N1 | | N2 | | N3 | |
| $\xi_3$ | p1 | p2 | p1 | p2 | p1 | p2 | p1 | p2 | p1 | p2 | p1 | p2 |
|---|---|---|---|---|---|---|---|---|---|---|---|---|
| 1.6 | 0.1616 | 0.0852 | 0.4948 | 0.0776 | 0.6868 | 0.0876 | 0.3240 | 0.0740 | 0.8632 | 0.1040 | 0.9692 | 0.2440 |
| 1.7 | 0.2760 | 0.1028 | 0.7000 | 0.1056 | 0.8680 | 0.1308 | 0.5116 | 0.0840 | 0.9472 | 0.1884 | 0.9932 | 0.3816 |
| 1.8 | 0.4252 | 0.1224 | 0.8432 | 0.1484 | 0.9612 | 0.2140 | 0.6852 | 0.1192 | 0.9780 | 0.3124 | 0.9996 | 0.5396 |
| 1.9 | 0.5832 | 0.1664 | 0.9160 | 0.2320 | 0.9856 | 0.3096 | 0.8092 | 0.1764 | 0.9948 | 0.4648 | 0.9996 | 0.6744 |
| 2.0 | 0.7148 | 0.2136 | 0.9600 | 0.3400 | 0.9952 | 0.4276 | 0.8944 | 0.2496 | 0.9988 | 0.5880 | 1.0000 | 0.7860 |

$(\eta_1^2,\eta_2^2,\eta_3^2)=(0.5,0.7,0.8)$

| | $(\alpha_1,\alpha_2,\alpha_3)=(2,3,4)$ | | | | | | $(\alpha_1,\alpha_2,\alpha_3)=(5,5,6)$ | | | | | |
| | N1 | | N2 | | N3 | | N1 | | N2 | | N3 | |
| $\xi_3$ | p1 | p2 | p1 | p2 | p1 | p2 | p1 | p2 | p1 | p2 | p1 | p2 |
|---|---|---|---|---|---|---|---|---|---|---|---|---|
| 1.6 | 0.1444 | 0.0840 | 0.4768 | 0.0548 | 0.7516 | 0.0620 | 0.2164 | 0.0560 | 0.7472 | 0.0524 | 0.9452 | 0.1352 |
| 1.7 | 0.2460 | 0.0920 | 0.6804 | 0.0660 | 0.8576 | 0.1072 | 0.3696 | 0.0692 | 0.8712 | 0.1208 | 0.9732 | 0.2684 |
| 1.8 | 0.3644 | 0.1108 | 0.8196 | 0.1144 | 0.9264 | 0.2104 | 0.5456 | 0.1000 | 0.9388 | 0.2296 | 0.9932 | 0.4448 |
| 1.9 | 0.4992 | 0.1412 | 0.8980 | 0.2104 | 0.9732 | 0.3532 | 0.6980 | 0.1456 | 0.9740 | 0.3932 | 0.9984 | 0.5952 |
| 2.0 | 0.6304 | 0.1956 | 0.9400 | 0.3448 | 0.9876 | 0.5040 | 0.8096 | 0.2212 | 0.9920 | 0.5412 | 1.0000 | 0.7420 |

$(\eta_1^2,\eta_2^2,\eta_3^2)=(0.6,0.8,0.8)$

| | $(\alpha_1,\alpha_2,\alpha_3)=(2,3,4)$ | | | | | | $(\alpha_1,\alpha_2,\alpha_3)=(5,5,6)$ | | | | | |
| | N1 | | N2 | | N3 | | N1 | | N2 | | N3 | |
| $\xi_3$ | p1 | p2 | p1 | p2 | p1 | p2 | p1 | p2 | p1 | p2 | p1 | p2 |
|---|---|---|---|---|---|---|---|---|---|---|---|---|
| 1.6 | 0.1396 | 0.0744 | 0.4476 | 0.0580 | 0.7252 | 0.0812 | 0.2208 | 0.0548 | 0.7288 | 0.0848 | 0.9384 | 0.2116 |
| 1.7 | 0.2428 | 0.0904 | 0.6484 | 0.0732 | 0.8420 | 0.1224 | 0.3720 | 0.0716 | 0.8664 | 0.1584 | 0.9720 | 0.3552 |
| 1.8 | 0.3588 | 0.1076 | 0.7996 | 0.1204 | 0.9144 | 0.2044 | 0.5396 | 0.1092 | 0.9408 | 0.2712 | 0.9928 | 0.5132 |
| 1.9 | 0.4860 | 0.1424 | 0.8864 | 0.2044 | 0.9676 | 0.3312 | 0.6880 | 0.1596 | 0.9744 | 0.4160 | 0.9984 | 0.6524 |
| 2.0 | 0.6100 | 0.1932 | 0.9276 | 0.3180 | 0.9824 | 0.4836 | 0.8012 | 0.2384 | 0.9920 | 0.5460 | 1.0000 | 0.7688 |

*Note:* $N1 = (30,40,40), N2 = (60,60,80), N3 = (80,100,120)$.

**Table 3.8:** Simulated powers of hypothesis testing problem (3.6) as $k = 5$, $\xi_1 = 1$, $\xi_2 = 1.1$, $\xi_3 = 1.2$, and $\xi_4 = 1.3$.

$(\eta_1^2,\eta_2^2,\eta_3^2,\eta_4^2,\eta_5^2)=(0.2,0.4,0.6,0.8,0.9)$

| | $(\alpha_1,\alpha_2,\alpha_3,\alpha_4,\alpha_5)=(3,4,4,5,6)$ | | | | | | $(\alpha_1,\alpha_2,\alpha_3,\alpha_4,\alpha_5)=(5,5,6,7,8)$ | | | | | |
| | N1 | | N2 | | N3 | | N1 | | N2 | | N3 | |
| $\xi_5$ | p1 | p2 | p1 | p2 | p1 | p2 | p1 | p2 | p1 | p2 | p1 | p2 |
|---|---|---|---|---|---|---|---|---|---|---|---|---|
| 1.4 | 0.3160 | 0.1952 | 0.6904 | 0.1792 | 0.9248 | 0.2264 | 0.3940 | 0.1760 | 0.8344 | 0.1916 | 0.9780 | 0.2516 |
| 1.5 | 0.4184 | 0.1760 | 0.7960 | 0.1600 | 0.9612 | 0.2012 | 0.5180 | 0.1528 | 0.8952 | 0.1672 | 0.9912 | 0.2184 |
| 1.6 | 0.5488 | 0.1652 | 0.8736 | 0.1352 | 0.9812 | 0.1608 | 0.6632 | 0.1332 | 0.9396 | 0.1384 | 0.9968 | 0.1776 |
| 1.7 | 0.6824 | 0.1476 | 0.9336 | 0.1100 | 0.9924 | 0.1224 | 0.7780 | 0.1204 | 0.9700 | 0.1008 | 0.9992 | 0.1300 |
| 1.8 | 0.7904 | 0.1432 | 0.9692 | 0.0912 | 0.9968 | 0.0940 | 0.8708 | 0.1128 | 0.9900 | 0.0828 | 0.9996 | 0.1024 |

$(\eta_1^2,\eta_2^2,\eta_3^2,\eta_4^2,\eta_5^2)=(0.3,0.4,0.5,0.8,0.9)$

| | $(\alpha_1,\alpha_2,\alpha_3,\alpha_4,\alpha_5)=(3,4,4,5,6)$ | | | | | | $(\alpha_1,\alpha_2,\alpha_3,\alpha_4,\alpha_5)=(5,5,6,7,8)$ | | | | | |
| | N1 | | N2 | | N3 | | N1 | | N2 | | N3 | |
| $\xi_5$ | p1 | p2 | p1 | p2 | p1 | p2 | p1 | p2 | p1 | p2 | p1 | p2 |
|---|---|---|---|---|---|---|---|---|---|---|---|---|
| 1.4 | 0.2524 | 0.1252 | 0.5248 | 0.1060 | 0.8504 | 0.1088 | 0.3216 | 0.1112 | 0.7248 | 0.0984 | 0.9500 | 0.1004 |
| 1.5 | 0.3328 | 0.1216 | 0.6484 | 0.0972 | 0.9092 | 0.0984 | 0.4280 | 0.1056 | 0.8136 | 0.0852 | 0.9726 | 0.0864 |
| 1.6 | 0.4496 | 0.1232 | 0.7588 | 0.0820 | 0.9440 | 0.0832 | 0.5572 | 0.0976 | 0.8832 | 0.0684 | 0.9884 | 0.0740 |
| 1.7 | 0.5744 | 0.1224 | 0.8484 | 0.0696 | 0.9676 | 0.0688 | 0.6972 | 0.0984 | 0.9384 | 0.0544 | 0.9956 | 0.0604 |
| 1.8 | 0.7048 | 0.1196 | 0.9064 | 0.0644 | 0.9836 | 0.0620 | 0.8152 | 0.0988 | 0.9712 | 0.0512 | 0.9980 | 0.0640 |

$(\eta_1^2,\eta_2^2,\eta_3^2,\eta_4^2,\eta_5^2)=(0.3,0.5,0.6,0.8,1.0)$

| | $(\alpha_1,\alpha_2,\alpha_3,\alpha_4,\alpha_5)=(3,4,4,5,6)$ | | | | | | $(\alpha_1,\alpha_2,\alpha_3,\alpha_4,\alpha_5)=(5,5,6,7,8)$ | | | | | |
| | N1 | | N2 | | N3 | | N1 | | N2 | | N3 | |
| $\xi_5$ | p1 | p2 | p1 | p2 | p1 | p2 | p1 | p2 | p1 | p2 | p1 | p2 |
|---|---|---|---|---|---|---|---|---|---|---|---|---|
| 1.4 | 0.1104 | 0.1748 | 0.1944 | 0.2092 | 0.5240 | 0.2764 | 0.0920 | 0.1788 | 0.3408 | 0.2324 | 0.7492 | 0.3336 |
| 1.5 | 0.1224 | 0.1700 | 0.2624 | 0.1988 | 0.6156 | 0.2588 | 0.1232 | 0.1716 | 0.4376 | 0.2216 | 0.8124 | 0.3120 |
| 1.6 | 0.1540 | 0.1600 | 0.3620 | 0.1780 | 0.7076 | 0.2368 | 0.1800 | 0.1556 | 0.5412 | 0.1924 | 0.8688 | 0.2764 |
| 1.7 | 0.2096 | 0.1456 | 0.4756 | 0.1524 | 0.7956 | 0.1960 | 0.2616 | 0.1372 | 0.6644 | 0.1636 | 0.9140 | 0.2308 |
| 1.8 | 0.3000 | 0.1364 | 0.6100 | 0.1208 | 0.8684 | 0.1532 | 0.3708 | 0.1152 | 0.7700 | 0.1280 | 0.9444 | 0.1836 |

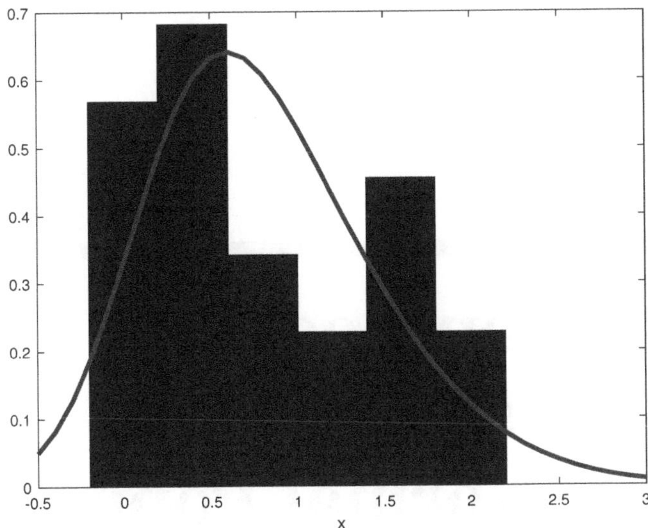

**Figure 3.1:** GDP histogram and probability density curve of Tianjin (1995–2018).

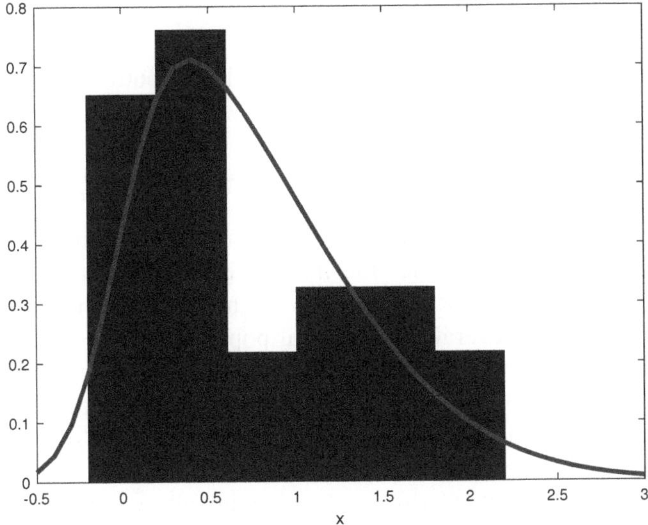

**Figure 3.2:** GDP histogram and probability density curve of Chongqing (1995–2017).

# Chapter 4

# Common Location Parameter of Skew-Normal Populations

The random variable $Y$ follows a skew-normal distribution with location parameter $\xi \in R$, scale parameter $\eta^2 \in R^+$ and skewness parameter $\lambda \in R$, denoted by $Y \sim SN(\xi, \eta^2, \lambda)$, and its density function is

$$f(y; \xi, \eta^2, \lambda) = 2\phi(y; \xi, \eta^2)\Phi[\lambda\eta^{-1}(y - \xi)]. \tag{4.1}$$

This chapter focuses on different skew-normal populations with the common location parameter, and studies the interval estimation and hypothesis testing problems of the location parameter with unknown scale and skewness parameters. First of all, for several skew-normal populations, the methods of moment estimation and maximum likelihood (ML) estimation are used for estimating the unknown parameters. Subsequently, the Bootstrap confidence intervals and Bootstrap test statistics for the common location parameter of several skew-normal populations with unknown scale parameters and skewness parameters are constructed. Then the Monte Carlo simulation results in two, three and five populations are presented. Finally, the proposed approaches are applied to the real data examples of regional gross domestic product (GDP) of China and bioavailability.

## 4.1 Parameter estimation

Referring to the estimation method in Chapter 3, this section extends one skew-normal population to k skew-normal populations with common location parameters. For $i = 1,\ldots,k$, suppose that $Y_{i1},\ldots,Y_{in_i}$ are a group of random samples with the distribution $SN(\xi,\eta_i^2,\lambda_i)$. Let $(\bar{Y}_i,S_{2i},S_{3i})$ be the sample mean, the second and third central moment, such that

$$\bar{Y}_i = \frac{1}{n_i}\sum_{j=1}^{n_i} Y_{ij},\ S_{2i} = \frac{1}{n_i}\sum_{j=1}^{n_i}(Y_{ij}-\bar{Y}_i)^2,\ S_{3i} = \frac{1}{n_i}\sum_{j=1}^{n_i}(Y_{ij}-\bar{Y}_i)^3,\ i=1,\ldots,k. \quad (4.2)$$

Similar to one population, we get the estimators of $(\eta_i^2,\lambda_i)$ in several skew-normal populations, $i = 1,\ldots,k$. From Theorem 3.2, the moment estimators of $(\eta_i^2,\lambda_i)$ can be expressed as

$$\hat{\eta}_i^2 = S_{2i} + c^2 S_{3i}^{2/3},\ \hat{\lambda}_i = \hat{\delta}_i/(1-\hat{\delta}_i^2)^{1/2},\ i=1,\ldots,k, \quad (4.3)$$

where

$$\hat{\delta}_i = \frac{cS_{3i}^{1/3}}{b\sqrt{S_{2i}+c^2 S_{3i}^{2/3}}}.$$

Then we obtain

$$E(\bar{Y}_i) = \xi + b\eta_i\delta_i,\ D(\bar{Y}_i) = \frac{\eta_i^2(1-b^2\delta_i^2)}{n_i},\ i=1,\ldots,k. \quad (4.4)$$

Note that if $(\eta_i^2,\delta_i)$ is known, the estimator of $\xi$ and its variance based on the *i*th sample are given by

$$\hat{\xi}^i\big|_{(\eta_i,\delta_i)} = \bar{Y}_i - b\eta_i\delta_i,\ D(\hat{\xi}^i\big|_{(\eta_i,\delta_i)}) = \frac{\eta_i^2(1-b^2\delta_i^2)}{n_i},\ i=1,\ldots,k.$$

Using the idea of Graybill-Deal estimation ( Graybill and Deal, 1959), we have

$$\hat{\xi} = \frac{\sum\limits_{i=1}^{k}\dfrac{1}{D(\hat{\xi}^i|_{(\eta_i,\delta_i)})}\hat{\xi}^i\big|_{(\eta_i,\delta_i)}}{\sum\limits_{i=1}^{k}\dfrac{1}{D(\hat{\xi}^i|_{(\eta_i,\delta_i)})}} = \bar{Y}_G - \frac{\sum\limits_{i=1}^{k}\dfrac{bn_i\delta_i}{\eta_i(1-b^2\delta_i^2)}}{\sum\limits_{i=1}^{k}\dfrac{n_i}{\eta_i^2(1-b^2\delta_i^2)}}, \quad (4.5)$$

where

$$\bar{Y}_G = \frac{\sum\limits_{i=1}^{k}\dfrac{n_i}{\eta_i^2(1-b^2\delta_i^2)}\bar{Y}_i}{\sum\limits_{i=1}^{k}\dfrac{n_i}{\eta_i^2(1-b^2\delta_i^2)}}.$$

Suppose $(\hat{\eta}_i^{*2}, \hat{\delta}_i^*, \hat{\lambda}_i^*)$ are the moment estimates corresponding to $(\hat{\eta}_i^2, \hat{\delta}_i, \hat{\lambda}_i)$, $i = 1, \ldots, k$. Then, replacing $(\eta_i, \delta_i)$ with $(\hat{\eta}_i^*, \hat{\delta}_i^*)$ in (4.5), we obtain the estimate of $\xi$, namely

$$\hat{\xi}^* = \bar{y}_{G1} - \frac{\displaystyle\sum_{i=1}^{k} \frac{b n_i \hat{\delta}_i^*}{\hat{\eta}_i^*(1 - b^2 \hat{\delta}_i^{*2})}}{\displaystyle\sum_{i=1}^{k} \frac{n_i}{\hat{\eta}_i^{*2}(1 - b^2 \hat{\delta}_i^{*2})}}, \tag{4.6}$$

where $\bar{y}_{G1}$ is the observed value of $\bar{Y}_{G1}$, and $\bar{Y}_{G1}$ is obtained by replacing $(\eta_i, \delta_i)$ with their moment estimators. By Theorem 3.4, the ML estimators $(\tilde{\xi}_i, \tilde{\eta}_i^2, \tilde{\delta}_i, \tilde{\lambda}_i)$ of $(\xi_i, \eta_i^2, \delta_i, \lambda_i)$ are obtained, $i = 1, \ldots, k$. Suppose $(\tilde{\xi}_i^*, \tilde{\eta}_i^{*2}, \tilde{\delta}_i^*, \tilde{\lambda}_i^*)$ are the ML estimates corresponding to $(\tilde{\xi}_i, \tilde{\eta}_i^2, \tilde{\delta}_i, \tilde{\lambda}_i), i = 1, \ldots, k$. Thus

$$\tilde{\xi}^* = \bar{y}_{G2} - \frac{\displaystyle\sum_{i=1}^{k} \frac{b n_i \tilde{\delta}_i^*}{\tilde{\eta}_i^*(1 - b^2 \tilde{\delta}_i^{*2})}}{\displaystyle\sum_{i=1}^{k} \frac{n_i}{\tilde{\eta}_i^{*2}(1 - b^2 \tilde{\delta}_i^{*2})}}, \tag{4.7}$$

where $\bar{y}_{G2}$ is the observed value of $\bar{Y}_{G2}$, and $\bar{Y}_{G2}$ is obtained by replacing $(\eta_i, \delta_i)$ with their ML estimators.

## 4.2 Bootstrap confidence interval

In this section, the confidence interval and hypothesis test for the common location parameter $\xi$ based on the Bootstrap approach is discussed. Using the central limit theorem, we have

$$Z = \sqrt{\sum_{i=1}^{k} \frac{n_i}{\eta_i^2(1 - b^2 \delta_i^2)}} \left( \bar{Y}_G - \xi - \frac{\displaystyle\sum_{i=1}^{k} \frac{b n_i \delta_i}{\eta_i(1 - b^2 \delta_i^2)}}{\displaystyle\sum_{i=1}^{k} \frac{n_i}{\eta_i^2(1 - b^2 \delta_i^2)}} \right). \tag{4.8}$$

Its well-known, when $n_i \to \infty, i = 1, \ldots, k$, the approximate distribution of $Z$ is the standard normal distribution $N(0, 1)$. Suppose that $U(\beta)$ is the $100\beta$ empirical percentile of $N(0, 1)$. Then the $1 - \alpha$ confidence interval for $\xi$ is given by

$$\left[ \bar{Y}_G - \frac{U(1 - \alpha/2)}{\sqrt{\displaystyle\sum_{i=1}^{k} \frac{n_i}{\eta_i^2(1 - b^2 \delta_i^2)}}} - \frac{\displaystyle\sum_{i=1}^{k} \frac{b n_i \delta_i}{\eta_i(1 - b^2 \delta_i^2)}}{\displaystyle\sum_{i=1}^{k} \frac{n_i}{\eta_i^2(1 - b^2 \delta_i^2)}}, \bar{Y}_G - \frac{U(\alpha/2)}{\sqrt{\displaystyle\sum_{i=1}^{k} \frac{n_i}{\eta_i^2(1 - b^2 \delta_i^2)}}} - \frac{\displaystyle\sum_{i=1}^{k} \frac{b n_i \delta_i}{\eta_i(1 - b^2 \delta_i^2)}}{\displaystyle\sum_{i=1}^{k} \frac{n_i}{\eta_i^2(1 - b^2 \delta_i^2)}} \right].$$

Whereas $(\eta_i, \delta_i)$ is often unknown in a practical problem, the pivotal quantities might be developed by replacing $(\eta_i, \delta_i)$ with their moment estimators and ML estimators in (4.8) respectively, $i = 1, \ldots, k$. Namely,

$$
Z_1 = \sqrt{\sum_{i=1}^{k} \frac{n_i}{\hat{\eta}_i^2 (1 - b^2 \hat{\delta}_i^2)}} \left( \bar{Y}_{G1} - \xi - \frac{\sum_{i=1}^{k} \frac{b n_i \hat{\delta}_i}{\hat{\eta}_i (1 - b^2 \hat{\delta}_i^2)}}{\sum_{i=1}^{k} \frac{n_i}{\hat{\eta}_i^2 (1 - b^2 \hat{\delta}_i^2)}} \right), \tag{4.9}
$$

and

$$
Z_2 = \sqrt{\sum_{i=1}^{k} \frac{n_i}{\tilde{\eta}_i^2 (1 - b^2 \tilde{\delta}_i^2)}} \left( \bar{Y}_{G2} - \xi - \frac{\sum_{i=1}^{k} \frac{b n_i \tilde{\delta}_i}{\tilde{\eta}_i (1 - b^2 \tilde{\delta}_i^2)}}{\sum_{i=1}^{k} \frac{n_i}{\tilde{\eta}_i^2 (1 - b^2 \tilde{\delta}_i^2)}} \right). \tag{4.10}
$$

Unfortunately, the exact distributions of $Z_1$ and $Z_2$ are unknown. Thus, it is impossible to find their exact quantile values. It motivates us to construct the confidence interval for the common location parameter $\xi$ by virtue of the Bootstrap approach. Define $Y_{BMij}$ as the Bootstrap sample from $SN(\hat{\xi}^*, \hat{\eta}_i^{*2}, \hat{\lambda}_i^*)$, $i = 1, \ldots, k$, $j = 1, \ldots, n_i$. $(\bar{Y}_{BMi}, S_{BM2i}, S_{BM3i})$ represents the sample mean, the second and third center moment of $Y_{BMij}$, $i = 1, \ldots, k$, $j = 1, \ldots, n_i$. From Theorem 3.2, the moment estimators of $(\eta_i^2, \delta_i)$ can be expressed as

$$
\hat{\eta}_{BMi}^2 = S_{BM2i} + c^2 S_{BM3i}^{2/3}, \quad \hat{\delta}_{BMi} = \frac{c S_{BM3i}^{1/3}}{b \sqrt{S_{BM2i} + c^2 S_{BM3i}^{2/3}}}, \quad i = 1, \ldots, k. \tag{4.11}
$$

For $i = 1, \ldots, k$, $j = 1, \ldots, n_i$, suppose $(\hat{\eta}_{BMi}^{*2}, \hat{\delta}_{BMi}^*)$ are the moment estimates corresponding to $(\hat{\eta}_{BMi}^2, \hat{\delta}_{BMi})$ and define $Y_{BLij}$ as the Bootstrap sample from $SN(\tilde{\xi}^*, \tilde{\eta}_i^{*2}, \tilde{\lambda}_i^*)$. $(\bar{Y}_{BLi}, S_{BL2i}, S_{BL3i})$ represents the sample mean, the second and third center moments of $Y_{BLij}$, $i = 1, \ldots, k$, $j = 1, \ldots, n_i$. Then the ML estimators $(\tilde{\eta}_{BLi}^2, \tilde{\delta}_{BLi})$ can be obtained by Theorem 3.4, $i = 1, \ldots, k$. Define

$$
\bar{Y}_{GB1} = \frac{\sum_{i=1}^{k} \frac{n_i}{\hat{\eta}_{BMi}^2 (1 - b^2 \hat{\delta}_{BMi}^2)} \bar{Y}_{BMi}}{\sum_{i=1}^{k} \frac{n_i}{\hat{\eta}_{BMi}^2 (1 - b^2 \hat{\delta}_{BMi}^2)}}, \tag{4.12}
$$

and

$$
\bar{Y}_{GB2} = \frac{\sum_{i=1}^{k} \frac{n_i}{\tilde{\eta}_{BLi}^2 (1 - b^2 \tilde{\delta}_{BLi}^2)} \bar{Y}_{BLi}}{\sum_{i=1}^{k} \frac{n_i}{\tilde{\eta}_{BLi}^2 (1 - b^2 \tilde{\delta}_{BLi}^2)}}. \tag{4.13}
$$

Similar to (4.9) and (4.10), the Bootstrap pivot quantities are constructed as follows

$$
Z_{B1} = \sqrt{\sum_{i=1}^{k} \frac{n_i}{\hat{\eta}_{BMi}^2(1-b^2\hat{\delta}_{BMi}^2)}} \left( \bar{Y}_{GB1} - \frac{\sum_{i=1}^{k} \frac{bn_i\hat{\delta}_{BMi}}{\hat{\eta}_{BMi}(1-b^2\hat{\delta}_{BMi}^2)}}{\sum_{i=1}^{k} \frac{n_i}{\hat{\eta}_{BMi}^2(1-b^2\hat{\delta}_{BMi}^2)}} - \left( \bar{y}_{G1} - \frac{\sum_{i=1}^{k} \frac{bn_i\hat{\delta}_i^*}{\hat{\eta}_i^*(1-b^2\hat{\delta}_i^{*2})}}{\sum_{i=1}^{k} \frac{n_i}{\hat{\eta}_i^{*2}(1-b^2\hat{\delta}_i^{*2})}} \right) \right),
$$

$$(4.14)$$

and

$$
Z_{B2} = \sqrt{\sum_{i=1}^{k} \frac{n_i}{\tilde{\eta}_{BLi}^2(1-b^2\tilde{\delta}_{BLi}^2)}} \left( \bar{Y}_{GB2} - \frac{\sum_{i=1}^{k} \frac{bn_i\tilde{\delta}_{BLi}}{\tilde{\eta}_{BLi}(1-b^2\tilde{\delta}_{BLi}^2)}}{\sum_{i=1}^{k} \frac{n_i}{\tilde{\eta}_{BLi}^2(1-b^2\tilde{\delta}_{BLi}^2)}} - \left( \bar{y}_{G2} - \frac{\sum_{i=1}^{k} \frac{bn_i\tilde{\delta}_i^*}{\tilde{\eta}_i^*(1-b^2\tilde{\delta}_i^{*2})}}{\sum_{i=1}^{k} \frac{n_i}{\tilde{\eta}_i^{*2}(1-b^2\tilde{\delta}_i^{*2})}} \right) \right).
$$

$$(4.15)$$

Suppose that $Z_{B1}(\beta)$ is the $100\beta$ empirical percentile of $Z_{B1}$. Then the $1-\alpha$ confidence interval for $\xi$ is given by

$$
\left[ \bar{y}_{G1} - \frac{Z_{B1}(1-\alpha/2)}{\sqrt{\sum_{i=1}^{k} \frac{n_i}{\hat{\eta}_i^{*2}(1-b^2\hat{\delta}_i^{*2})}}} - \frac{\sum_{i=1}^{k} \frac{bn_i\hat{\delta}_i^*}{\hat{\eta}_i^*(1-b^2\hat{\delta}_i^{*2})}}{\sum_{i=1}^{k} \frac{n_i}{\hat{\eta}_i^{*2}(1-b^2\hat{\delta}_i^{*2})}}, \bar{y}_{G1} - \frac{Z_{B1}(\alpha/2)}{\sqrt{\sum_{i=1}^{k} \frac{n_i}{\hat{\eta}_i^{*2}(1-b^2\hat{\delta}_i^{*2})}}} - \frac{\sum_{i=1}^{k} \frac{bn_i\hat{\delta}_i^*}{\hat{\eta}_i^*(1-b^2\hat{\delta}_i^{*2})}}{\sum_{i=1}^{k} \frac{n_i}{\hat{\eta}_i^{*2}(1-b^2\hat{\delta}_i^{*2})}} \right].
$$

Similarly, the $1-\alpha$ Bootstrap confidence interval is obtained based on $Z_{B2}$.

**Remark 4.1.** *For $i = 1,\ldots,k$, the moment estimator and ML estimator of $\eta_i^2$ are equal to each other when $\lambda_i = 0$, that is $S_{2i}$. Thus, $\hat{\xi}$ given in (4.5) is the Graybill-Deal estimator of $\xi$, and the Bootstrap confidence interval of $\xi$ degenerates to the result of Xu (2016).*

Next, the Bootstrap approach for the hypothesis testing problem of the common location parameter $\xi$ in several skew-normal populations is proposed. Specifically, the hypothesis of interest is

$$
H_0 : \xi = \xi_0 \qquad versus \qquad H_1 : \xi \neq \xi_0 , \qquad (4.16)
$$

where $\xi_0$ is a specified value. Using the central limit theorem, under $H_0$ in (4.16) we have

$$
Z^* = \sqrt{\sum_{i=1}^{k} \frac{n_i}{\eta_i^2(1-b^2\delta_i^2)}} \left( \bar{Y}_G - \xi_0 - \frac{\sum_{i=1}^{k} \frac{bn_i\delta_i}{\eta_i(1-b^2\delta_i^2)}}{\sum_{i=1}^{k} \frac{n_i}{\eta_i^2(1-b^2\delta_i^2)}} \right). \qquad (4.17)
$$

If $(\eta_i, \delta_i)$ is known, then $Z^*$ is a natural test statistic for hypothesis testing problem (4.16). In fact, $(\eta_i, \delta_i)$ is often unknown. Thus, the test statistics might be developed by replacing $(\eta_i, \delta_i)$ with their moment estimators and ML estimators in (4.17) respectively. Then the test statistics can be written as

$$Z_1^* = \sqrt{\sum_{i=1}^{k} \frac{n_i}{\hat{\eta}_i^2(1-b^2\hat{\delta}_i^2)}} \left( \bar{Y}_{G1} - \xi_0 - \frac{\sum_{i=1}^{k} \frac{bn_i\hat{\delta}_i}{\hat{\eta}_i(1-b^2\hat{\delta}_i^2)}}{\sum_{i=1}^{k} \frac{n_i}{\hat{\eta}_i^2(1-b^2\hat{\delta}_i^2)}} \right),$$

and

$$Z_2^* = \sqrt{\sum_{i=1}^{k} \frac{n_i}{\tilde{\eta}_i^2(1-b^2\tilde{\delta}_i^2)}} \left( \bar{Y}_{G2} - \xi_0 - \frac{\sum_{i=1}^{k} \frac{bn_i\tilde{\delta}_i}{\tilde{\eta}_i(1-b^2\tilde{\delta}_i^2)}}{\sum_{i=1}^{k} \frac{n_i}{\tilde{\eta}_i^2(1-b^2\tilde{\delta}_i^2)}} \right).$$

Similar to $Z_1$ and $Z_2$, the exact distributions of $Z_1^*$ and $Z_2^*$ are also unknown. To this end, the Bootstrap approach will be used to construct test statistics for the hypothesis testing problem (4.16) as follows.

$$Z_{B1}^* = \sqrt{\sum_{i=1}^{k} \frac{n_i}{\hat{\eta}_{BMi}^2(1-b^2\hat{\delta}_{BMi}^2)}} \left( \bar{Y}_{GB1} - \xi_0 - \frac{\sum_{i=1}^{k} \frac{bn_i\hat{\delta}_{BMi}}{\hat{\eta}_{BMi}(1-b^2\hat{\delta}_{BMi}^2)}}{\sum_{i=1}^{k} \frac{n_i}{\hat{\eta}_{BMi}^2(1-b^2\hat{\delta}_{BMi}^2)}} \right), \qquad (4.18)$$

and

$$Z_{B2}^* = \sqrt{\sum_{i=1}^{k} \frac{n_i}{\tilde{\eta}_{BLi}^2(1-b^2\tilde{\delta}_{BLi}^2)}} \left( \bar{Y}_{GB2} - \xi_0 - \frac{\sum_{i=1}^{k} \frac{bn_i\tilde{\delta}_{BLi}}{\tilde{\eta}_{BLi}(1-b^2\tilde{\delta}_{BLi}^2)}}{\sum_{i=1}^{k} \frac{n_i}{\tilde{\eta}_{BLi}^2(1-b^2\tilde{\delta}_{BLi}^2)}} \right). \qquad (4.19)$$

Then the Bootstrap p-values for the hypothesis testing problem (4.16) are computed as

$$p_i = 2\min\{P(Z_{Bi}^* > z_i^*), P(Z_{Bi}^* < z_i^*)\}, i = 1, 2, \qquad (4.20)$$

where $z_1^*$ and $z_2^*$ are observed values of $Z_1^*$ and $Z_2^*$ respectively. The null hypothesis $H_0$ in (4.16) is rejected whenever the above p-values are less than the nominal significance level of $\alpha$, which means that the difference between $\xi$ and $\xi_0$ is significant.

**Remark 4.2.** *If $\lambda_1 = \lambda_2 = \cdots = \lambda_k = 0$, then we can obtain $p_1 = p_2$. Thus, the above Bootstrap p-value in (4.16) degenerates to the result of Xu (2016).*

In addition, the second Bootstrap confidence interval is constructed based on different weights. Let $\bar{Y} = \sum_{i=1}^{k} n_i \bar{Y}_i / \tilde{n}$ with $\tilde{n} = \sum_{i=1}^{k} n_i$. By replacing $\bar{Y}_G$ with $\bar{Y}$ in (4.8) and combining with the central limit theorem, we obtain

$$
T = \frac{\bar{Y} - \sum_{i=1}^{k} n_i (\xi + b \eta_i \delta_i) / \tilde{n}}{\sqrt{\sum_{i=1}^{k} n_i \eta_i^2 (1 - b^2 \delta_i^2) / \tilde{n}^2}}.
\tag{4.21}
$$

By replacing $(\eta_i^2, \delta_i)$ with their moment estimators and ML estimators in (4.21), we gain

$$
T_1 = \frac{\bar{Y}_1 - \sum_{i=1}^{k} n_i (\xi + b \hat{\eta}_i \hat{\delta}_i) / \tilde{n}}{\sqrt{\sum_{i=1}^{k} n_i \hat{\eta}_i^2 (1 - b^2 \hat{\delta}_i^2) / \tilde{n}^2}},
$$

and

$$
T_2 = \frac{\bar{Y}_2 - \sum_{i=1}^{k} n_i (\xi + b \tilde{\eta}_i \tilde{\delta}_i) / \tilde{n}}{\sqrt{\sum_{i=1}^{k} n_i \tilde{\eta}_i^2 (1 - b^2 \tilde{\delta}_i^2) / \tilde{n}^2}}.
$$

Similar to $Z_{B1}$ and $Z_{B2}$, we have

$$
T_{B1} = \frac{\bar{Y}_{B1} - \sum_{i=1}^{k} n_i \left( \left( \sum_{i=1}^{k} n_i \bar{y}_i / \tilde{n} - \sum_{i=1}^{k} b n_i \hat{\eta}_i^* \hat{\delta}_i^* / \tilde{n} \right) + b \hat{\eta}_{BMi} \hat{\delta}_{BMi} \right) / \tilde{n}}{\sqrt{\sum_{i=1}^{k} n_i \hat{\eta}_{BMi}^2 (1 - b^2 \hat{\delta}_{BMi}^2) / \tilde{n}^2}},
\tag{4.22}
$$

and

$$
T_{B2} = \frac{\bar{Y}_{B2} - \sum_{i=1}^{k} n_i \left( \left( \sum_{i=1}^{k} n_i \bar{y}_i / \tilde{n} - \sum_{i=1}^{k} b n_i \tilde{\eta}_i^* \tilde{\delta}_i^* / \tilde{n} \right) + b \tilde{\eta}_{BLi} \tilde{\delta}_{BLi} \right) / \tilde{n}}{\sqrt{\sum_{i=1}^{k} n_i \tilde{\eta}_{BLi}^2 (1 - b^2 \tilde{\delta}_{BLi}^2) / \tilde{n}^2}}.
\tag{4.23}
$$

Suppose that $T_{B1}(\beta)$ is the $100\beta$ empirical percentile of $T_{B1}$. Then the $1-\alpha$ Bootstrap confidence interval for $\xi$ is given by

$$\left[ U - \frac{T_{B1}(1-\alpha/2)\sqrt{\sum_{i=1}^{k} n_i \hat{\eta}_i^{*2}(1-b^2\hat{\delta}_i^{*2})}}{\tilde{n}}, U - \frac{T_{B1}(\alpha/2)\sqrt{\sum_{i=1}^{k} n_i \hat{\eta}_i^{*2}(1-b^2\hat{\delta}_i^{*2})}}{\tilde{n}} \right],$$

where

$$U = \bar{y}_1 - \sum_{i=1}^{k} \frac{bn_i \hat{\eta}_i^* \hat{\delta}_i^*}{\tilde{n}}.$$

Similarly, the $1-\alpha$ Bootstrap confidence interval is derived based on $T_{B2}$.

Under $H_0$ in (4.16), similar to (4.21), the test statistics are defined as

$$T_1^* = \frac{\bar{Y}_1 - \sum_{i=1}^{k} n_i(\xi_0 + b\hat{\eta}_i\hat{\delta}_i)/\tilde{n}}{\sqrt{\sum_{i=1}^{k} n_i \hat{\eta}_i^2(1-b^2\hat{\delta}_i^2)/\tilde{n}^2}},$$

and

$$T_2^* = \frac{\bar{Y}_2 - \sum_{i=1}^{k} n_i(\xi_0 + b\tilde{\eta}_i\tilde{\delta}_i)/\tilde{n}}{\sqrt{\sum_{i=1}^{k} n_i \tilde{\eta}_i^2(1-b^2\tilde{\delta}_i^2)/\tilde{n}^2}}.$$

Analogous to $Z_{B1}^*$ and $Z_{B2}^*$, the Bootstrap test statistics $T_{B1}^*$ and $T_{B2}^*$ are constructed. Then the Bootstrap p-values are computed as

$$p_i^* = 2\min\{P(T_{Bi}^* > t_i), P(T_{Bi}^* < t_i)\}, i = 1,2, \tag{4.24}$$

where $t_1$ and $t_2$ denote the observed values of $T_1^*$ and $T_2^*$, respectively. The null hypothesis $H_0$ in (4.16) is rejected whenever the above p-values are less than the nominal significance level of $\alpha$, which means that the difference between $\xi$ and $\xi_0$ is significant.

## 4.3  Monte Carlo simulation

In this section, the Monte Carlo simulation is adopted to numerically investigate properties of the above confidence intervals from the aspects of the coverage probability and expected length. For convenience, we only provide the main steps of the Bootstrap approach based on the moment estimators for the confidence interval of $\xi$.

**Step 1:** For a given $(n_i, \xi_0, \eta_i^2, \lambda_i)$, generate a group of random samples $Y_{ij} \sim SN(\xi_0, \eta_i^2, \lambda_i)$, and $(\bar{Y}_i, S_{2i}, S_{3i})$ is computed by (4.2), $i = 1, \ldots, k$, $j = 1, \ldots, n_i$.

**Step 2:** Using (4.3) and (4.5), $(\hat{\xi}^*, \hat{\eta}_i^{*2}, \hat{\lambda}_i^*)$, the feasible estimates of $(\xi, \eta_i^2, \lambda_i)$ are computed, $i = 1, \ldots, k$.

**Step 3:** Generate a group of Bootstrap samples $Y_{BMij} \sim SN(\hat{\xi}^*, \hat{\eta}_i^{*2}, \hat{\lambda}_i^*)$, and compute $(\bar{Y}_{BMi}, S_{2BMi}, S_{3BMi})$ for $i = 1, \ldots, k$, $j = 1, \ldots, n_i$.

**Step 4:** From (4.2), $(\hat{\eta}_{BMi}^{*2}, \hat{\lambda}_{BMi}^*)$, the moment estimates of $(\eta^2, \lambda)$ from the Bootstrap samples are computed, $i = 1, \ldots, k$. Then $Z_{B1}$ and $T_{B1}$ are obtained by (4.14) and (4.22) respectively.

**Step 5:** Repeat steps 3–4 $n_1$ times and get $n_1$ values of $Z_{B1}$ and $T_{B1}$. Then, the $1 - \alpha$ Bootstrap confidence interval of $\xi$ is obtained.

**Step 6:** Repeat steps 1–5 $n_2$ times and obtain $n_2$ confidence intervals of $\xi$. The percentage of times these intervals contain $\xi$ is computed and reported as an estimate of the coverage probability. The expected length of confidence limits is estimated by the average length of the above confidence intervals.

In this simulation, the parameters and sample sizes are set as follows. Initially, let the nominal confidence level be 95%, the number of inner loops $n_1$ and number of outer loops $n_2$ with both equal to 2500, and $\xi_0 = 2$. Subsequently, for the Bootstrap confidence interval of two populations, we set $\eta_1^2 = (0.1^2, 1^2), \eta_2^2 = (0.3^2, 2.5^2), \eta_3^2 = (0.5^2, 4^2), \eta_4^2 = (0.7^2, 7^2), \eta_5^2 = (0.9^2, 10^2)$, $(\lambda_1, \lambda_2) = (3, 4), (5, 6), (8, 9)$, and $(n_1, n_2) = (30, 40), (40, 60), (60, 80), (90, 120), (120, 150), (150, 200)$.

For the Bootstrap confidence interval of three populations, we set $\eta^2_1 = (0.3^2, 0.9^2, 3^2), \eta_2^2 = (0.4^2, 1.1^2, 4^2), \eta_3^2 = (0.5^2, 1.2^2, 5^2), \eta_4^2 = (0.7^2, 1.5^2, 7^2), \eta_5^2 = (0.9^2, 2.1^2, 9^2), (\lambda_1, \lambda_2, \lambda_3) = (3, 3, 4), (5, 5, 6), (6, 8, 9)$, and $(n_1, n_2, n_3) = (30, 40, 40), (40, 50, 60), (60, 80, 90), (90, 100, 120), (120, 150, 180), (150, 200, 240)$.

For five populations, we set $\eta_1^2 = (0.3^2, 0.9^2 2^2, 3^2, 3^2), \eta^2_2 = (0.4^2, 1.2^2, 4^2, 4^2, 5^2), \eta_3^2 = (0.5^2, 1.8^2, 6^2, 5^2, 7^2), \eta_4^2 = (0.7^2, 3^2, 8^2, 7^2, 9^2), \eta_5^2 = (0.9^2, 5.4^2, 10^2, 9^2, 11^2), (\lambda_1, \lambda_2, \lambda_3, \lambda_4, \lambda_5) = (3, 3, 4, 4, 5), (4, 4, 5, 5, 6), (7, 7, 8, 8, 9)$, and $(n_1, n_2, n_3, n_4, n_5) = (30, 40, 40, 50, 50), (50, 50, 60, 60, 80), (70, 70, 90, 90, 100), (90, 90, 90, 120, 120), (100, 120, 120, 150, 150), (150, 150, 200, 200, 200)$.

Similar to the proposed approaches in Section 4.2, we add two Bootstrap confidence intervals based on the maximum penalized likelihood estimators (mple) (Azzalini and Arellano-Valle, 2013) in simulation study, and denote them by $Z_{mple}$ and $T_{mple}$.

For Bootstrap confidence intervals of two populations, Tables 4.1 and 4.4 respectively present the simulated coverage probabilities and expected lengths of six Bootstrap confidence intervals. In terms of coverage probability, $Z_{mple}$, $Z_{mle}$ and $Z_{mm}$ are liberal relatively when the skewness parameters are small. This result is significantly improved with sample sizes and skewness parameters increasing. The actual confidence levels of $T_{mple}$, $T_{mle}$ and $T_{mm}$ are close to 95% nominal confidence level and perform well, but their performances are slightly conservative as the skewness parameters increase. The expected lengths of six Bootstrap confidence intervals increase with scale parameters increasing, but decrease with sample sizes increasing. However, $Z_{mple}$, $Z_{mle}$ and $Z_{mm}$ perform significantly better than $T_{mple}$, $T_{mle}$ and $T_{mm}$ regardless of the methods of moment estimation or ML estimation.

Tables 4.2 and 4.3 respectively present the simulated coverage probabilities of six Bootstrap confidence intervals for three and five populations. Tables 4.5 and 4.6 present the expected lengths. In terms of coverage probability, $Z_{mple}$, $Z_{mle}$, $Z_{mm}$ and $T_{mle}$ are liberal when the skewness parameters and sample sizes are small. With the increase of skewness parameters and sample sizes, the actual confidence level of $Z_{mple}$ and $Z_{mm}$ is significantly improved regardless of three or five populations, and gradually get closer to a 95% nominal confidence level. The performance of $T_{mle}$ is similar to $Z_{mm}$ only in three populations. $T_{mple}$ and $T_{mm}$ performs well generally, but becomes slightly conservative with skewness parameters increasing. In addition, the simulation results for the expected lengths in three and five populations are similar to those of two populations.

**Remark 4.3.** *According to the Bootstrap confidence intervals of $Z_{mple}$, $Z_{mle}$, $Z_{mm}$, $T_{mple}$, $T_{mle}$, and $T_{mm}$, the Bootstrap test statistics of the hypothesis test problem (4.16) can be established. Tables 4.1–4.3 present that $Z_{mple}$, $Z_{mle}$, $Z_{mm}$ and $T_{mle}$ have low coverage probabilities under certain parameter settings. Therefore, these approaches cannot control the Type I error probability effectively. Conversely, $T_{mple}$ and $T_{mm}$ can control the Type I error probability effectively in the overall situation. But with the increase of the skewness parameters, $T_{mple}$ and $T_{mm}$ behave slightly conservative.*

**Table 4.1:** Simulated coverage probabilities of six Bootstrap confidence intervals in two populations.

$(\lambda_1,\lambda_2)=(3,4)$

| | N1 | | | | | | N2 | | | | | |
|---|---|---|---|---|---|---|---|---|---|---|---|---|
| | Zmple | Zmle | Zmm | Tmple | Tmle | Tmm | Zmple | Zmle | Zmm | Tmple | Tmle | Tmm |
| $\eta_1^2$ | 0.8616 | 0.8552 | 0.8740 | 0.9488 | 0.9532 | 0.9460 | 0.9012 | 0.8984 | 0.8980 | 0.9500 | 0.9540 | 0.9548 |
| $\eta_2^2$ | 0.8636 | 0.8564 | 0.8748 | 0.9492 | 0.9528 | 0.9464 | 0.9008 | 0.8968 | 0.8980 | 0.9508 | 0.9536 | 0.9548 |
| $\eta_3^2$ | 0.8636 | 0.8564 | 0.8752 | 0.9492 | 0.9524 | 0.9472 | 0.9012 | 0.8948 | 0.8988 | 0.9508 | 0.9536 | 0.9548 |
| $\eta_4^2$ | 0.8616 | 0.8552 | 0.8740 | 0.9488 | 0.9532 | 0.9460 | 0.9012 | 0.8984 | 0.8980 | 0.9500 | 0.9540 | 0.9548 |
| $\eta_5^2$ | 0.8612 | 0.8552 | 0.8736 | 0.9484 | 0.9532 | 0.9460 | 0.9008 | 0.9000 | 0.8980 | 0.9500 | 0.9548 | 0.9536 |

| | N3 | | | | | | N4 | | | | | |
|---|---|---|---|---|---|---|---|---|---|---|---|---|
| | Zmple | Zmle | Zmm | Tmple | Tmle | Tmm | Zmple | Zmle | Zmm | Tmple | Tmle | Tmm |
| $\eta_1^2$ | 0.9388 | 0.9224 | 0.9248 | 0.9464 | 0.9544 | 0.9588 | 0.9260 | 0.9324 | 0.9396 | 0.9492 | 0.9544 | 0.9532 |
| $\eta_2^2$ | 0.9392 | 0.9196 | 0.9256 | 0.9464 | 0.9536 | 0.9600 | 0.9260 | 0.9292 | 0.9400 | 0.9492 | 0.9532 | 0.9532 |
| $\eta_3^2$ | 0.9396 | 0.9196 | 0.9260 | 0.9464 | 0.9536 | 0.9600 | 0.9260 | 0.9284 | 0.9404 | 0.9488 | 0.9528 | 0.9532 |
| $\eta_4^2$ | 0.9388 | 0.9224 | 0.9248 | 0.9464 | 0.9544 | 0.9588 | 0.9260 | 0.9324 | 0.9396 | 0.9492 | 0.9544 | 0.9532 |
| $\eta_5^2$ | 0.9388 | 0.9224 | 0.9252 | 0.9464 | 0.9548 | 0.9588 | 0.9260 | 0.9332 | 0.9396 | 0.9492 | 0.9544 | 0.9532 |

| | N5 | | | | | | N6 | | | | | |
|---|---|---|---|---|---|---|---|---|---|---|---|---|
| | Zmple | Zmle | Zmm | Tmple | Tmle | Tmm | Zmple | Zmle | Zmm | Tmple | Tmle | Tmm |
| $\eta_1^2$ | 0.9236 | 0.9376 | 0.9404 | 0.9412 | 0.9492 | 0.9520 | 0.9284 | 0.9336 | 0.9400 | 0.9472 | 0.9536 | 0.9576 |
| $\eta_2^2$ | 0.9240 | 0.9348 | 0.9404 | 0.9408 | 0.9472 | 0.9512 | 0.9288 | 0.9300 | 0.9408 | 0.9468 | 0.9536 | 0.9576 |
| $\eta_3^2$ | 0.9244 | 0.9336 | 0.9404 | 0.9408 | 0.9472 | 0.9512 | 0.9288 | 0.9292 | 0.9408 | 0.9472 | 0.9528 | 0.9576 |
| $\eta_4^2$ | 0.9236 | 0.9376 | 0.9404 | 0.9412 | 0.9492 | 0.9520 | 0.9284 | 0.9336 | 0.9400 | 0.9472 | 0.9536 | 0.9576 |
| $\eta_5^2$ | 0.9228 | 0.9392 | 0.9404 | 0.9412 | 0.9496 | 0.9520 | 0.9284 | 0.9348 | 0.9400 | 0.9472 | 0.9540 | 0.9576 |

$(\lambda_1,\lambda_2)=(5,6)$

| | N1 | | | | | | N2 | | | | | |
|---|---|---|---|---|---|---|---|---|---|---|---|---|
| | Zmple | Zmle | Zmm | Tmple | Tmle | Tmm | Zmple | Zmle | Zmm | Tmple | Tmle | Tmm |
| $\eta_1^2$ | 0.9312 | 0.9312 | 0.9400 | 0.9652 | 0.9688 | 0.9656 | 0.9548 | 0.9532 | 0.9584 | 0.9656 | 0.9684 | 0.9724 |
| $\eta_2^2$ | 0.9320 | 0.9312 | 0.9408 | 0.9652 | 0.9688 | 0.9660 | 0.9556 | 0.9504 | 0.9592 | 0.9656 | 0.9680 | 0.9724 |
| $\eta_3^2$ | 0.9328 | 0.9304 | 0.9408 | 0.9652 | 0.9688 | 0.9660 | 0.9556 | 0.9496 | 0.9596 | 0.9656 | 0.9680 | 0.9728 |
| $\eta_4^2$ | 0.9312 | 0.9312 | 0.9400 | 0.9652 | 0.9688 | 0.9656 | 0.9548 | 0.9532 | 0.9584 | 0.9656 | 0.9684 | 0.9724 |
| $\eta_5^2$ | 0.9312 | 0.9324 | 0.9400 | 0.9652 | 0.9688 | 0.9656 | 0.9548 | 0.9536 | 0.9580 | 0.9660 | 0.9684 | 0.9720 |

| | N3 | | | | | | N4 | | | | | |
|---|---|---|---|---|---|---|---|---|---|---|---|---|
| | Zmple | Zmle | Zmm | Tmple | Tmle | Tmm | Zmple | Zmle | Zmm | Tmple | Tmle | Tmm |
| $\eta_1^2$ | 0.9680 | 0.9572 | 0.9660 | 0.9612 | 0.9652 | 0.9724 | 0.9584 | 0.9584 | 0.9680 | 0.9648 | 0.9696 | 0.9716 |
| $\eta_2^2$ | 0.9680 | 0.9548 | 0.9660 | 0.9620 | 0.9640 | 0.9724 | 0.9588 | 0.9552 | 0.9680 | 0.9648 | 0.9684 | 0.9716 |
| $\eta_3^2$ | 0.9676 | 0.9544 | 0.9664 | 0.9616 | 0.9640 | 0.9724 | 0.9588 | 0.9544 | 0.9680 | 0.9648 | 0.9684 | 0.9716 |
| $\eta_4^2$ | 0.9680 | 0.9572 | 0.9660 | 0.9612 | 0.9652 | 0.9724 | 0.9584 | 0.9584 | 0.9680 | 0.9648 | 0.9696 | 0.9716 |
| $\eta_5^2$ | 0.9676 | 0.9592 | 0.9656 | 0.9612 | 0.9652 | 0.9728 | 0.9576 | 0.9588 | 0.9680 | 0.9648 | 0.9704 | 0.9716 |

**Table 4.1** (continued)

| $(\lambda_1,\lambda_2)=(5,6)$ | | | | | | | | | | | |
| N5 | | | | | | N6 | | | | | |
| Zmple | Zmle | Zmm | Tmple | Tmle | Tmm | Zmple | Zmle | Zmm | Tmple | Tmle | Tmm |
|---|---|---|---|---|---|---|---|---|---|---|---|
| $\eta_1^2$ 0.9532 | 0.9668 | 0.9680 | 0.9620 | 0.9676 | 0.9724 | 0.9564 | 0.9560 | 0.9668 | 0.9588 | 0.9708 | 0.9692 |
| $\eta_2^2$ 0.9524 | 0.9640 | 0.9680 | 0.9616 | 0.9672 | 0.9724 | 0.9568 | 0.9524 | 0.9664 | 0.9588 | 0.9688 | 0.9692 |
| $\eta_3^2$ 0.9524 | 0.9636 | 0.9680 | 0.9616 | 0.9672 | 0.9728 | 0.9564 | 0.9520 | 0.9668 | 0.9588 | 0.9680 | 0.9692 |
| $\eta_4^2$ 0.9532 | 0.9668 | 0.9680 | 0.9620 | 0.9676 | 0.9724 | 0.9564 | 0.9560 | 0.9668 | 0.9588 | 0.9708 | 0.9692 |
| $\eta_5^2$ 0.9536 | 0.9672 | 0.9676 | 0.9620 | 0.9684 | 0.9720 | 0.9564 | 0.9580 | 0.9672 | 0.9588 | 0.9716 | 0.9692 |

| $(\lambda_1,\lambda_2)=(8,9)$ | | | | | | | | | | | |
| N1 | | | | | | N2 | | | | | |
| Zmple | Zmle | Zmm | Tmple | Tmle | Tmm | Zmple | Zmle | Zmm | Tmple | Tmle | Tmm |
|---|---|---|---|---|---|---|---|---|---|---|---|
| $\eta_1^2$ 0.9548 | 0.9564 | 0.9620 | 0.9736 | 0.9752 | 0.9720 | 0.9680 | 0.9664 | 0.9720 | 0.9724 | 0.9744 | 0.9776 |
| $\eta_2^2$ 0.9548 | 0.9556 | 0.9628 | 0.9736 | 0.9752 | 0.9716 | 0.9684 | 0.9656 | 0.9728 | 0.9724 | 0.9744 | 0.9776 |
| $\eta_3^2$ 0.9548 | 0.9552 | 0.9628 | 0.9736 | 0.9752 | 0.9716 | 0.9684 | 0.9656 | 0.9736 | 0.9724 | 0.9744 | 0.9780 |
| $\eta_4^2$ 0.9548 | 0.9564 | 0.9620 | 0.9736 | 0.9752 | 0.9720 | 0.9680 | 0.9664 | 0.9720 | 0.9724 | 0.9744 | 0.9776 |
| $\eta_5^2$ 0.9548 | 0.9576 | 0.9624 | 0.9736 | 0.9756 | 0.9720 | 0.9680 | 0.9664 | 0.9720 | 0.9724 | 0.9748 | 0.9776 |

| N3 | | | | | | N4 | | | | | |
| Zmple | Zmle | Zmm | Tmple | Tmle | Tmm | Zmple | Zmle | Zmm | Tmple | Tmle | Tmm |
|---|---|---|---|---|---|---|---|---|---|---|---|
| $\eta_1^2$ 0.9764 | 0.9676 | 0.9764 | 0.9668 | 0.9708 | 0.9776 | 0.9716 | 0.9680 | 0.9772 | 0.9704 | 0.9764 | 0.9796 |
| $\eta_2^2$ 0.9764 | 0.9660 | 0.9764 | 0.9672 | 0.9704 | 0.9772 | 0.9720 | 0.9648 | 0.9776 | 0.9700 | 0.9756 | 0.9800 |
| $\eta_3^2$ 0.9764 | 0.9656 | 0.9764 | 0.9672 | 0.9704 | 0.9772 | 0.9716 | 0.9640 | 0.9776 | 0.9700 | 0.9752 | 0.9800 |
| $\eta_4^2$ 0.9764 | 0.9676 | 0.9764 | 0.9668 | 0.9708 | 0.9776 | 0.9716 | 0.9680 | 0.9772 | 0.9704 | 0.9764 | 0.9796 |
| $\eta_5^2$ 0.9760 | 0.9684 | 0.9764 | 0.9668 | 0.9716 | 0.9776 | 0.9704 | 0.9696 | 0.9772 | 0.9704 | 0.9768 | 0.9796 |

| N5 | | | | | | N6 | | | | | |
| Zmple | Zmle | Zmm | Tmple | Tmle | Tmm | Zmple | Zmle | Zmm | Tmple | Tmle | Tmm |
|---|---|---|---|---|---|---|---|---|---|---|---|
| $\eta_1^2$ 0.9692 | 0.9748 | 0.9780 | 0.9704 | 0.9748 | 0.9772 | 0.9692 | 0.9772 | 0.9836 | 0.9684 | 0.9788 | 0.9736 |
| $\eta_2^2$ 0.9696 | 0.9732 | 0.9784 | 0.9700 | 0.9736 | 0.9772 | 0.9656 | 0.9760 | 0.9876 | 0.9680 | 0.9768 | 0.9736 |
| $\eta_3^2$ 0.9696 | 0.9732 | 0.9784 | 0.9704 | 0.9736 | 0.9772 | 0.9656 | 0.9764 | 0.9809 | 0.9680 | 0.9768 | 0.9736 |
| $\eta_4^2$ 0.9692 | 0.9748 | 0.9780 | 0.9704 | 0.9748 | 0.9772 | 0.9692 | 0.9772 | 0.9863 | 0.9684 | 0.9788 | 0.9736 |
| $\eta_5^2$ 0.9696 | 0.9756 | 0.9784 | 0.9704 | 0.9756 | 0.9772 | 0.9700 | 0.9772 | 0.9868 | 0.9684 | 0.9800 | 0.9732 |

*Note:* $\eta_1^2=(0.1^2,1^2)$, $\eta_2^2=(0.3^2,2.5^2)$, $\eta_3^2=(0.5^2,4^2)$, $\eta_4^2=(0.7^2,7^2)$, $\eta_5^2=(0.9^2,10^2)$; $N1=(30,40)$, $N2=(40,60)$, $N3=(60,80)$, $N4=(90,120)$, $N5=(120,150)$, $N6=(150,200)$.

**Table 4.2:** Simulated coverage probabilities of six Bootstrap confidence intervals in three populations.

$(\lambda_1,\lambda_2,\lambda_3)=(3,3,4)$

|  | N1 | | | | | | N2 | | | | | |
|---|---|---|---|---|---|---|---|---|---|---|---|---|
|  | Zmple | Zmle | Zmm | Tmple | Tmle | Tmm | Zmple | Zmle | Zmm | Tmple | Tmle | Tmm |
| $\eta_1^2$ | 0.8655 | 0.8396 | 0.8668 | 0.9330 | 0.9144 | 0.9428 | 0.9085 | 0.8744 | 0.9080 | 0.9580 | 0.9388 | 0.9620 |
| $\eta_2^2$ | 0.8675 | 0.8380 | 0.8668 | 0.9335 | 0.9180 | 0.9424 | 0.9080 | 0.8724 | 0.9076 | 0.9565 | 0.9432 | 0.9608 |
| $\eta_3^2$ | 0.8685 | 0.8348 | 0.8668 | 0.9310 | 0.9216 | 0.9408 | 0.9065 | 0.8708 | 0.9084 | 0.9560 | 0.9480 | 0.9620 |
| $\eta_4^2$ | 0.8690 | 0.8340 | 0.8672 | 0.9320 | 0.9248 | 0.9396 | 0.9080 | 0.8708 | 0.9104 | 0.9550 | 0.9492 | 0.9620 |
| $\eta_5^2$ | 0.8690 | 0.8336 | 0.8676 | 0.9315 | 0.9228 | 0.9412 | 0.9060 | 0.8712 | 0.9088 | 0.9560 | 0.9484 | 0.9620 |

|  | N3 | | | | | | N4 | | | | | |
|---|---|---|---|---|---|---|---|---|---|---|---|---|
|  | Zmple | Zmle | Zmm | Tmple | Tmle | Tmm | Zmple | Zmle | Zmm | Tmple | Tmle | Tmm |
| $\eta_1^2$ | 0.9230 | 0.8804 | 0.9324 | 0.9580 | 0.9320 | 0.9624 | 0.9400 | 0.8988 | 0.9416 | 0.9615 | 0.9336 | 0.9664 |
| $\eta_2^2$ | 0.9205 | 0.8736 | 0.9344 | 0.9570 | 0.9380 | 0.9624 | 0.9415 | 0.8976 | 0.9412 | 0.9605 | 0.9352 | 0.9664 |
| $\eta_3^2$ | 0.9275 | 0.8708 | 0.9340 | 0.9560 | 0.9436 | 0.9624 | 0.9420 | 0.8964 | 0.9420 | 0.9605 | 0.9436 | 0.9676 |
| $\eta_4^2$ | 0.9295 | 0.8696 | 0.9340 | 0.9545 | 0.9464 | 0.9620 | 0.9445 | 0.8944 | 0.9432 | 0.9590 | 0.9484 | 0.9672 |
| $\eta_5^2$ | 0.9275 | 0.8720 | 0.9336 | 0.9560 | 0.9448 | 0.9620 | 0.9435 | 0.8964 | 0.9428 | 0.9605 | 0.9452 | 0.9672 |

|  | N5 | | | | | | N6 | | | | | |
|---|---|---|---|---|---|---|---|---|---|---|---|---|
|  | Zmple | Zmle | Zmm | Tmple | Tmle | Tmm | Zmple | Zmle | Zmm | Tmple | Tmle | Tmm |
| $\eta_1^2$ | 0.9415 | 0.8904 | 0.9448 | 0.9345 | 0.9000 | 0.9456 | 0.9450 | 0.8752 | 0.9420 | 0.9380 | 0.8924 | 0.9448 |
| $\eta_2^2$ | 0.9430 | 0.8844 | 0.9452 | 0.9335 | 0.9088 | 0.9448 | 0.9450 | 0.8684 | 0.9420 | 0.9385 | 0.9016 | 0.9452 |
| $\eta_3^2$ | 0.9450 | 0.8772 | 0.9448 | 0.9335 | 0.9200 | 0.9456 | 0.9465 | 0.8604 | 0.9424 | 0.9400 | 0.9112 | 0.9452 |
| $\eta_4^2$ | 0.9440 | 0.8740 | 0.9448 | 0.9340 | 0.9252 | 0.9452 | 0.9445 | 0.8528 | 0.9424 | 0.9410 | 0.9188 | 0.9448 |
| $\eta_5^2$ | 0.9445 | 0.8768 | 0.9440 | 0.9335 | 0.9228 | 0.9452 | 0.9460 | 0.8588 | 0.9424 | 0.9405 | 0.9136 | 0.9448 |

$(\lambda_1,\lambda_2,\lambda_3)=(5,5,6)$

|  | N1 | | | | | | N2 | | | | | |
|---|---|---|---|---|---|---|---|---|---|---|---|---|
|  | Zmple | Zmle | Zmm | Tmple | Tmle | Tmm | Zmple | Zmle | Zmm | Tmple | Tmle | Tmm |
| $\eta_1^2$ | 0.9410 | 0.9036 | 0.9444 | 0.9595 | 0.9388 | 0.9664 | 0.9550 | 0.9128 | 0.9588 | 0.9670 | 0.9540 | 0.9756 |
| $\eta_2^2$ | 0.9415 | 0.9004 | 0.9440 | 0.9595 | 0.9436 | 0.9664 | 0.9560 | 0.9072 | 0.9596 | 0.9665 | 0.9576 | 0.9756 |
| $\eta_3^2$ | 0.9415 | 0.8936 | 0.9448 | 0.9590 | 0.9476 | 0.9656 | 0.9580 | 0.9016 | 0.9608 | 0.9670 | 0.9616 | 0.9752 |
| $\eta_4^2$ | 0.9395 | 0.8892 | 0.9452 | 0.9580 | 0.9516 | 0.9644 | 0.9565 | 0.8948 | 0.9616 | 0.9670 | 0.9620 | 0.9744 |
| $\eta_5^2$ | 0.9415 | 0.8920 | 0.9444 | 0.9590 | 0.9484 | 0.9652 | 0.9575 | 0.9016 | 0.9612 | 0.9670 | 0.9616 | 0.9752 |

|  | N3 | | | | | | N4 | | | | | |
|---|---|---|---|---|---|---|---|---|---|---|---|---|
|  | Zmple | Zmle | Zmm | Tmple | Tmle | Tmm | Zmple | Zmle | Zmm | Tmple | Tmle | Tmm |
| $\eta_1^2$ | 0.9630 | 0.8964 | 0.9704 | 0.9735 | 0.9432 | 0.9796 | 0.9650 | 0.8976 | 0.9704 | 0.9735 | 0.9444 | 0.9796 |
| $\eta_2^2$ | 0.9635 | 0.8852 | 0.9704 | 0.9725 | 0.9492 | 0.9800 | 0.9655 | 0.8904 | 0.9688 | 0.9740 | 0.9516 | 0.9796 |
| $\eta_3^2$ | 0.9650 | 0.8672 | 0.9704 | 0.9730 | 0.9576 | 0.9804 | 0.9655 | 0.8760 | 0.9696 | 0.9745 | 0.9588 | 0.9792 |
| $\eta_4^2$ | 0.9625 | 0.8608 | 0.9692 | 0.9720 | 0.9620 | 0.9800 | 0.9650 | 0.8660 | 0.9708 | 0.9745 | 0.9628 | 0.9784 |
| $\eta_5^2$ | 0.9645 | 0.8652 | 0.9692 | 0.9730 | 0.9604 | 0.9800 | 0.9650 | 0.8744 | 0.9692 | 0.9745 | 0.9604 | 0.9788 |

**Table 4.2** (continued)

| $(\lambda_1,\lambda_2,\lambda_3)=(5,5,6)$ | | | | | | | | | | | |
| --- | --- | --- | --- | --- | --- | --- | --- | --- | --- | --- | --- |
| N5 | | | | | | N6 | | | | | |
| Zmple | Zmle | Zmm | Tmple | Tmle | Tmm | Zmple | Zmle | Zmm | Tmple | Tmle | Tmm |
| $\eta_1^2$ 0.9665 | 0.8680 | 0.9716 | 0.9520 | 0.9200 | 0.9696 | 0.9595 | 0.8388 | 0.9672 | 0.9595 | 0.9060 | 0.9660 |
| $\eta_2^2$ 0.9650 | 0.8536 | 0.9724 | 0.9510 | 0.9292 | 0.9696 | 0.9595 | 0.8196 | 0.9688 | 0.9585 | 0.9192 | 0.9660 |
| $\eta_3^2$ 0.9650 | 0.8336 | 0.9712 | 0.9515 | 0.9364 | 0.9688 | 0.9620 | 0.7944 | 0.9688 | 0.9585 | 0.9312 | 0.9656 |
| $\eta_4^2$ 0.9660 | 0.8248 | 0.9688 | 0.9520 | 0.9404 | 0.9688 | 0.9625 | 0.7784 | 0.9676 | 0.9585 | 0.9380 | 0.9668 |
| $\eta_5^2$ 0.9655 | 0.8312 | 0.9700 | 0.9520 | 0.9380 | 0.9692 | 0.9620 | 0.7900 | 0.9684 | 0.9585 | 0.9320 | 0.9664 |

| $(\lambda_1,\lambda_2,\lambda_3)=(6,8,9)$ | | | | | | | | | | | |
| --- | --- | --- | --- | --- | --- | --- | --- | --- | --- | --- | --- |
| N1 | | | | | | N2 | | | | | |
| Zmple | Zmle | Zmm | Tmple | Tmle | Tmm | Zmple | Zmle | Zmm | Tmple | Tmle | Tmm |
| $\eta_1^2$ 0.9510 | 0.9116 | 0.9568 | 0.9650 | 0.9484 | 0.9728 | 0.9625 | 0.9184 | 0.9656 | 0.9765 | 0.9620 | 0.9816 |
| $\eta_2^2$ 0.9510 | 0.9104 | 0.9560 | 0.9650 | 0.9524 | 0.9732 | 0.9620 | 0.9108 | 0.9656 | 0.9755 | 0.9628 | 0.9812 |
| $\eta_3^2$ 0.9525 | 0.9016 | 0.9552 | 0.9650 | 0.9572 | 0.9728 | 0.9640 | 0.9060 | 0.9660 | 0.9735 | 0.9660 | 0.9816 |
| $\eta_4^2$ 0.9510 | 0.8952 | 0.9548 | 0.9655 | 0.9612 | 0.9724 | 0.9640 | 0.9000 | 0.9664 | 0.9730 | 0.9684 | 0.9800 |
| $\eta_5^2$ 0.9530 | 0.9008 | 0.9548 | 0.9650 | 0.9588 | 0.9728 | 0.9645 | 0.9048 | 0.9664 | 0.9730 | 0.9660 | 0.9816 |

| N3 | | | | | | N4 | | | | | |
| --- | --- | --- | --- | --- | --- | --- | --- | --- | --- | --- | --- |
| Zmple | Zmle | Zmm | Tmple | Tmle | Tmm | Zmple | Zmle | Zmm | Tmple | Tmle | Tmm |
| $\eta_1^2$ 0.9685 | 0.8964 | 0.9748 | 0.9780 | 0.9568 | 0.9820 | 0.9705 | 0.9036 | 0.9744 | 0.9785 | 0.9560 | 0.9828 |
| $\eta_2^2$ 0.9695 | 0.8868 | 0.9756 | 0.9785 | 0.9604 | 0.9824 | 0.9705 | 0.8928 | 0.9740 | 0.9785 | 0.9616 | 0.9824 |
| $\eta_3^2$ 0.9695 | 0.8660 | 0.9756 | 0.9775 | 0.9672 | 0.9820 | 0.9705 | 0.8744 | 0.9744 | 0.9780 | 0.9664 | 0.9824 |
| $\eta_4^2$ 0.9695 | 0.8560 | 0.9760 | 0.9775 | 0.9704 | 0.9820 | 0.9695 | 0.8652 | 0.9756 | 0.9780 | 0.9704 | 0.9824 |
| $\eta_5^2$ 0.9695 | 0.8644 | 0.9756 | 0.9775 | 0.9668 | 0.9820 | 0.9705 | 0.8728 | 0.9740 | 0.9780 | 0.9672 | 0.9828 |

| N5 | | | | | | N6 | | | | | |
| --- | --- | --- | --- | --- | --- | --- | --- | --- | --- | --- | --- |
| Zmple | Zmle | Zmm | Tmple | Tmle | Tmm | Zmple | Zmle | Zmm | Tmple | Tmle | Tmm |
| $\eta_1^2$ 0.9720 | 0.8676 | 0.9776 | 0.9630 | 0.9324 | 0.9768 | 0.9665 | 0.8388 | 0.9736 | 0.9690 | 0.9224 | 0.9716 |
| $\eta_2^2$ 0.9715 | 0.8516 | 0.9772 | 0.9630 | 0.9372 | 0.9768 | 0.9660 | 0.8068 | 0.9744 | 0.9690 | 0.9320 | 0.9708 |
| $\eta_3^2$ 0.9705 | 0.8300 | 0.9776 | 0.9610 | 0.9468 | 0.9764 | 0.9680 | 0.7800 | 0.9732 | 0.9695 | 0.9428 | 0.9708 |
| $\eta_4^2$ 0.9700 | 0.8156 | 0.9752 | 0.9620 | 0.9520 | 0.9768 | 0.9670 | 0.7604 | 0.9724 | 0.9685 | 0.9492 | 0.9696 |
| $\eta_5^2$ 0.9700 | 0.8272 | 0.9772 | 0.9610 | 0.9476 | 0.9756 | 0.9675 | 0.7748 | 0.9728 | 0.9695 | 0.9452 | 0.9704 |

*Note:* $\eta_1^2=(0.3^2,0.9^2,3^2)$, $\eta_2^2=(0.4^2,1.1^2,4^2)$, $\eta_3^2=(0.5^2,1.2^2,5^2)$, $\eta_4^2=(0.7^2,1.5^2,7^2)$, $\eta_5^2=(0.9^2,2.1^2,9^2)$; $N1=(30,40,40)$, $N2=(40,50,60)$, $N3=(60,80,90)$, $N4=(90,100,120)$, $N5=(120,150,180)$, $N6=(150,200,240)$.

**Table 4.3:** Simulated coverage probabilities of six Bootstrap confidence intervals in five populations.

$(\lambda_1,\lambda_2,\lambda_3,\lambda_4,\lambda_5)=(3,3,4,4,5)$

| | N1 | | | | | | N2 | | | | | |
|---|---|---|---|---|---|---|---|---|---|---|---|---|
| | Zmple | Zmle | Zmm | Tmple | Tmle | Tmm | Zmple | Zmle | Zmm | Tmple | Tmle | Tmm |
| $\eta_1^2$ | 0.8720 | 0.8332 | 0.8700 | 0.9600 | 0.9280 | 0.9596 | 0.9210 | 0.8760 | 0.9220 | 0.9655 | 0.9220 | 0.9664 |
| $\eta_2^2$ | 0.8690 | 0.8368 | 0.8664 | 0.9545 | 0.9144 | 0.9560 | 0.9190 | 0.8836 | 0.9192 | 0.9615 | 0.9148 | 0.9656 |
| $\eta_3^2$ | 0.8670 | 0.8412 | 0.8644 | 0.9500 | 0.9088 | 0.9544 | 0.9165 | 0.8868 | 0.9188 | 0.9635 | 0.9112 | 0.9660 |
| $\eta_4^2$ | 0.8655 | 0.8440 | 0.8632 | 0.9525 | 0.9196 | 0.9552 | 0.9175 | 0.8900 | 0.9168 | 0.9640 | 0.9228 | 0.9648 |
| $\eta_5^2$ | 0.8595 | 0.8504 | 0.8644 | 0.9500 | 0.9280 | 0.9516 | 0.9135 | 0.8948 | 0.9144 | 0.9645 | 0.9224 | 0.9636 |

| | N3 | | | | | | N4 | | | | | |
|---|---|---|---|---|---|---|---|---|---|---|---|---|
| | Zmple | Zmle | Zmm | Tmple | Tmle | Tmm | Zmple | Zmle | Zmm | Tmple | Tmle | Tmm |
| $\eta_1^2$ | 0.9300 | 0.8784 | 0.9352 | 0.9630 | 0.9132 | 0.9728 | 0.9405 | 0.8888 | 0.9400 | 0.9535 | 0.9016 | 0.9608 |
| $\eta_2^2$ | 0.9290 | 0.8896 | 0.9324 | 0.9650 | 0.9056 | 0.9712 | 0.9390 | 0.8988 | 0.9388 | 0.9545 | 0.8796 | 0.9624 |
| $\eta_3^2$ | 0.9270 | 0.8964 | 0.9316 | 0.9655 | 0.8936 | 0.9700 | 0.9395 | 0.9032 | 0.9396 | 0.9625 | 0.8632 | 0.9644 |
| $\eta_4^2$ | 0.9260 | 0.8996 | 0.9316 | 0.9635 | 0.9152 | 0.9704 | 0.9390 | 0.9084 | 0.9376 | 0.9615 | 0.8916 | 0.9648 |
| $\eta_5^2$ | 0.9240 | 0.9096 | 0.9296 | 0.9640 | 0.9164 | 0.9712 | 0.9380 | 0.9164 | 0.9344 | 0.9615 | 0.8964 | 0.9652 |

| | N5 | | | | | | N6 | | | | | |
|---|---|---|---|---|---|---|---|---|---|---|---|---|
| | Zmple | Zmle | Zmm | Tmple | Tmle | Tmm | Zmple | Zmle | Zmm | Tmple | Tmle | Tmm |
| $\eta_1^2$ | 0.9480 | 0.8772 | 0.9444 | 0.9660 | 0.9040 | 0.9672 | 0.9450 | 0.8688 | 0.9380 | 0.9630 | 0.8732 | 0.9640 |
| $\eta_2^2$ | 0.9480 | 0.8844 | 0.9440 | 0.9670 | 0.8788 | 0.9700 | 0.9445 | 0.8780 | 0.9376 | 0.9580 | 0.8484 | 0.9620 |
| $\eta_3^2$ | 0.9455 | 0.8976 | 0.9420 | 0.9680 | 0.8588 | 0.9692 | 0.9420 | 0.8944 | 0.9376 | 0.9565 | 0.8328 | 0.9572 |
| $\eta_4^2$ | 0.9445 | 0.9048 | 0.9416 | 0.9685 | 0.8896 | 0.9692 | 0.9410 | 0.9016 | 0.9364 | 0.9565 | 0.8708 | 0.9580 |
| $\eta_5^2$ | 0.9450 | 0.9152 | 0.9412 | 0.9640 | 0.8928 | 0.9684 | 0.9410 | 0.9096 | 0.9364 | 0.9590 | 0.8816 | 0.9588 |

$(\lambda_1,\lambda_2,\lambda_3,\lambda_4,\lambda_5)=(4,4,5,5,6)$

| | N1 | | | | | | N2 | | | | | |
|---|---|---|---|---|---|---|---|---|---|---|---|---|
| | Zmple | Zmle | Zmm | Tmple | Tmle | Tmm | Zmple | Zmle | Zmm | Tmple | Tmle | Tmm |
| $\eta_1^2$ | 0.9250 | 0.8764 | 0.9248 | 0.9645 | 0.9248 | 0.9668 | 0.9535 | 0.8948 | 0.9568 | 0.9695 | 0.9172 | 0.9740 |
| $\eta_2^2$ | 0.9235 | 0.8808 | 0.9232 | 0.9575 | 0.9096 | 0.9616 | 0.9530 | 0.9016 | 0.9552 | 0.9680 | 0.9088 | 0.9740 |
| $\eta_3^2$ | 0.9220 | 0.8900 | 0.9216 | 0.9565 | 0.9012 | 0.9608 | 0.9505 | 0.9124 | 0.9532 | 0.9710 | 0.9036 | 0.9736 |
| $\eta_4^2$ | 0.9195 | 0.8940 | 0.9212 | 0.9575 | 0.9144 | 0.9604 | 0.9515 | 0.9168 | 0.9516 | 0.9685 | 0.9164 | 0.9720 |
| $\eta_5^2$ | 0.9160 | 0.9016 | 0.9212 | 0.9570 | 0.9188 | 0.9588 | 0.9500 | 0.9252 | 0.9516 | 0.9705 | 0.9188 | 0.9720 |

| | N3 | | | | | | N4 | | | | | |
|---|---|---|---|---|---|---|---|---|---|---|---|---|
| | Zmple | Zmle | Zmm | Tmple | Tmle | Tmm | Zmple | Zmle | Zmm | Tmple | Tmle | Tmm |
| $\eta_1^2$ | 0.9540 | 0.8812 | 0.9608 | 0.9675 | 0.9052 | 0.9756 | 0.9555 | 0.8800 | 0.9596 | 0.9620 | 0.8912 | 0.9720 |
| $\eta_2^2$ | 0.9545 | 0.8968 | 0.9612 | 0.9700 | 0.8960 | 0.9780 | 0.9565 | 0.8924 | 0.9588 | 0.9580 | 0.8700 | 0.9672 |
| $\eta_3^2$ | 0.9525 | 0.9076 | 0.9596 | 0.9710 | 0.8836 | 0.9764 | 0.9545 | 0.9072 | 0.9572 | 0.9645 | 0.8496 | 0.9680 |
| $\eta_4^2$ | 0.9490 | 0.9140 | 0.9568 | 0.9700 | 0.9096 | 0.9772 | 0.9530 | 0.9156 | 0.9568 | 0.9640 | 0.8808 | 0.9704 |
| $\eta_5^2$ | 0.9450 | 0.9288 | 0.9564 | 0.9705 | 0.9076 | 0.9772 | 0.9530 | 0.9272 | 0.9536 | 0.9650 | 0.8880 | 0.9708 |

**Table 4.3** (continued)

| $(\lambda_1,\lambda_2,\lambda_3,\lambda_4,\lambda_5)=(4,4,5,5,6)$ | | | | | | | | | | | |
|---|---|---|---|---|---|---|---|---|---|---|---|
| N5 | | | | | | N6 | | | | | |
| Zmple | Zmle | Zmm | Tmple | Tmle | Tmm | Zmple | Zmle | Zmm | Tmple | Tmle | Tmm |
| $\eta_1^2$ 0.9655 | 0.8628 | 0.9640 | 0.9695 | 0.8952 | 0.9692 | 0.9545 | 0.8284 | 0.9536 | 0.9645 | 0.8544 | 0.9684 |
| $\eta_2^2$ 0.9640 | 0.8712 | 0.9632 | 0.9720 | 0.8648 | 0.9736 | 0.9540 | 0.8524 | 0.9532 | 0.9600 | 0.8264 | 0.9624 |
| $\eta_3^2$ 0.9625 | 0.8948 | 0.9632 | 0.9715 | 0.8472 | 0.9748 | 0.9535 | 0.8780 | 0.9516 | 0.9580 | 0.8032 | 0.9584 |
| $\eta_4^2$ 0.9625 | 0.9080 | 0.9620 | 0.9715 | 0.8752 | 0.9748 | 0.9530 | 0.8892 | 0.9528 | 0.9590 | 0.8532 | 0.9596 |
| $\eta_5^2$ 0.9610 | 0.9256 | 0.9608 | 0.9690 | 0.8792 | 0.9744 | 0.9515 | 0.9064 | 0.9504 | 0.9570 | 0.8632 | 0.9608 |

| $(\lambda_1,\lambda_2,\lambda_3,\lambda_4,\lambda_5)=(7,7,8,8,9)$ | | | | | | | | | | | |
|---|---|---|---|---|---|---|---|---|---|---|---|
| N1 | | | | | | N2 | | | | | |
| Zmple | Zmle | Zmm | Tmple | Tmle | Tmm | Zmple | Zmle | Zmm | Tmple | Tmle | Tmm |
| $\eta_1^2$ 0.9615 | 0.9072 | 0.9656 | 0.9710 | 0.9228 | 0.9756 | 0.9740 | 0.9080 | 0.9764 | 0.9770 | 0.9176 | 0.9808 |
| $\eta_2^2$ 0.9595 | 0.9152 | 0.9644 | 0.9680 | 0.9060 | 0.9712 | 0.9725 | 0.9172 | 0.9760 | 0.9760 | 0.9100 | 0.9804 |
| $\eta_3^2$ 0.9585 | 0.9236 | 0.9616 | 0.9665 | 0.8972 | 0.9684 | 0.9710 | 0.9308 | 0.9752 | 0.9765 | 0.9048 | 0.9800 |
| $\eta_4^2$ 0.9575 | 0.9308 | 0.9624 | 0.9660 | 0.9120 | 0.9692 | 0.9690 | 0.9400 | 0.9732 | 0.9770 | 0.9156 | 0.9800 |
| $\eta_5^2$ 0.9560 | 0.9372 | 0.9620 | 0.9655 | 0.9132 | 0.9700 | 0.9670 | 0.9516 | 0.9716 | 0.9755 | 0.9168 | 0.9792 |

| N3 | | | | | | N4 | | | | | |
|---|---|---|---|---|---|---|---|---|---|---|---|
| Zmple | Zmle | Zmm | Tmple | Tmle | Tmm | Zmple | Zmle | Zmm | Tmple | Tmle | Tmm |
| $\eta_1^2$ 0.9750 | 0.8956 | 0.9800 | 0.9755 | 0.9016 | 0.9820 | 0.9735 | 0.8924 | 0.9764 | 0.9675 | 0.8852 | 0.9780 |
| $\eta_2^2$ 0.9735 | 0.9104 | 0.9792 | 0.9765 | 0.8888 | 0.9828 | 0.9735 | 0.9064 | 0.9768 | 0.9670 | 0.8664 | 0.9792 |
| $\eta_3^2$ 0.9705 | 0.9268 | 0.9796 | 0.9750 | 0.8796 | 0.9820 | 0.9725 | 0.9252 | 0.9756 | 0.9725 | 0.8432 | 0.9780 |
| $\eta_4^2$ 0.9695 | 0.9356 | 0.9800 | 0.9745 | 0.9040 | 0.9816 | 0.9715 | 0.9328 | 0.9740 | 0.9725 | 0.8752 | 0.9788 |
| $\eta_5^2$ 0.9670 | 0.9532 | 0.9780 | 0.9750 | 0.9048 | 0.9816 | 0.9695 | 0.9436 | 0.9732 | 0.9725 | 0.8796 | 0.9808 |

| N5 | | | | | | N6 | | | | | |
|---|---|---|---|---|---|---|---|---|---|---|---|
| Zmple | Zmle | Zmm | Tmple | Tmle | Tmm | Zmple | Zmle | Zmm | Tmple | Tmle | Tmm |
| $\eta_1^2$ 0.9780 | 0.8640 | 0.9800 | 0.9735 | 0.8916 | 0.9748 | 0.9720 | 0.8320 | 0.9764 | 0.9635 | 0.8320 | 0.9732 |
| $\eta_2^2$ 0.9775 | 0.8808 | 0.9800 | 0.9735 | 0.8584 | 0.9768 | 0.9715 | 0.8580 | 0.9756 | 0.9660 | 0.8120 | 0.9696 |
| $\eta_3^2$ 0.9770 | 0.9100 | 0.9792 | 0.9760 | 0.8352 | 0.9800 | 0.9705 | 0.8940 | 0.9748 | 0.9630 | 0.7788 | 0.9680 |
| $\eta_4^2$ 0.9760 | 0.9244 | 0.9792 | 0.9765 | 0.8652 | 0.9812 | 0.9700 | 0.9148 | 0.9736 | 0.9635 | 0.8380 | 0.9692 |
| $\eta_5^2$ 0.9760 | 0.9448 | 0.9776 | 0.9760 | 0.8648 | 0.9800 | 0.9705 | 0.9316 | 0.9728 | 0.9620 | 0.8496 | 0.9692 |

*Note:* $\eta_1^2 = (0.3^2, 0.9^2, 2^2, 3^2, 3^2)$, $\eta_2^2=(0.4^2, 1.2^2, 4^2, 4^2, 5^2)$, $\eta_3^2=(0.5^2, 1.8^2, 6^2, 5^2, 7^2)$, $\eta_4^2=(0.7^2, 3^2, 8^2, 7^2, 9^2)$, $\eta_5^2=(0.9^2, 5.4^2, 10^2, 9^2, 11^2)$; $N1 = (30, 40, 40, 50, 50)$, $N2 = (50, 50, 60, 60, 80)$, $N3 = (70, 70, 90, 90, 100)$, $N4 = (90, 90, 90, 120, 120)$, $N5 = (100, 120, 120, 150, 150)$, $N6 = (150, 150, 200, 200, 200)$.

**Table 4.4:** Simulated expected lengths of six Bootstrap confidence intervals in two populations.

|  | $\eta_1^2$ | $\eta_2^2$ | $\eta_3^2$ | $\eta_4^2$ | $\eta_5^2$ | $\eta_1^2$ | $\eta_2^2$ | $\eta_3^2$ | $\eta_4^2$ | $\eta_5^2$ |
|---|---|---|---|---|---|---|---|---|---|---|
| | | | | | $(\lambda_1,\lambda_2)=(3,4)$ | | | | | |
| | | | N1 | | | | | N2 | | |
| *Zmple* | 0.0411 | 0.1802 | 0.4284 | 0.8817 | 1.3595 | 0.0275 | 0.1553 | 0.4068 | 0.8903 | 1.4416 |
| *Zmle* | 0.0221 | 0.1991 | 0.5529 | 1.0838 | 1.7916 | 0.0201 | 0.1808 | 0.5022 | 0.9845 | 1.6275 |
| *Zmm* | 0.0154 | 0.1384 | 0.3845 | 0.7537 | 1.2460 | 0.0137 | 0.1236 | 0.6729 | 1.1124 | 0.0112 |
| *Tmple* | 1.2987 | 4.9169 | 13.9794 | 36.8349 | 74.1995 | 1.0710 | 4.1442 | 10.8372 | 32.5810 | 61.4367 |
| *Tmle* | 1.0654 | 6.6592 | 17.0478 | 52.2064 | 106.5424 | 0.9018 | 5.6363 | 14.4292 | 44.1873 | 90.1772 |
| *Tmm* | 0.6986 | 4.3665 | 11.1784 | 34.2320 | 69.8603 | 0.5738 | 3.5863 | 9.1810 | 28.1151 | 57.3771 |
| | | | N3 | | | | | N4 | | |
| *Zmple* | 0.0252 | 0.1485 | 0.3626 | 0.5683 | 1.2108 | 0.0383 | 0.1147 | 0.2774 | 0.5835 | 0.8832 |
| *Zmle* | 0.0171 | 0.1539 | 0.4274 | 0.8377 | 1.3848 | 0.0129 | 0.1164 | 0.3235 | 0.6340 | 1.0481 |
| *Zmm* | 0.0112 | 0.1009 | 0.2802 | 0.5493 | 0.9080 | 0.0083 | 0.0746 | 0.2072 | 0.4062 | 0.6715 |
| *Tmple* | 0.8519 | 3.2747 | 9.6313 | 26.9447 | 48.5261 | 0.5550 | 2.5189 | 6.4404 | 21.0352 | 32.1665 |
| *Tmle* | 0.7178 | 4.4861 | 11.4847 | 35.1702 | 71.7750 | 0.5160 | 3.2254 | 8.2571 | 25.2859 | 51.6033 |
| *Tmm* | 0.4647 | 2.9044 | 7.4355 | 22.7699 | 46.4686 | 0.3071 | 1.9195 | 4.9140 | 15.0482 | 30.7102 |
| | | | N5 | | | | | N6 | | |
| *Zmple* | 0.0336 | 0.0935 | 0.2080 | 0.4737 | 0.8088 | 0.0345 | 0.1076 | 0.2012 | 0.3902 | 0.6367 |
| *Zmle* | 0.0110 | 0.0986 | 0.2740 | 0.5371 | 0.8878 | 0.0092 | 0.0826 | 0.2295 | 0.4499 | 0.7437 |
| *Zmm* | 0.0068 | 0.0615 | 0.1708 | 0.3349 | 0.5536 | 0.0056 | 0.0503 | 0.1397 | 0.2739 | 0.4527 |
| *Tmple* | 0.6014 | 1.8589 | 5.7627 | 13.8291 | 27.4740 | 0.4908 | 1.7424 | 5.5726 | 13.5280 | 21.7438 |
| *Tmle* | 0.3940 | 2.4626 | 6.3043 | 19.3065 | 39.4007 | 0.3422 | 2.1391 | 5.4763 | 16.7701 | 34.2241 |
| *Tmm* | 0.2379 | 1.4867 | 3.8061 | 11.6555 | 23.7863 | 0.2053 | 1.2834 | 3.2856 | 10.0614 | 20.5332 |
| | | | | | $(\lambda_1,\lambda_2)=(5,6)$ | | | | | |
| | | | N1 | | | | | N2 | | |
| *Zmple* | 0.0394 | 0.1646 | 0.3848 | 0.7964 | 1.2185 | 0.0255 | 0.1372 | 0.3566 | 0.7917 | 1.2786 |
| *Zmle* | 0.0210 | 0.1887 | 0.5242 | 1.0275 | 1.6985 | 0.0183 | 0.1645 | 0.4568 | 0.8955 | 1.4804 |
| *Zmm* | 0.0138 | 0.1243 | 0.3452 | 0.6766 | 1.1185 | 0.0118 | 0.1064 | 0.2956 | 0.5795 | 0.9579 |
| *Tmple* | 1.2360 | 4.5252 | 12.9767 | 33.7643 | 67.9331 | 0.9932 | 3.6578 | 9.5920 | 28.7679 | 53.6549 |
| *Tmle* | 1.0023 | 6.2645 | 16.0372 | 49.1118 | 100.2271 | 0.8023 | 5.0143 | 12.8368 | 39.3111 | 80.2260 |
| *Tmm* | 0.6375 | 3.9848 | 10.2012 | 31.2397 | 63.7537 | 0.5009 | 3.1310 | 8.0154 | 24.5460 | 50.0932 |
| | | | N3 | | | | | N4 | | |
| *Zmple* | 0.0228 | 0.1275 | 0.3042 | 0.4537 | 1.0214 | 0.0361 | 0.0952 | 0.2233 | 0.4774 | 0.7079 |
| *Zmle* | 0.0143 | 0.1287 | 0.3575 | 0.7008 | 1.1585 | 0.0098 | 0.0879 | 0.2441 | 0.4785 | 0.7911 |
| *Zmm* | 0.0089 | 0.0803 | 0.2231 | 0.4373 | 0.7229 | 0.0061 | 0.0545 | 0.1515 | 0.2969 | 0.4908 |
| *Tmple* | 0.7857 | 2.8605 | 8.5709 | 23.6974 | 41.8990 | 0.5066 | 2.2166 | 5.6665 | 18.6652 | 27.3300 |
| *Tmle* | 0.6215 | 3.8848 | 9.9451 | 30.4554 | 62.1532 | 0.4393 | 2.7457 | 7.0291 | 21.5255 | 43.9289 |
| *Tmm* | 0.3957 | 2.4733 | 6.3316 | 19.3897 | 39.5704 | 0.2632 | 1.6448 | 4.2107 | 12.8946 | 26.3153 |

**Table 4.4** (continued)

| | $(\lambda_1,\lambda_2)=(5,6)$ | | | | | | | | | |
|---|---|---|---|---|---|---|---|---|---|---|
| | N5 | | | | | N6 | | | | |
| | $\eta_1^2$ | $\eta_2^2$ | $\eta_3^2$ | $\eta_4^2$ | $\eta_5^2$ | $\eta_1^2$ | $\eta_2^2$ | $\eta_3^2$ | $\eta_4^2$ | $\eta_5^2$ |
| *Zmple* | 0.0319 | 0.0777 | 0.1642 | 0.3879 | 0.6670 | 0.0331 | 0.0953 | 0.1670 | 0.3232 | 0.5259 |
| *Zmle* | 0.0080 | 0.0724 | 0.2010 | 0.3939 | 0.6512 | 0.0068 | 0.0616 | 0.1712 | 0.3355 | 0.5546 |
| *Zmm* | 0.0049 | 0.0444 | 0.1233 | 0.2416 | 0.3994 | 0.0042 | 0.0375 | 0.1042 | 0.2043 | 0.3377 |
| *Tmple* | 0.5740 | 1.6875 | 5.3241 | 12.4861 | 24.7334 | 0.4703 | 1.6146 | 5.2454 | 12.5257 | 19.6984 |
| *Tmle* | 0.3437 | 2.1483 | 5.4997 | 16.8425 | 34.3722 | 0.3005 | 1.8781 | 4.8079 | 14.7231 | 30.0466 |
| *Tmm* | 0.2114 | 1.3215 | 3.3830 | 10.3598 | 21.1422 | 0.1874 | 1.1713 | 2.9985 | 9.1822 | 18.7387 |

| | $(\lambda_1,\lambda_2)=(8,9)$ | | | | | | | | | |
|---|---|---|---|---|---|---|---|---|---|---|
| | N1 | | | | | N2 | | | | |
| | $\eta_1^2$ | $\eta_2^2$ | $\eta_3^2$ | $\eta_4^2$ | $\eta_5^2$ | $\eta_1^2$ | $\eta_2^2$ | $\eta_3^2$ | $\eta_4^2$ | $\eta_5^2$ |
| *Zmple* | 0.0386 | 0.1578 | 0.3660 | 0.7595 | 1.1574 | 0.0246 | 0.1297 | 0.3357 | 0.7508 | 1.2110 |
| *Zmle* | 0.0204 | 0.1837 | 0.5103 | 1.0002 | 1.6535 | 0.0174 | 0.1563 | 0.4342 | 0.8511 | 1.4069 |
| *Zmm* | 0.0131 | 0.1180 | 0.3279 | 0.6427 | 1.0625 | 0.0109 | 0.0984 | 0.2733 | 0.5357 | 0.8856 |
| *Tmple* | 1.2039 | 4.3248 | 12.4635 | 32.1929 | 64.7261 | 0.9618 | 3.4612 | 9.0888 | 27.2271 | 50.5105 |
| *Tmle* | 0.9676 | 6.0474 | 15.4815 | 47.4100 | 96.7542 | 0.7591 | 4.7443 | 12.1456 | 37.1946 | 75.9066 |
| *Tmm* | 0.6056 | 3.7849 | 9.6895 | 29.6727 | 60.5558 | 0.4681 | 2.9255 | 7.4894 | 22.9350 | 46.8056 |

| | N3 | | | | | N4 | | | | |
|---|---|---|---|---|---|---|---|---|---|---|
| | $\eta_1^2$ | $\eta_2^2$ | $\eta_3^2$ | $\eta_4^2$ | $\eta_5^2$ | $\eta_1^2$ | $\eta_2^2$ | $\eta_3^2$ | $\eta_4^2$ | $\eta_5^2$ |
| *Zmple* | 0.0219 | 0.1190 | 0.2806 | 0.4076 | 0.9453 | 0.0355 | 0.0897 | 0.2080 | 0.4473 | 0.6581 |
| *Zmle* | 0.0131 | 0.1178 | 0.3272 | 0.6413 | 1.0601 | 0.0088 | 0.0788 | 0.2188 | 0.4288 | 0.7089 |
| *Zmm* | 0.0080 | 0.0721 | 0.2004 | 0.3927 | 0.6492 | 0.0054 | 0.0486 | 0.1351 | 0.2648 | 0.4378 |
| *Tmple* | 0.7570 | 2.6816 | 8.1129 | 22.2950 | 39.0370 | 0.4892 | 2.1073 | 5.3869 | 17.8090 | 25.5826 |
| *Tmle* | 0.5777 | 3.6109 | 9.2440 | 28.3083 | 57.7713 | 0.4095 | 2.5595 | 6.5525 | 20.0658 | 40.9500 |
| *Tmm* | 0.3643 | 2.2768 | 5.8287 | 17.8497 | 36.4275 | 0.2485 | 1.5533 | 3.9764 | 12.1772 | 24.8510 |

| | N5 | | | | | N6 | | | | |
|---|---|---|---|---|---|---|---|---|---|---|
| | $\eta_1^2$ | $\eta_2^2$ | $\eta_3^2$ | $\eta_4^2$ | $\eta_5^2$ | $\eta_1^2$ | $\eta_2^2$ | $\eta_3^2$ | $\eta_4^2$ | $\eta_5^2$ |
| *Zmple* | 0.0314 | 0.0738 | 0.1535 | 0.3669 | 0.6322 | 0.0329 | 0.0928 | 0.1599 | 0.3092 | 0.5028 |
| *Zmle* | 0.0072 | 0.0651 | 0.1809 | 0.3546 | 0.5862 | 0.0063 | 0.0564 | 0.1566 | 0.3069 | 0.5073 |
| *Zmm* | 0.0045 | 0.0404 | 0.1123 | 0.2201 | 0.3639 | 0.0039 | 0.0347 | 0.0965 | 0.1891 | 0.3126 |
| *Tmple* | 0.5646 | 1.6289 | 5.1740 | 12.0263 | 23.7951 | 0.4632 | 1.5702 | 5.1318 | 12.1779 | 18.9885 |
| *Tmle* | 0.3261 | 2.0381 | 5.2176 | 15.9787 | 32.6094 | 0.2855 | 1.7846 | 4.5686 | 13.9902 | 28.5507 |
| *Tmm* | 0.2034 | 1.2713 | 3.2545 | 9.9664 | 20.3393 | 0.1814 | 1.1336 | 2.9020 | 8.8866 | 18.1355 |

*Note:* $\eta_1^2=(0.1^2,1^2), \eta_2^2=(0.3^2,2.5^2), \eta_3^2=(0.5^2,4^2), \eta_4^2=(0.7^2,7^2), \eta_5^2=(0.9^2,10^2); N1=(30,40), N2=(40,60), N3=(60,80), N4=(90,120), N5=(120,150), N6=(150,200)$.

**Table 4.5:** Simulated expected lengths of six Bootstrap confidence intervals in three populations.

| $(\lambda_1,\lambda_2,\lambda_3)=(3,3,4)$ | | | | | | | | | |
|---|---|---|---|---|---|---|---|---|---|
| N1 | | | | | N2 | | | | |
| $\eta_1^2$ | $\eta_2^2$ | $\eta_3^2$ | $\eta_4^2$ | $\eta_5^2$ | $\eta_1^2$ | $\eta_2^2$ | $\eta_3^2$ | $\eta_4^2$ | $\eta_5^2$ |
| Zmple 0.1558 | 0.3006 | 0.4433 | 1.0154 | 1.5271 | 0.1325 | 0.2495 | 0.4046 | 0.7806 | 1.3446 |
| Zmle 0.1979 | 0.3512 | 0.5465 | 1.0665 | 1.7688 | 0.1794 | 0.3182 | 0.4949 | 0.9649 | 1.6015 |
| Zmm 0.1365 | 0.2418 | 0.3751 | 0.7290 | 1.2130 | 0.1215 | 0.2154 | 0.3343 | 0.6497 | 1.0812 |
| Tmple 4.3721 | 7.7139 | 13.3325 | 26.7962 | 40.0428 | 3.7023 | 6.4917 | 12.2296 | 24.4722 | 35.8804 |
| Tmle 6.2373 | 11.0764 | 17.2881 | 33.8652 | 56.0040 | 5.2625 | 9.3478 | 14.5935 | 28.5907 | 47.2769 |
| Tmm 4.0877 | 7.2551 | 11.3168 | 22.1617 | 36.6571 | 3.3734 | 5.9910 | 9.3507 | 18.3170 | 30.2912 |
| N3 | | | | | N4 | | | | |
| $\eta_1^2$ | $\eta_2^2$ | $\eta_3^2$ | $\eta_4^2$ | $\eta_5^2$ | $\eta_1^2$ | $\eta_2^2$ | $\eta_3^2$ | $\eta_4^2$ | $\eta_5^2$ |
| Zmple 0.1100 | 0.2372 | 0.3379 | 0.5451 | 1.2405 | 0.0906 | 0.1882 | 0.2753 | 0.5376 | 0.8750 |
| Zmle 0.1527 | 0.2708 | 0.4209 | 0.8201 | 1.3619 | 0.1159 | 0.2057 | 0.3204 | 0.6261 | 1.0374 |
| Zmm 0.0994 | 0.1761 | 0.2729 | 0.5295 | 0.8823 | 0.0733 | 0.1300 | 0.2019 | 0.3929 | 0.6532 |
| Tmple 3.0012 | 4.7556 | 9.1752 | 16.6665 | 25.6048 | 2.3937 | 3.8212 | 6.8204 | 12.8209 | 19.8941 |
| Tmle 3.9181 | 6.9595 | 10.8646 | 21.2852 | 35.1967 | 3.0532 | 5.4245 | 8.4705 | 16.5977 | 27.4422 |
| Tmm 2.4516 | 4.3525 | 6.7914 | 13.3020 | 21.9996 | 1.8877 | 3.3539 | 5.2370 | 10.2607 | 16.9660 |
| N5 | | | | | N6 | | | | |
| $\eta_1^2$ | $\eta_2^2$ | $\eta_3^2$ | $\eta_4^2$ | $\eta_5^2$ | $\eta_1^2$ | $\eta_2^2$ | $\eta_3^2$ | $\eta_4^2$ | $\eta_5^2$ |
| Zmple 0.0770 | 0.1658 | 0.2416 | 0.4589 | 0.8659 | 0.0687 | 0.1298 | 0.1859 | 0.4102 | 0.6102 |
| Zmle 0.0981 | 0.1740 | 0.2708 | 0.5281 | 0.8764 | 0.0822 | 0.1459 | 0.2270 | 0.4424 | 0.7345 |
| Zmm 0.0608 | 0.1077 | 0.1668 | 0.3235 | 0.5392 | 0.0494 | 0.0875 | 0.1356 | 0.2631 | 0.4385 |
| Tmple 1.9892 | 2.8175 | 5.6525 | 10.3481 | 13.4808 | 1.8176 | 2.7334 | 5.1862 | 10.0297 | 14.6270 |
| Tmle 2.3561 | 4.1868 | 6.5386 | 12.8113 | 21.1830 | 2.0390 | 3.6225 | 5.6567 | 11.0841 | 18.3261 |
| Tmm 1.4262 | 2.5327 | 3.9525 | 7.7421 | 12.8039 | 1.2296 | 2.1837 | 3.4092 | 6.6801 | 11.0449 |
| $(\lambda_1,\lambda_2,\lambda_3)=(5,5,6)$ | | | | | | | | | |
| N1 | | | | | N2 | | | | |
| $\eta_1^2$ | $\eta_2^2$ | $\eta_3^2$ | $\eta_4^2$ | $\eta_5^2$ | $\eta_1^2$ | $\eta_2^2$ | $\eta_3^2$ | $\eta_4^2$ | $\eta_5^2$ |
| Zmple 0.1407 | 0.2739 | 0.4017 | 0.9341 | 1.3924 | 0.1151 | 0.2185 | 0.3563 | 0.6866 | 1.1886 |
| Zmle 0.1878 | 0.3332 | 0.5182 | 1.0101 | 1.6771 | 0.1632 | 0.2894 | 0.4498 | 0.8763 | 1.4554 |
| Zmm 0.1222 | 0.2165 | 0.3357 | 0.6519 | 1.0854 | 0.1041 | 0.1845 | 0.2864 | 0.5565 | 0.9262 |
| Tmple 4.0248 | 7.0974 | 12.3715 | 24.9148 | 36.9300 | 3.2368 | 5.6653 | 10.9406 | 21.9479 | 31.7051 |
| Tmle 5.8983 | 10.4754 | 16.3519 | 32.0333 | 52.9723 | 4.6661 | 8.2891 | 12.9415 | 25.3549 | 41.9254 |
| Tmm 3.7440 | 6.6448 | 10.3646 | 20.2967 | 33.5725 | 2.9283 | 5.2006 | 8.1174 | 15.9014 | 26.2962 |
| N3 | | | | | N4 | | | | |
| $\eta_1^2$ | $\eta_2^2$ | $\eta_3^2$ | $\eta_4^2$ | $\eta_5^2$ | $\eta_1^2$ | $\eta_2^2$ | $\eta_3^2$ | $\eta_4^2$ | $\eta_5^2$ |
| Zmple 0.0887 | 0.1993 | 0.2792 | 0.4309 | 1.0506 | 0.0700 | 0.1517 | 0.2185 | 0.4269 | 0.6914 |
| Zmle 0.1279 | 0.2269 | 0.3524 | 0.6860 | 1.1400 | 0.0875 | 0.1552 | 0.2419 | 0.4728 | 0.7832 |
| Zmm 0.0788 | 0.1396 | 0.2163 | 0.4192 | 0.6993 | 0.0532 | 0.0943 | 0.1463 | 0.2844 | 0.4732 |
| Tmple 2.6180 | 4.0753 | 8.1131 | 14.5853 | 22.1638 | 2.1090 | 3.3151 | 6.0298 | 11.2715 | 17.3326 |
| Tmle 3.3553 | 5.9608 | 9.3072 | 18.2361 | 30.1523 | 2.6020 | 4.6228 | 7.2186 | 14.1454 | 23.3868 |
| Tmm 2.0751 | 3.6841 | 5.7488 | 11.2604 | 18.6226 | 1.6216 | 2.8811 | 4.4990 | 8.8144 | 14.5749 |

**Table 4.5** (continued)

| | | | | $(\lambda_1,\lambda_2,\lambda_3)=(5,5,6)$ | | | | | | |
| | | N5 | | | | | N6 | | |
| | $\eta_1^2$ | $\eta_2^2$ | $\eta_3^2$ | $\eta_4^2$ | $\eta_5^2$ | $\eta_1^2$ | $\eta_2^2$ | $\eta_3^2$ | $\eta_4^2$ | $\eta_5^2$ |
|---|---|---|---|---|---|---|---|---|---|---|
| *Zmple* | 0.0593 | 0.1345 | 0.1932 | 0.3651 | 0.7096 | 0.0558 | 0.1069 | 0.1503 | 0.3410 | 0.4951 |
| *Zmle* | 0.0720 | 0.1277 | 0.1988 | 0.3879 | 0.6436 | 0.0614 | 0.1089 | 0.1695 | 0.3304 | 0.5484 |
| *Zmm* | 0.0437 | 0.0774 | 0.1197 | 0.2319 | 0.3869 | 0.0369 | 0.0654 | 0.1013 | 0.1963 | 0.3276 |
| *Tmple* | 1.8513 | 2.5730 | 5.2713 | 9.6019 | 12.2461 | 1.7059 | 2.5355 | 4.8778 | 9.4261 | 13.6283 |
| *Tmle* | 2.0602 | 3.6615 | 5.7193 | 11.2065 | 18.5292 | 1.8071 | 3.2111 | 5.0149 | 9.8271 | 16.2471 |
| *Tmm* | 1.2781 | 2.2697 | 3.5423 | 6.9387 | 11.4749 | 1.1257 | 1.9992 | 3.1219 | 6.1179 | 10.1146 |

| | | | | $(\lambda_1,\lambda_2,\lambda_3)=(6,8,9)$ | | | | | | |
| | | N1 | | | | | N2 | | |
| | $\eta_1^2$ | $\eta_2^2$ | $\eta_3^2$ | $\eta_4^2$ | $\eta_5^2$ | $\eta_1^2$ | $\eta_2^2$ | $\eta_3^2$ | $\eta_4^2$ | $\eta_5^2$ |
|---|---|---|---|---|---|---|---|---|---|---|
| *Zmple* | 0.1374 | 0.2679 | 0.3922 | 0.9154 | 1.3617 | 0.1115 | 0.2122 | 0.3464 | 0.6669 | 1.1564 |
| *Zmle* | 0.1851 | 0.3283 | 0.5104 | 0.9943 | 1.6516 | 0.1595 | 0.2828 | 0.4395 | 0.8558 | 1.4220 |
| *Zmm* | 0.1190 | 0.2107 | 0.3265 | 0.6336 | 1.0557 | 0.1006 | 0.1783 | 0.2767 | 0.5375 | 0.8948 |
| *Tmple* | 3.8328 | 6.7565 | 11.8395 | 23.8733 | 35.2072 | 3.0461 | 5.3267 | 10.4123 | 20.9130 | 29.9936 |
| *Tmle* | 5.6934 | 10.1120 | 15.7855 | 30.9242 | 51.1376 | 4.4063 | 7.8279 | 12.2221 | 23.9460 | 39.5952 |
| *Tmm* | 3.5617 | 6.3209 | 9.8587 | 19.3057 | 31.9339 | 2.7456 | 4.8761 | 7.6110 | 14.9098 | 24.6560 |

| | | N3 | | | | | N4 | | |
| | $\eta_1^2$ | $\eta_2^2$ | $\eta_3^2$ | $\eta_4^2$ | $\eta_5^2$ | $\eta_1^2$ | $\eta_2^2$ | $\eta_3^2$ | $\eta_4^2$ | $\eta_5^2$ |
|---|---|---|---|---|---|---|---|---|---|---|
| *Zmple* | 0.1374 | 0.2679 | 0.3922 | 0.9154 | 1.3617 | 0.1115 | 0.2122 | 0.3464 | 0.6669 | 1.1564 |
| *Zmle* | 0.1851 | 0.3283 | 0.5104 | 0.9943 | 1.6516 | 0.1595 | 0.2828 | 0.4395 | 0.8558 | 1.4220 |
| *Zmm* | 0.1190 | 0.2107 | 0.3265 | 0.6336 | 1.0557 | 0.1006 | 0.1783 | 0.2767 | 0.5375 | 0.8948 |
| *Tmple* | 3.8328 | 6.7565 | 11.8395 | 23.8733 | 35.2072 | 3.0461 | 5.3267 | 10.4123 | 20.9130 | 29.9936 |
| *Tmle* | 5.6934 | 10.1120 | 15.7855 | 30.9242 | 51.1376 | 4.4063 | 7.8279 | 12.2221 | 23.9460 | 39.5952 |
| *Tmm* | 3.5617 | 6.3209 | 9.8587 | 19.3057 | 31.9339 | 2.7456 | 4.8761 | 7.6110 | 14.9098 | 24.6560 |

| | | N5 | | | | | N6 | | |
| | $\eta_1^2$ | $\eta_2^2$ | $\eta_3^2$ | $\eta_4^2$ | $\eta_5^2$ | $\eta_1^2$ | $\eta_2^2$ | $\eta_3^2$ | $\eta_4^2$ | $\eta_5^2$ |
|---|---|---|---|---|---|---|---|---|---|---|
| *Zmple* | 0.0571 | 0.1306 | 0.1871 | 0.3531 | 0.6897 | 0.0543 | 0.1043 | 0.1462 | 0.3329 | 0.4818 |
| *Zmle* | 0.0680 | 0.1207 | 0.1879 | 0.3666 | 0.6083 | 0.0586 | 0.1040 | 0.1618 | 0.3155 | 0.5237 |
| *Zmm* | 0.0415 | 0.0734 | 0.1136 | 0.2198 | 0.3669 | 0.0355 | 0.0630 | 0.0976 | 0.1889 | 0.3154 |
| *Tmple* | 1.8026 | 2.4866 | 5.1367 | 9.3385 | 11.8101 | 1.6661 | 2.4648 | 4.7677 | 9.2105 | 13.2715 |
| *Tmle* | 1.9617 | 3.4866 | 5.4466 | 10.6722 | 17.6458 | 1.7271 | 3.0692 | 4.7936 | 9.3939 | 15.5304 |
| *Tmm* | 1.2330 | 2.1896 | 3.4172 | 6.6937 | 11.0699 | 1.0921 | 1.9394 | 3.0287 | 5.9356 | 9.8127 |

*Note:* $\eta_1^2=(0.3^2, 0.9^2, 3^2)$, $\eta_2^2=(0.4^2, 1.1^2, 4^2)$, $\eta_3^2=(0.5^2, 1.2^2, 5^2)$, $\eta_4^2=(0.7^2, 1.5^2, 7^2)$, $\eta_5^2=(0.9^2, 2.1^2, 9^2)$; $N1=(30, 40, 40), N2=(40, 50, 60), N3=(60, 80, 90), N4=(90, 100, 120), N5=(120, 150, 180), N6=(150, 200, 240)$.

**Table 4.6:** Simulated expected lengths of six Bootstrap confidence intervals in five populations.

$(\lambda_1,\lambda_2,\lambda_3,\lambda_4,\lambda_5)=(3,3,4,4,5)$

| | N1 | | | | | N2 | | | | |
|---|---|---|---|---|---|---|---|---|---|---|
| | $\eta_1^2$ | $\eta_2^2$ | $\eta_3^2$ | $\eta_4^2$ | $\eta_5^2$ | $\eta_1^2$ | $\eta_2^2$ | $\eta_3^2$ | $\eta_4^2$ | $\eta_5^2$ |
| *Zmple* | 0.1557 | 0.2734 | 0.4387 | 1.0438 | 1.4713 | 0.1216 | 0.2131 | 0.3928 | 0.7844 | 1.2714 |
| *Zmle* | 0.1978 | 0.3518 | 0.5513 | 1.0821 | 1.7906 | 0.1617 | 0.2876 | 0.4504 | 0.8838 | 1.4625 |
| *Zmm* | 0.1363 | 0.2424 | 0.3804 | 0.7472 | 1.2372 | 0.1078 | 0.1917 | 0.3005 | 0.5901 | 0.9766 |
| *Tmple* | 3.4939 | 8.2839 | 17.0336 | 29.4770 | 44.0148 | 2.8773 | 6.2643 | 13.6951 | 25.7350 | 37.1142 |
| *Tmle* | 4.6909 | 11.5465 | 22.4545 | 38.7087 | 60.0451 | 3.4579 | 8.7179 | 17.0843 | 29.3646 | 45.4880 |
| *Tmm* | 3.2412 | 7.9518 | 15.4017 | 26.8397 | 41.9806 | 2.3837 | 5.9407 | 11.6810 | 20.3567 | 31.8257 |

| | N3 | | | | | N4 | | | | |
|---|---|---|---|---|---|---|---|---|---|---|
| | $\eta_1^2$ | $\eta_2^2$ | $\eta_3^2$ | $\eta_4^2$ | $\eta_5^2$ | $\eta_1^2$ | $\eta_2^2$ | $\eta_3^2$ | $\eta_4^2$ | $\eta_5^2$ |
| *Zmple* | 0.1027 | 0.2213 | 0.3330 | 0.5100 | 0.9985 | 0.0935 | 0.1706 | 0.2479 | 0.5928 | 0.8089 |
| *Zmle* | 0.1398 | 0.2485 | 0.3895 | 0.7648 | 1.2659 | 0.1159 | 0.2060 | 0.3226 | 0.6331 | 1.0476 |
| *Zmm* | 0.0902 | 0.1604 | 0.2515 | 0.4939 | 0.8175 | 0.0733 | 0.1304 | 0.2044 | 0.4013 | 0.6642 |
| *Tmple* | 2.5296 | 5.2675 | 10.8420 | 21.4102 | 26.7238 | 1.8318 | 4.2271 | 9.5049 | 17.7956 | 22.7187 |
| *Tmle* | 2.8396 | 7.0858 | 13.8792 | 24.0453 | 37.3193 | 2.4289 | 5.9759 | 11.5423 | 20.1387 | 31.3854 |
| *Tmm* | 1.9479 | 4.7783 | 9.3431 | 16.3943 | 25.6653 | 1.6117 | 3.9423 | 7.6441 | 13.4950 | 21.2205 |

| | N5 | | | | | N6 | | | | |
|---|---|---|---|---|---|---|---|---|---|---|
| | $\eta_1^2$ | $\eta_2^2$ | $\eta_3^2$ | $\eta_4^2$ | $\eta_5^2$ | $\eta_1^2$ | $\eta_2^2$ | $\eta_3^2$ | $\eta_4^2$ | $\eta_5^2$ |
| *Zmple* | 0.0822 | 0.1728 | 0.2729 | 0.5130 | 0.7733 | 0.0628 | 0.1143 | 0.1815 | 0.4510 | 0.5895 |
| *Zmle* | 0.1093 | 0.1943 | 0.3044 | 0.5974 | 0.9888 | 0.0822 | 0.1462 | 0.2290 | 0.4493 | 0.7434 |
| *Zmm* | 0.0687 | 0.1221 | 0.1915 | 0.3761 | 0.6224 | 0.0494 | 0.0879 | 0.1378 | 0.2705 | 0.4476 |
| *Tmple* | 1.7325 | 3.6881 | 8.6829 | 16.8130 | 24.5885 | 1.6502 | 3.3868 | 8.1659 | 14.5028 | 16.8295 |
| *Tmle* | 2.0830 | 5.0325 | 9.8244 | 17.2494 | 26.9702 | 1.6998 | 4.1695 | 8.2079 | 14.2889 | 22.2257 |
| *Tmm* | 1.3409 | 3.3183 | 6.4719 | 11.4077 | 17.9168 | 1.0693 | 2.6306 | 5.2124 | 9.0520 | 14.1171 |

$(\lambda_1,\lambda_2,\lambda_3,\lambda_4,\lambda_5)=(4,4,5,5,6)$

| | N1 | | | | | N2 | | | | |
|---|---|---|---|---|---|---|---|---|---|---|
| | $\eta_1^2$ | $\eta_2^2$ | $\eta_3^2$ | $\eta_4^2$ | $\eta_5^2$ | $\eta_1^2$ | $\eta_2^2$ | $\eta_3^2$ | $\eta_4^2$ | $\eta_5^2$ |
| *Zmple* | 0.1462 | 0.2565 | 0.4124 | 0.9921 | 1.3857 | 0.1088 | 0.1904 | 0.3571 | 0.7145 | 1.1556 |
| *Zmle* | 0.1915 | 0.3406 | 0.5337 | 1.0475 | 1.7332 | 0.1479 | 0.2630 | 0.4118 | 0.8081 | 1.3371 |
| *Zmm* | 0.1272 | 0.2263 | 0.3552 | 0.6977 | 1.1552 | 0.0948 | 0.1686 | 0.2644 | 0.5192 | 0.8594 |
| *Tmple* | 3.2911 | 7.8440 | 16.2008 | 27.9733 | 41.6062 | 2.7034 | 5.8552 | 12.8877 | 24.2983 | 34.8158 |
| *Tmle* | 4.4496 | 11.0346 | 21.4728 | 36.9794 | 57.3327 | 3.2557 | 8.2163 | 16.0774 | 27.6426 | 42.8044 |
| *Tmm* | 3.0456 | 7.5213 | 14.5817 | 25.3735 | 39.6393 | 2.2115 | 5.5371 | 10.8849 | 18.9434 | 29.5654 |

| | N3 | | | | | N4 | | | | |
|---|---|---|---|---|---|---|---|---|---|---|
| | $\eta_1^2$ | $\eta_2^2$ | $\eta_3^2$ | $\eta_4^2$ | $\eta_5^2$ | $\eta_1^2$ | $\eta_2^2$ | $\eta_3^2$ | $\eta_4^2$ | $\eta_5^2$ |
| *Zmple* | 0.0880 | 0.1951 | 0.2919 | 0.4294 | 0.8652 | 0.0791 | 0.1449 | 0.2077 | 0.5139 | 0.6784 |
| *Zmle* | 0.1214 | 0.2159 | 0.3383 | 0.6643 | 1.0995 | 0.0964 | 0.1714 | 0.2684 | 0.5266 | 0.8714 |
| *Zmm* | 0.0758 | 0.1348 | 0.2114 | 0.4151 | 0.6871 | 0.0591 | 0.1051 | 0.1648 | 0.3234 | 0.5352 |
| *Tmple* | 2.3754 | 4.9387 | 10.1844 | 20.2033 | 24.7762 | 1.7105 | 3.9676 | 8.9952 | 16.8518 | 21.1760 |

**Table 4.6** (continued)

|  | N3 | | | | | N4 | | | | |
|---|---|---|---|---|---|---|---|---|---|---|
|  | $\eta_1^2$ | $\eta_2^2$ | $\eta_3^2$ | $\eta_4^2$ | $\eta_5^2$ | $\eta_1^2$ | $\eta_2^2$ | $\eta_3^2$ | $\eta_4^2$ | $\eta_5^2$ |
| *Tmle* | 2.6513 | 6.6647 | 13.0444 | 22.5874 | 35.0130 | 2.2721 | 5.6446 | 10.9070 | 19.0010 | 29.5517 |
| *Tmm* | 1.7957 | 4.4483 | 8.6890 | 15.1945 | 23.7310 | 1.4887 | 3.6908 | 7.1541 | 12.5837 | 19.7318 |

|  | N5 | | | | | N6 | | | | |
|---|---|---|---|---|---|---|---|---|---|---|
|  | $\eta_1^2$ | $\eta_2^2$ | $\eta_3^2$ | $\eta_4^2$ | $\eta_5^2$ | $\eta_1^2$ | $\eta_2^2$ | $\eta_3^2$ | $\eta_4^2$ | $\eta_5^2$ |
| *Zmple* | 0.0696 | 0.1504 | 0.2378 | 0.4440 | 0.6591 | 0.0532 | 0.0973 | 0.1548 | 0.3986 | 0.5028 |
| *Zmle* | 0.0912 | 0.1622 | 0.2540 | 0.4984 | 0.8249 | 0.0672 | 0.1195 | 0.1872 | 0.3673 | 0.6077 |
| *Zmm* | 0.0561 | 0.0998 | 0.1565 | 0.3073 | 0.5084 | 0.0400 | 0.0712 | 0.1116 | 0.2191 | 0.3626 |
| *Tmple* | 1.6539 | 3.5044 | 8.3027 | 16.1106 | 23.4391 | 1.6002 | 3.2736 | 7.9416 | 14.0896 | 16.1526 |
| *Tmle* | 1.9649 | 4.7685 | 9.2860 | 16.2937 | 25.4566 | 1.6103 | 3.9771 | 7.8271 | 13.6050 | 21.1227 |
| *Tmm* | 1.2599 | 3.1352 | 6.0901 | 10.7029 | 16.7651 | 1.0197 | 2.5161 | 4.9874 | 8.6378 | 13.4314 |

$(\lambda_1,\lambda_2,\lambda_3,\lambda_4,\lambda_5)=(7,7,8,8,9)$

|  | N1 | | | | | N2 | | | | |
|---|---|---|---|---|---|---|---|---|---|---|
|  | $\eta_1^2$ | $\eta_2^2$ | $\eta_3^2$ | $\eta_4^2$ | $\eta_5^2$ | $\eta_1^2$ | $\eta_2^2$ | $\eta_3^2$ | $\eta_4^2$ | $\eta_5^2$ |
| *Zmple* | 0.1355 | 0.2374 | 0.3824 | 0.9334 | 1.2886 | 0.0949 | 0.1657 | 0.3185 | 0.6387 | 1.0302 |
| *Zmle* | 0.1836 | 0.3266 | 0.5116 | 1.0040 | 1.6610 | 0.1315 | 0.2338 | 0.3661 | 0.7184 | 1.1885 |
| *Zmm* | 0.1170 | 0.2081 | 0.3267 | 0.6417 | 1.0626 | 0.0811 | 0.1442 | 0.2264 | 0.4446 | 0.7359 |
| *Tmple* | 3.0581 | 7.3303 | 15.2237 | 26.2275 | 38.8013 | 2.5129 | 5.4125 | 11.9978 | 22.7218 | 32.3204 |
| *Tmle* | 4.1632 | 10.4187 | 20.2877 | 34.9196 | 54.0965 | 3.0279 | 7.6619 | 14.9555 | 25.7450 | 39.8907 |
| *Tmm* | 2.8178 | 7.0135 | 13.6218 | 23.6569 | 36.9026 | 2.0208 | 5.1002 | 10.0096 | 17.3886 | 27.1060 |

|  | N3 | | | | | N4 | | | | |
|---|---|---|---|---|---|---|---|---|---|---|
|  | $\eta_1^2$ | $\eta_2^2$ | $\eta_3^2$ | $\eta_4^2$ | $\eta_5^2$ | $\eta_1^2$ | $\eta_2^2$ | $\eta_3^2$ | $\eta_4^2$ | $\eta_5^2$ |
| *Zmple* | 0.0747 | 0.1715 | 0.2548 | 0.3566 | 0.7446 | 0.0685 | 0.1260 | 0.1780 | 0.4556 | 0.5819 |
| *Zmle* | 0.1028 | 0.1827 | 0.2864 | 0.5624 | 0.9308 | 0.0801 | 0.1424 | 0.2230 | 0.4376 | 0.7240 |
| *Zmm* | 0.0627 | 0.1114 | 0.1748 | 0.3432 | 0.5684 | 0.0486 | 0.0865 | 0.1356 | 0.2662 | 0.4405 |
| *Tmple* | 2.2214 | 4.6076 | 9.5321 | 18.9937 | 22.8372 | 1.5998 | 3.7212 | 8.5029 | 15.9378 | 19.6857 |
| *Tmle* | 2.4616 | 6.2369 | 12.1893 | 21.1033 | 32.6800 | 2.1215 | 5.3159 | 10.2646 | 17.8566 | 27.7385 |
| *Tmm* | 1.6481 | 4.1287 | 8.0624 | 14.0387 | 21.8718 | 1.3816 | 3.4558 | 6.6820 | 11.7123 | 18.3212 |

|  | N5 | | | | | N6 | | | | |
|---|---|---|---|---|---|---|---|---|---|---|
|  | $\eta_1^2$ | $\eta_2^2$ | $\eta_3^2$ | $\eta_4^2$ | $\eta_5^2$ | $\eta_1^2$ | $\eta_2^2$ | $\eta_3^2$ | $\eta_4^2$ | $\eta_5^2$ |
| *Zmple* | 0.0593 | 0.1321 | 0.2092 | 0.3879 | 0.5663 | 0.0476 | 0.0873 | 0.1391 | 0.3678 | 0.4518 |
| *Zmle* | 0.0757 | 0.1346 | 0.2109 | 0.4137 | 0.6848 | 0.0571 | 0.1015 | 0.1589 | 0.3118 | 0.5158 |
| *Zmm* | 0.0464 | 0.0825 | 0.1294 | 0.2540 | 0.4202 | 0.0347 | 0.0617 | 0.0967 | 0.1899 | 0.3143 |
| *Tmple* | 1.5813 | 3.3250 | 7.9352 | 15.4452 | 22.3662 | 1.5523 | 3.1667 | 7.7241 | 13.7053 | 15.5373 |
| *Tmle* | 1.8492 | 4.5016 | 8.7334 | 15.3345 | 23.9540 | 1.5169 | 3.7736 | 7.4248 | 12.8871 | 19.9767 |
| *Tmm* | 1.1884 | 2.9623 | 5.7341 | 10.0587 | 15.7304 | 0.9747 | 2.4147 | 4.7839 | 8.2708 | 12.8403 |

*Note:* $\eta_1^2 = (0.3^2, 0.9^2, 2^2, 3^2, 3^2)$, $\eta_2^2=(0.4^2, 1.2^2, 4^2, 4^2, 5^2)$, $\eta_3^2=(0.5^2, 1.8^2, 6^2, 5^2, 7^2)$, $\eta_4^2=(0.7^2, 3^2, 8^2, 7^2, 9^2)$, $\eta_5^2=(0.9^2, 5.4^2, 10^2, 9^2, 11^2)$; $N1 = (30, 40, 40, 50, 50)$, $N2 = (50, 50, 60, 60, 80)$, $N3 = (70, 70, 90, 90, 100)$, $N4 = (90, 90, 90, 120, 120)$, $N5 = (100, 120, 120, 150, 150)$, $N6 = (150, 150, 200, 200, 200)$.

## 4.4 Illustrative examples

In this section, to verify the reasonableness and effectiveness of the proposed approaches, the examples of regional GDP of China and bioavailability data are presented.

**Example 4.1** The above approaches are applied to the GDP data of Fujian Province and Hubei Province from 1995 to 2017. As in Figures 4.1 and 4.2, the distributions of the GDPs of Fujian and Hubei don't follow the normal distribution but show asymmetric and right-skewed characteristics. To confirm the conclusion, we first conduct the normality test for these data sets. It turns out that the p-values of the Shapiro-Wilk test, Anderson-Darling test and Kolmogorov-Smirnov test for Fujian's GDP are 0.0046, 0.0031 and 0.0337, and for Hubei's GDP are 0.0021, 0.0010 and 0.0181. Hence, the GDPs of Fujian and Hubei are not normally distributed at the nominal significance level of 5%. In addition, we should prove whether the distributions of the GDPs of Fujian and Hubei Province are skew-normal by the chi-square goodness-of-fit test. By calculation, the fitted value of Fujian is $\chi_f^2 = 3.4012 < \chi_3^2(0.95) = 7.8147$, and the fitted value of Hubei is $\chi_h^2 = 5.5185 < \chi_3^2(0.95) = 7.8147$. Therefore, the GDPs of Fujian and Hubei from 1995 to 2017 follow the skew-normal distributions $SN(\xi_f, \eta_f^2, \lambda_f)$ and $SN(\xi_h, \eta_h^2, \lambda_h)$ respectively at the nominal significance level of 5%.

According to Ye et al. (2022), we consider the hypothesis testing problem

$$H_0 : \xi_f = \xi_h \qquad versus \qquad H_1 : \xi_f \neq \xi_h .$$

The p-value of Bootstrap test statistics is 0.8984. Thus, the null hypothesis $H_0$ can not be rejected at the nominal significance level of 5%, which means that there is no significant difference between the location parameters of the GDPs of Fujian and Hubei from 1995 to 2017. Therefore, the Bootstrap confidence intervals of common location parameter $\xi$ based on $Z_{mple}$, $Z_{mle}$, $Z_{mm}$, $T_{mple}$, $T_{mle}$, and $T_{mm}$ are (-1.5286e+4, 2.3504e+3), (-2.6774e+4, 2.9020e+3), (-1.5336e+4, 2.5805e+3), (-1.4132e+4, 2.5262e+3), (-2.3826e+4, 3.0783e+3), and (-1.4180e+4, 2.7639e+3) respectively. At the same time, we consider the hypothesis testing problem

$$H_0 : \xi = 267 \qquad versus \qquad H_1 : \xi \neq 267 .$$

The p-values of Bootstrap test statistics of $Z_{B1}^*$, $Z_{B2}^*$, $Z_{B3}^*$, $T_{B1}^*$, $T_{B2}^*$ and $T_{B3}^*$ are 0.3006, 0.9176, 0.9247, 0.2676, 0.8982 and 0.9075 respectively, where two Bootstrap test statistics $Z_{B3}^*$ and $T_{B3}^*$ are constructed based on a sample similar to that used to calculate $Z_{B1}^*$ and $T_{B1}^*$. Hence, the null hypothesis $H_0$ can not be rejected at the nominal significance level of 5%, that is, the common location parameter $\xi$ of the GDPs of Fujian and Hubei from 1995 to 2017 is 267.

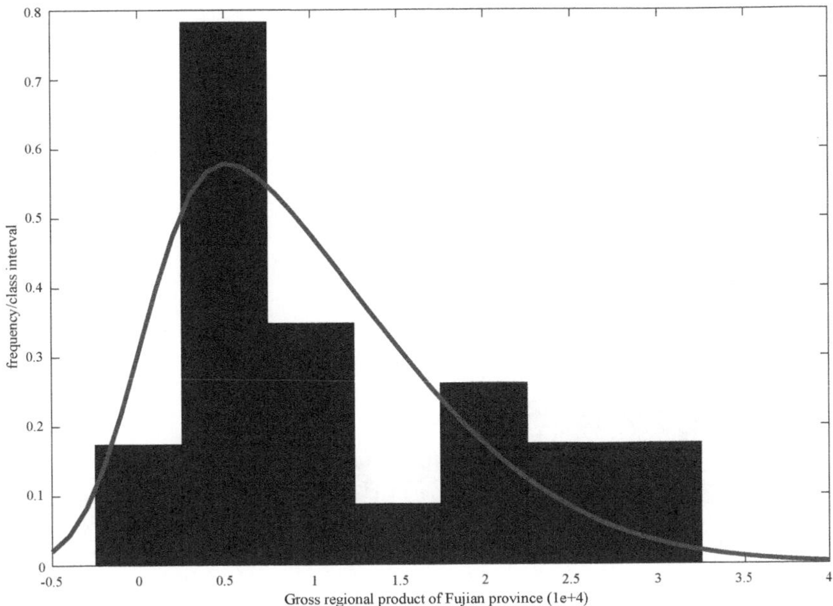


**Figure 4.1:** GDP histogram and probability density curve of Fujian Province (1995–2017).

**Example 4.2** The data of bioavailability is analyzed in this example. Wu et al. (2002) studied the characteristics of the max concentration (Cmax) data of two groups, named X and Y respectively, and considered that the distribution of Cmax data was highly positively skewed. Furthermore, to verify the skew-normality of Cmax data, we intend to test the null hypothesis $H_0$: the Cmax data of X and Y is skew-normally distributed. It can be obtained by calculation that the fitted values of X and Y are $\chi_x^2 = 2.0812 < \chi_1^2(0.95) = 3.8400$, and $\chi_y^2 = 7.6045 < \chi_3^2(0.95) = 7.8147$. Therefore, the Cmax data of X and Y follow the skew-normal distributions $SN(\xi_x, \eta_x^2, \lambda_x)$ and $SN(\xi_y, \eta_y^2, \lambda_y)$ respectively at the nominal significance level of 5% .

Consider the hypothesis testing problem

$$H_0 : \xi_x = \xi_y \qquad versus \qquad H_1 : \xi_x \neq \xi_y \ .$$

The p-value of the Bootstrap test statistics is 0.4606. Therefore, the null hypothesis $H_0$ can not be rejected at the nominal significance level of 5%, which means that there is no significant difference between the location parameters of the Cmax data of X and Y. Similar to Example 4.1, the Bootstrap confidence intervals of common location parameter $\xi$ based on $Z_{mple}$, $Z_{mle}$, $Z_{mm}$, $T_{mple}$, $T_{mle}$, and $T_{mm}$ are (-7.1913e+2, 3.2911e+2), (-1.3289e+3, 2.9597e+2),

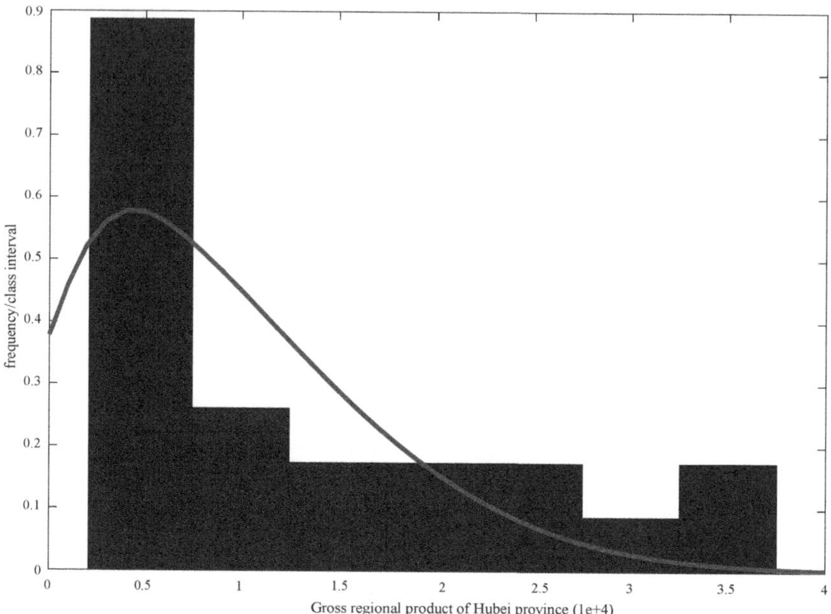


**Figure 4.2:** GDP histogram and probability density curve of Hubei Province (1995–2017).

(-7.1686e+2, 3.2305e+2), (-1.6733e+3, 1.9553e+2), (-2.7322e+3, 1.2537e+2), and (-1.6693e+3, 1.8460e+2) respectively. Further, we consider the hypothesis testing problem

$$H_0 : \xi = 112 \qquad versus \qquad H_1 : \xi \neq 112 .$$

The p-values of the Bootstrap test statistics of $Z_{B1}^*$, $Z_{B2}^*$, $Z_{B3}^*$, $T_{B1}^*$, $T_{B2}^*$ and $T_{B3}^*$ are 0.5519, 0.6428, 0.6181, 0.2501, 0.6922 and 0.6773 respectively. Hence, the null hypothesis $H_0$ can not be rejected at the nominal significance level of 5%, that is, the common location parameter $\xi$ of the Cmax data of X and Y is 112.

# Chapter 5

# One-Way Classification Model with Skew-Normal Random Effects

The one-way classification model with skew-normal random effects is a special skew-normal mixed effects model, which is often used to compare the size of two or more factors. It has been widely used in econometrics, market research, social sciences, among others. Therefore, this chapter considers the one-way classification model with skew-normal random effects given by

$$Y = 1_{ab}\mu + (I_a \otimes 1_b)\varepsilon_1 + \varepsilon_0, \tag{5.1}$$

where $Y$ is a $ab \times 1$ observed variable, $\mu$ is a real number of fixed effect, $\varepsilon_1$ is a $a \times 1$ vector of random effects, and $\varepsilon_0$ is a $ab \times 1$ vector of random errors. $1_m$ is a $m \times 1$ vector with each component equal to 1, $I_m$ is an identity matrix of order m, and $\otimes$ represents the Kronecher product. We assume that $\varepsilon_1 \sim SN_a(0, \sigma_1^2 I_a, \alpha)$, $\varepsilon_0 \sim N_{ab}(0, \sigma_0^2 I_{ab})$, and $\varepsilon_1$ and $\varepsilon_0$ are mutually independent, where $SN_m(\mu_0, \Sigma_0, \alpha_0)$ denotes the $m$-dimensional skew-normal distribution, with location parameter $\mu_0$, scale parameter $\Sigma_0$, and skewness parameter $\alpha_0$. When $\mu_0 = 0$ and covariance matrix $\Sigma_0 = I_m$, $SN_m(\mu_0, \Sigma_0, \alpha_0)$ is reduced to standard skew-normal distribution $SN_m(\alpha_0)$. When $\alpha_0 = 0$, model (5.1) is reduced to the usual normal one-way classification model with random effects.

For convenience, let $M_{n \times k}$ be the set of all $n \times k$ matrices over the real field $R$ and $R^n = M_{n \times 1}$. For any $B \in M_{n \times k}$, use $B'$ to denote the transpose. Let $P_B = B(B'B)^- B'$. For any non-negative definite matrix $T \in M_{n \times n}$ and $m > 0$, we use $rk(T)$ and $tr(T)$ to denote the rank and trace of matrix $T$, respectively, and use $T^m$ and $T^{-m}$ to denote the $m$th non-negative definite roots of $T$ and $T^+$, respectively. Also for $B \in M_{m \times n}$ and $C \in M_{p \times q}$, use $B \otimes C$ to denote the kronecker product of $B$ and $C$. In this chapter, hypothesis testing and interval estimation problems of fixed effect and variance component function are considered for model (5.1). Firstly, the distribution characteristics of model (5.1) are studied, such as moment generation function (MGF), density function, distributions of linear function and quadratic form. Secondly, based on the EM algorithm, we get a maximum likelihood estimate of fixed effect and unbiased estimate of variance component. Thirdly, the Bootstrap test statistic is constructed for the two-sided hypothesis testing problem of fixed effect. Furthermore, the test statistics and confidence intervals of the variance component functions are constructed. On this basis, Monte Carlo simulation results of the fixed effect and variance component functions are given. Finally, the above method is applied to the case analysis of birth rate and leaf area index.

## 5.1 Model properties

For model (5.1), the following theorems are easily obtained. Due to the simple proof process, they are omitted, which can be referred to Ye and Luo (2016).

**Theorem 5.1.** *For the model (5.1), we get,*

*(i) The MGF of Y,*

$$M_Y(t) = 2\exp(t'\mu_y + \frac{t'\Sigma_y t}{2})\Phi\{\frac{\sigma_1 \alpha'(I_a \otimes 1_b')t}{(1+\alpha'\alpha)^{1/2}}\}, t \in R^n, \tag{5.2}$$

*where $\mu_y = 1_{ab}\mu$ and $\Sigma_y = \sigma_0^2 I_n + \sigma_1^2(I_a \otimes (1_b 1_b'))$.*

*(ii) The density function of Y,*

$$f_y(x; \mu_y, \Sigma_y, \alpha_1) = 2\phi_n(x; \mu_y, \Sigma_y)\Phi(\alpha_1'\Sigma_y^{-1/2}(x - \mu_y)), x \in R^n, \tag{5.3}$$

*where $\alpha_1 = \dfrac{\sigma_1 \Sigma_y^{-1/2}(I_a \otimes 1_b)\alpha}{[1+\alpha'(I_a - \sigma_1^2(I_a \otimes 1_b)'\Sigma_y^{-1}(I_a \otimes 1_b))\alpha]^{1/2}}$. We denote $Y \sim SN_n(\mu_y, \Sigma_y, \alpha_1)$.*

*(iii) The mean vector and covariance matrix of Y are*

$$E(Y) = \mu_y + \sqrt{\frac{2}{\pi}}\frac{\Sigma_y^{1/2}\alpha_1}{(1+\alpha_1'\alpha_1)^{1/2}}, Cov(Y) = \Sigma_y^{1/2}\left[I_n - \frac{2\alpha_1\alpha_1'}{\pi(1+\alpha_1'\alpha_1)}\right]\Sigma_y^{1/2}. \tag{5.4}$$

**Theorem 5.2.** *For the model* (5.1), *let* $Y = \mu^* + \Sigma^{1/2}V$, *where* $V \sim SN_n(0, I_n, \alpha)$ *and* $\Sigma$ *is a positive definite matrix. Then* $Y \sim SN_n(\mu^*, \Sigma, \alpha)$.

**Theorem 5.3.** *For the model* (5.1), *let* $Q = Y'AY/\sigma^2$ *with symmetric* $A \in M_{n \times n}$, $m = rk(A)$, *and* $\sigma^2 = \frac{1}{m}\left[\sigma_0^2 tr(A) + \sigma_1^2 tr(A(I_a \otimes (1_b 1_b')))\right]$. *Then the necessary and sufficient conditions under which* $Q \sim S\chi_m^2(\lambda, \delta_1, \delta_2)$, *for some* $\delta_1 \in R$ *including* $\delta_1 = 0$, *are:*

*(i)* $\Omega A$ *is idempotent of rank m,*

*(ii)* $\lambda = \mu_y' A \mu_y / \sigma^2$,

*(iii)* $\delta_1 = \alpha_1' \Omega^{1/2} A \mu_y / (d\sigma)$, *and*

*(iv)* $\delta_2 = \alpha_1' P_1 P_1' \alpha_1 / d^2$,

*where* $\alpha_1 = \dfrac{\sigma_1 \Sigma_y^{-1/2}(I_a \otimes 1_b)\alpha}{\left[1 + \alpha'(I_a - \sigma_1^2(I_a \otimes 1_b)' \Sigma_y^{-1}(I_a \otimes 1_b))\alpha\right]^{1/2}}$, $d = (1 + \alpha' P_2 P_2' \alpha)^{1/2}$, $\mu_y = 1_{ab}\mu$, $\Sigma_y = \sigma_0^2 I_n + \sigma_1^2(I_a \otimes (1_b 1_b')) = \sigma^2 \Omega$, *and* $P = (P_1, P_2)$ *is an orthogonal matrix in* $M_{n \times n}$ *such that*

$$\Omega^{1/2} A \Omega^{1/2} = P \begin{pmatrix} I_m & 0 \\ 0 & 0 \end{pmatrix} P' = P_1 P_1'.$$

*In particular, if either* $\mu_y = 0$ *or* $\alpha_1 = 0$, *then* $Q \sim \chi_m^2(\lambda)$.

**Theorem 5.4.** *For the model* (5.1), *let* $X = 1_{ab}, Z = (I_a \otimes 1_b)$. *We can easily obtain* $P_X ZZ' = ZZ' P_X, ZZ' = bP_Z$. *Then*

*(i)* $Y'(P_{(X:Z)} - P_X)Y/\sigma_2^2 \sim \chi_{n_1}^2$,

*(ii)* $Y'(I_n - P_{(X:Z)})Y/\sigma_0^2 \sim \chi_{n_2}^2$,

*(iii)* $Y'(P_{(X:Z)} - P_X)Y$ *and* $Y'(I_n - P_{(X:Z)})Y$ *are mutually independent,*

*where* $\sigma_2^2 = \sigma_0^2 + b\sigma_1^2, n_1 = rk(X:Z) - rk(X) = a - 1, n_2 = n - rk(X:Z) = a(b - 1), n = ab$.

## 5.2  Parameter estimation

Firstly, model (5.1) is expressed as component form as follows.

$$y_j = \mu_j + 1_b \varepsilon_{1j} + \varepsilon_{0j}, j = 1, 2, \cdots, a, \tag{5.5}$$

where $\mu_j = 1_b \mu$, $\varepsilon_{1j} \sim SN(0, \sigma_1^2, \alpha^*)$ and $\varepsilon_{0j} \sim N_b(0, \sigma_0^2 I_b)$.

By Proposition 2.2 (Ye et al., 2019), we can obtain the following result

$$\varepsilon_{1j} = \sigma_1 \delta t_j + \sigma_1 (1 - \delta^2)^{1/2} X_j,$$

where $\delta = \alpha^*/\sqrt{1+\alpha^*\alpha^*}$, $t_j = |x_j|$, $x_j \sim N(0,1)$, $X_j \sim N(0,1)$, and $t_j$ and $X_j$ are mutually independent. Therefore, the model (5.5) can be expressed as

$$y_j = \mu_j + 1_b\varepsilon_{1j} + \varepsilon_{0j} = \mu_j + 1_b\sigma_1\delta t_j + r_j, \tag{5.6}$$

where $r_j = 1_b\sigma_1(1-\delta^2)^{1/2}X_j + \varepsilon_{0j}$ and $r_j \sim N_b(0, \sigma_0^2 I_b + 1_b 1_b' \sigma_1^2(1-\delta^2))$.

When the EM algorithm is applied, the hidden variable is $t_j$. Let $\Psi = \sigma_0^2 I_b + 1_b 1_b' \sigma_1^2(1-\delta^2)$, we get,

$$y_j|t_j \sim N_b(\mu_j + 1_b\sigma_1\delta t_j, \Psi). \tag{5.7}$$

Let $\theta = (\mu, \sigma_1, \sigma_0)'$, the estimated parameters of the model (5.5) are $\theta$ and $\delta$. By Proposition 2.3 (Ye et al., 2019) and (5.7), it follows that the joint density function of $Y_j$ and $t_j$ are given by

$$\begin{aligned}
f_{y_j,t_j}(y_j',t_j|\theta,\delta) &= 2\phi_b(y_j|\mu_j + 1_b\sigma_1\delta t_j, \Psi)\phi(t_j)\mathrm{II}\{t_j > 0\} \\
&= 2\phi_b(y_j|\mu_j, \sigma_0^2 I_b + \sigma_1^2 1_b 1_b')\phi(t_j|\eta_j, \tau_j^2)\mathrm{II}\{t_j > 0\},
\end{aligned}$$

where $\eta_j = \frac{(1_b\sigma_1\delta)'\Psi^{-1}(y_j-\mu_j)}{1+(1_b\sigma_1\delta)'\Psi^{-1}(1_b\sigma_1\delta)}$, $\tau_j^2 = \frac{1}{1+(1_b\sigma_1\delta)'\Psi^{-1}(1_b\sigma_1\delta)}$, and II is an indicator function.

By the above joint density function, we can find the logarithmic likelihood function involving $Y_j$ and hidden variable $t_j$.

$$l(\theta,\delta) \propto -\frac{1}{2}\sum_{j=1}^{a}\ln|\Psi| - \frac{1}{2}\sum_{j=1}^{a}(y_j-\mu_j)'\Sigma^{-1}(y_j-\mu_j) - \frac{1}{2}\sum_{j=1}^{a}\frac{(t_j-\eta_j)^2}{\tau_j^2}, \tag{5.8}$$

where $\Sigma = \sigma_0^2 I_b + \sigma_1^2 1_b 1_b'$.

At the same time, the conditional density function, first order and second order origin moments of $t_j$ about $y_j$ can be obtained as follows.

$$f_{t_j|y_j}(t_j|y_j) = 2\phi(t_j|\eta_j, \tau_j^2)\mathrm{II}\{t_j > 0\},$$

$$E[t_j|y_j] = \eta_j + \frac{\phi(\eta_j/\tau_j)}{\Phi(\eta_j/\tau_j)}\tau_j, \tag{5.9}$$

$$E[t_j^2|y_j] = \eta_j^2 + \tau_j^2 + \frac{\phi(\eta_j/\tau_j)}{\Phi(\eta_j/\tau_j)}\tau_j\eta_j.$$

Therefore, the EM algorithm can be used to estimate the parameters of model (5.5) as follows.

**E-step**: Given $y_j$ and the parameters of the last iteration $(\hat{\theta}, \hat{\delta})$, using (5.9) we obtain

$$\hat{t}_j = \hat{\eta}_j + \frac{\phi(\hat{\eta}_j/\hat{\tau}_j)}{\Phi(\hat{\eta}_j/\hat{\tau}_j)}\hat{\tau}_j,$$

$$\hat{t}_j^2 = \hat{\eta}_j^2 + \hat{\tau}_j^2 + \frac{\phi(\hat{\eta}_j/\hat{\tau}_j)}{\Phi(\hat{\eta}_j/\hat{\tau}_j)}\hat{\tau}_j\hat{\eta}_j,$$

**M-step**: By maximizing the likelihood function, namly, $\frac{\partial l(\theta,\delta)}{\partial \mu} = 0$, we obtain

$$\hat{\mu} = \left\{\sum_{j=1}^{a} 1_b' \left[\hat{\Sigma}^{-1} + \hat{\tau}_j^2\hat{\Psi}^{-1}1_b\hat{\sigma}_1\hat{\delta}(1_b\hat{\sigma}_1\hat{\delta})'\hat{\Psi}^{-1}\right]1_b\right\}^{-1} \times$$

$$\sum_{j=1}^{a}\left\{1_b'\left[\hat{\Sigma}^{-1} + \hat{\tau}_j^2\hat{\Psi}^{-1}1_b\hat{\sigma}_1\hat{\delta}(1_b\hat{\sigma}_1\hat{\delta})'\hat{\Psi}^{-1}\right]y_j - \hat{t}_j1_b'\hat{\Psi}^{-1}1_b\hat{\sigma}_1\hat{\delta}\right\},$$

where $\hat{\sigma}_1, \hat{\sigma}_0$ and $\hat{\delta}$ are obtained according to the last iteration. Then, the maximum likelihood estimates of $(\theta, \delta)$ can be obtained by substituting $\hat{\mu}$ into $l(\theta, \delta)$ and using the numerical algorithm to maximize it. Given the initial values of the parameters to be estimated, repeat the above two steps until convergence to obtain the maximum likelihood estimates of the parameters.

For the model (5.1), $\varepsilon_1 = (\varepsilon_{11}, \varepsilon_{12}, \cdots, \varepsilon_{1a})' \sim SN_a(0, \sigma_1^2 I_a, \alpha)$. Let $l = (1, 0, \ldots, 0)'$ be a $a \times 1$ vector. Thus, $l'\varepsilon_1 = \varepsilon_{11} \sim SN(0, \sigma_1^2, \alpha^*)$, where

$$\alpha^* = \frac{l'\alpha}{[1 + \alpha'(I_a - l'l)\alpha]^{1/2}}. \tag{5.10}$$

In particular, when all elements of the skewness parameter $\alpha$ in model (5.1) are equal, $\varepsilon_{1j}$ is independently and identically distributed in $SN(0, \sigma_1^2, \alpha^*)$, where $\alpha^*$ is as shown in Equation (5.10).

In addition, according to Theorem 5.4, the unbiased estimators of $\sigma_0^2$ and $\sigma_1^2$ are $\hat{\sigma}_0^2 = T_2/N_2$ and $\hat{\sigma}_1^2 = \frac{T_1/n_1 - T_2/n_2}{b}$, respectively, where $T_1 = Y'(P_{(X:Z)} - P_X)Y$, $T_2 = Y'(I_n - P_{(X:Z)})Y$.

## 5.3    Bootstrap inference of fixed effect

Based on the above parameter estimation method, this section uses the parametric Bootstrap (PB) approach to construct the exact test of fixed effect in model (5.1). First, consider the following hypothesis testing problem:

$$H_0 : \mu = d \quad \text{versus} \quad H_1 : \mu \neq d. \tag{5.11}$$

By Theorem 5.3, we know that

$$Q = \frac{Y'AY}{\sigma^2} \sim S\chi_m^2(\lambda, \delta_1, \delta_2), \tag{5.12}$$

where $A = I_a \otimes (1_b 1_b'/b)$, $\sigma^2 = \sigma_0^2 + b\sigma_1^2$, $\lambda = \mu_y' A \mu_y / \sigma^2$, $\delta_1 = \alpha_1' \Omega^{1/2} A \mu_y / (d\sigma)$, $\delta_2 = \alpha_1' P_1 P_1' \alpha_1 / d^2$. Meanwhile, $\Omega$, $d$, $P_1$ and $\alpha_1$ are defined in Theorem 5.3. In particular, when $d = 0$, $Q$ is degenerated into chi-square distribution, namely,

$$Q = \frac{Y'AY}{\sigma^2} \sim \chi_m^2. \tag{5.13}$$

Define

$$Q^* = \sigma^2 Q = Y'AY \sim \sigma^2 S\chi_m^2(\lambda, \delta_1, \delta_2). \tag{5.14}$$

If $\alpha$, $\sigma_1^2$ and $\sigma_0^2$ are known, then $Q^*$ can be a test statistic for hypothesis testing problem (5.11). Thus the null hypothesis $H_0$ is rejected at significance level $\beta$ whenever

$$Q^* = Y'AY > \sigma^2 S\chi_{m,\beta}^2(\lambda, \delta_1, \delta_2). \tag{5.15}$$

In fact, the skewness parameter $\alpha$ and variance components $\sigma_1^2$ and $\sigma_0^2$ are unknown. In this case, a test statistic can be obtained by replacing $\alpha$, $\sigma_1^2$ and $\sigma_0^2$ with $\hat{\alpha}$, $\hat{\sigma}_1^2$ and $\hat{\sigma}_0^2$ in Section 5.2, and is given by

$$Q^* = Y'AY \sim \hat{\sigma}^2 S\chi_m^2(\hat{\lambda}, \hat{\delta}_1, \hat{\delta}_2). \tag{5.16}$$

The PB approach involves sampling from the estimated model. That is, samples or sample statistics are generated from the model with the parameters replaced by their estimates. Under the null hypothesis $H_0$ in (5.11), we can generate $\widetilde{Q}^*$ as

$$\widetilde{Q}^* \sim \hat{\sigma}^2 S\chi_m^2(\hat{\lambda}, \hat{\delta}_1, \hat{\delta}_2). \tag{5.17}$$

Therefore, for a given significance level $\beta$, the PB test rejects $H_0$ in (5.11) when

$$p = P(\widetilde{Q}^* > Q^* = Y'AY) < \beta. \tag{5.18}$$

For given $\alpha$, $\sigma_1^2$ and $\sigma_0^2$, the above $p$-value does not depend on any unknown parameters. Thus, it can be estimated by Monte Carlo simulation given in Algorithm 5.1.

**Algorithm 5.1** For a given $\alpha$, $\sigma_1^2$ and $\sigma_0^2$ :

Compute $Q^* = Y'AY$

For $k = 1, 2, \cdots, n$

Generate $U \sim SN_m(v, I_m, \alpha)$ and $T = U'U \sim S\chi_m^2(\hat{\lambda}, \hat{\delta}_1, \hat{\delta}_2)$ with $\hat{\lambda} = v'v$, $\hat{\delta}_1 = \alpha'v$ and $\hat{\delta}_2 = \alpha'\alpha$.

Compute $\widetilde{Q}^*$, where $\widetilde{Q}^* = \hat{\sigma}^2 T$

If $\widetilde{Q}^* > Q^*$, set $W_k = 1$

(end loop)

$1/m \sum_{k=1}^{m} W_k$ is an estimate of $p$-value in (5.18) by using Monte Carlo simulation.

## 5.4 Inference on variance component functions

### 5.4.1 Inference on the single variance component

In this section, we employ the Bootstrap approach and generalized approach to test the variance component $\sigma_1^2$ in the model (5.1). We consider the one-sided hypothesis

$$H_0 : \sigma_1^2 \leqslant \delta_0^* \quad versus \quad H_1 : \sigma_1^2 > \delta_0^*, \tag{5.19}$$

where $\delta_0^*$ is a specified value.

#### 5.4.1.1 Bootstrap approach

For hypothesis testing problem (5.19), we first construct the Bootstrap test statistic. It is defined as follows.

$$F_1 = \frac{T_1}{\sigma_0^2 + b\sigma_1^2} \sim \chi_{n_1}^2. \tag{5.20}$$

If $\sigma_0^2$ is known, then $F_1$ in (5.20) serves as the test statistic for the hypothesis testing problem (5.19). However, $\sigma_0^2$ is often unknown in the applications. Therefore, under the null hypothesis $H_0$, $\sigma_0^2$ can be replaced by an unbiased estimator $\hat{\sigma}_0^2$. Then the test statistic is constructed as

$$F_1 = \frac{T_1}{T_2/n_2 + b\delta_0^*}. \tag{5.21}$$

Clearly, the exact distribution of $F_1$ is difficult to obtain, so we can not establish the exact testing method for hypothesis testing problem (5.19). Hence, the Bootstrap approach is used to construct the test statistic. Thus, based on (5.21), the

Bootstrap test statistic has the form

$$F_{1B} = \frac{T_{1B}}{T_{2B}/n_2 + b\delta_0^*},$$ (5.22)

where $T_{1B} \sim (t_2/n_2 + b\delta_0^*)\chi_{n_1}^2$, $T_{2B} \sim (t_2/n_2)\chi_{n_2}^2$, and $t_1$ and $t_2$ are the obversed values of $T_1$ and $T_2$, respectively. Therefore, for hypothesis testing problem (5.19), the Bootstrap p-value is computed by $F_{1B}$ in (5.22) as

$$p_1 = P(F_{1B} > f_1 | H_0),$$ (5.23)

where $f_1$ denotes the observed value of $F_1$ in (5.21). Let $\beta$ be the nominal significance level. If $p_1 \leqslant \beta$, then we reject the null hypothesis $H_0$ at the nominal significance level of $\beta$.

**Remark 5.1.** *When the skewness parameter $\alpha = 0$, the Bootstrap test statistic (5.22) degenerates into the one given by Yang et al. (2012).*

**Remark 5.2.** *Based on $F_{1B}$, we construct the Bootstrap pivot quantity of $\sigma_1^2$, denoted by $\tilde{F}_{1B}$. Let $\tilde{F}_{1B}(\gamma)$ be the $100\gamma$ empirical percentile of $\tilde{F}_{1B}$. Then, the $1 - \beta$ Bootstrap confidence interval for $\sigma_1^2$ is*

$$\left[ \frac{t_1}{b\tilde{F}_{1B}(1-\beta/2)} - \frac{t_2}{bn_2}, \frac{t_1}{b\tilde{F}_{1B}(\beta/2)} - \frac{t_2}{bn_2} \right].$$ (5.24)

### 5.4.1.2 Generalized approach

Let $V_1 = \frac{T_1}{\sigma^2} \sim \chi_{n_1}^2$, $V_2 = \frac{T_2}{\sigma_0^2} \sim \chi_{n_2}^2$. For hypothesis testing problem (5.19), the generalized test variable is

$$F_2 = V_1(1/V_2 + b\sigma_1^2/t_2).$$ (5.25)

It is apparent that the observed value $f_2 = t_1/t_2$ of $F_2$ is free of unknown parameters. And the distribution of $F_2$ is free of nuisance parameters. By (5.25), $F_2$ is stochastically monotonic increasing in $\sigma_1^2$. Namely, $F_2$ is a generalized test variable for hypothesis testing problem (5.19). Based on $F_2$, the generalized $p$-value is given by

$$
\begin{aligned}
p_2 &= P(F_2 \geqslant t_1/t_2 | H_0) = P\left( V_1 \geqslant \frac{t_1}{t_2/V_2 + b\delta_0^*} \right) \\
&= 1 - E_{V_2}\left[ F_{\chi_{n_1}^2}\left( \frac{t_1}{t_2/V_2 + b\delta_0^*} \right) \right],
\end{aligned}
$$ (5.26)

where $F_{\chi_{n_1}^2}$ represents the cumulative distribution function of the $\chi^2$ distribution with $n_1$ degrees of freedom. The expectation in (5.26) is taken with respect to the statistic $V_2$. The null hypothesis $H_0$ will be rejected if $p_3$ is less than the nominal significance level of $\beta$.

**Remark 5.3.** *If the skewness parameter* $\alpha = 0$, *the generalized test variable* (5.25) *degenerates into the one given by Weerahandi (1991).*

*Next, to obtain the generalized confidence interval of* $\sigma_1^2$, *we define*

$$F_2^* = \frac{1}{b}\left[\frac{t_1(\sigma_0^2 + b\sigma_1^2)}{T_1} - \frac{t_2\sigma_0^2}{T_2}\right].$$

*Apparently, the distribution of* $F_2^*$ *is free of any unknown parameters. The observed value of* $F_2^*$ *is* $\sigma_1^2$, *which is free of nuisance parameters. Thus,* $F_2^*$ *is a generalized pivot quantity. By the quantile of* $F_2^*$, *the generalized upper confidence limit and lower confidence limit of* $\sigma_1^2$ *are obtained at the confidence level of* $1 - \beta$, *which are written as* $F_2^*(1 - \beta/2)$ *and* $F_2^*(\beta/2)$ *respectively.*

**Remark 5.4.** *If the skewness parameter* $\alpha = 0$, *the generalized confidence interval* $[F_2^*(\beta/2), F_2^*(1 - \beta/2)]$ *degenerates into the one given by Weerahandi (1993).*

### 5.4.2  Inference on the sum of variance components

In this section, we employ the Bootstrap approach and generalized approach to test sum of variance components $\sigma_1^2 + \sigma_0^2$ in the model (5.1). We consider the one-sided hypothesis

$$H_0 : \sigma_1^2 + \sigma_0^2 \leqslant \delta_1^* \quad versus \quad H_1 : \sigma_1^2 + \sigma_0^2 > \delta_1^*, \tag{5.27}$$

where $\delta_1^*$ is a specified value.

#### 5.4.2.1  Bootstrap approach

For hypothesis testing problem (5.27), we first construct the Bootstrap test statistic. Define

$$F_3 = \frac{T_1}{\sigma_0^2 + b\sigma_1^2} \sim \chi_{n_1}^2. \tag{5.28}$$

If $\sigma_0^2$ is known, then $F_3$ in (5.28) serves as the test statistic for the hypothesis testing problem (5.27). However, $\sigma_0^2$ is often unknown in the applications. Therefore, under the null hypothesis $H_0$, $\sigma_0^2$ can be replaced by an unbiased estimator $\hat{\sigma}_0^2$. Then the test statistic is constructed as

$$F_3 = \frac{T_1}{b\delta_1^* - (b-1)T_2/n_2}. \tag{5.29}$$

Clearly, the exact distribution of $F_3$ is difficult to obtain. Hence, the Bootstrap approach is used to construct the test statistic. Thus, based on (5.29), the Bootstrap test statistic is given by

$$F_{3B} = \frac{T_{1B}}{b\delta_1^* - (b-1)T_{2B}/n_2}, \tag{5.30}$$

where $T_{1B} \sim (b\delta_1^* - (b-1)t_2/n_2)\chi_{n_1}^2$, $T_{2B} \sim (t_2/n_2)\chi_{n_2}^2$. Therefore, for hypothesis testing problem (5.27), the Bootstrap p-value is computed by $F_{3B}$ in (5.30) as

$$p_3 = P(F_{3B} > f_3|H_0), \qquad (5.31)$$

where $f_3$ denotes the observed value of $F_3$ in (5.29). If $p_3 \leqslant \beta$, then we reject the null hypothesis $H_0$ at the nominal significance level of $\beta$.

**Remark 5.5.** *Based on $F_{3B}$, we construct the Bootstrap pivot quantity of $\sigma_1^2 + \sigma_0^2$, denoted by $\tilde{F}_{3B}$. Let $\tilde{F}_{3B}(\gamma)$ be the $100\gamma$ empirical percentile of $\tilde{F}_{3B}$. Then, the $1 - \beta$ Bootstrap confidence interval for $\sigma_1^2 + \sigma_0^2$ is*

$$\left[ \frac{t_1}{b\tilde{F}_{3B}(1 - \beta/2)} + \frac{(b-1)t_2}{bn_2}, \frac{t_1}{b\tilde{F}_{3B}(\beta/2)} + \frac{(b-1)t_2}{bn_2} \right]. \qquad (5.32)$$

### 5.4.2.2  Generalized approach

For hypothesis testing problem (5.27), the generalized test variable is

$$F_4 = \frac{t_1}{bV_1} + \frac{(b-1)t_2}{bV_2} - (\sigma_1^2 + \sigma_0^2). \qquad (5.33)$$

It is apparent that the observed value $f_4 = 0$ for $F_4$ is free of unknown parameters. Since the distributions of $V_1$ and $V_2$ are known, the distribution of $F_4$ is free of nuisance parameters. By (5.33), $F_4$ is stochastically monotonically decreasing in $\sigma_1^2 + \sigma_0^2$. Therefore, $F_4$ is a generalized test variable for the hypothesis testing problem (5.27). Based on $F_4$, the generalized $p$-value is given by

$$p_4 = P(F_4 \leqslant 0|H_0) = 1 - E_{V_2}\left[ F_{\chi_{n_1}^2}\left( \left( \frac{b\delta_1^*}{t_1} - \frac{(b-1)t_2}{V_2 t_1} \right)^{-1} \right) \right]. \qquad (5.34)$$

The null hypothesis $H_0$ will be rejected if $p_4$ is less than the nominal significance level of $\beta$.

To obtain the generalized confidence interval of $\sigma_1^2 + \sigma_0^2$, we define

$$F_4^* = \frac{t_1}{bV_1} + \frac{(b-1)t_2}{bV_2}.$$

Let $F_4^*(\gamma)$ be the $100\gamma$ empirical percentile of $F_4^*$. Then, $[F_4^*(\beta/2), F_4^*(1 - \beta/2)]$ is the $1 - \beta$ generalized confidence interval for $\sigma_1^2 + \sigma_0^2$.

## 5.4.3  Inference on the ratio of variance components

In this section, we consider the one-sided hypothesis

$$H_0 : \sigma_1^2/\sigma_0^2 \leqslant \delta_2^* \quad versus \quad H_1 : \sigma_1^2/\sigma_0^2 > \delta_2^*, \qquad (5.35)$$

where $\delta_2^*$ is a specified value.

### 5.4.3.1 Bootstrap approach

For hypothesis testing problem (5.35), we first construct the Bootstrap test statistic. Define

$$F_5 = \frac{T_1}{\sigma_0^2 + b\sigma_1^2} \sim \chi_{n_1}^2. \tag{5.36}$$

Under the null hypothesis $H_0$, replace $\sigma_0^2$ with $\hat{\sigma}_0^2$. Then we have

$$F_5 = \frac{T_1}{(b\delta_2^* + 1)T_2/n_2}. \tag{5.37}$$

Since it is not easy to get the exact distribution of $F_5$, the Bootstrap approach is employed to set up the test statistic. Thus, based on (5.37), the Bootstrap test statistic is defined as

$$F_{5B} = \frac{T_{1B}}{(b\delta_2^* + 1)T_{2B}/n_2}, \tag{5.38}$$

where $T_{1B} \sim (b\delta_2^* + 1)(t_2/n_2)\chi_{n_1}^2$, $T_{2B} \sim (t_2/n_2)\chi_{n_2}^2$. Therefore, for hypothesis testing problem (5.35), the Bootstrap p-value is computed by $F_{5B}$ in (5.38) as

$$p_5 = P(F_{5B} > f_5 | H_0), \tag{5.39}$$

where $f_5$ denotes the observed value of $F_5$ in (5.37). If $p_5 \leqslant \beta$, then we reject the null hypothesis $H_0$ at the nominal significance level of $\beta$.

**Remark 5.6.** *Based on $F_{5B}$, we construct the Bootstrap pivot quantity of $\sigma_1^2/\sigma_0^2$, denoted by $\tilde{F}_{5B}$. Let $\tilde{F}_{5B}(\gamma)$ be the $100\gamma$ empirical percentile of $\tilde{F}_{5B}$. Then, the $1 - \beta$ Bootstrap confidence interval for $\sigma_1^2/\sigma_0^2$ is*

$$\left[ \frac{t_1 n_2}{b\tilde{F}_{5B}(1 - \beta/2)t_2} - \frac{1}{b}, \frac{t_1 n_2}{b\tilde{F}_{5B}(\beta/2)t_2} - \frac{1}{b} \right]. \tag{5.40}$$

### 5.4.3.2 Generalized approach

For hypothesis testing problem (5.35), the generalized test variable is defined as

$$F_6 = \frac{V_2 t_1}{bV_1 t_2} - \frac{1}{b} - \frac{\sigma_1^2}{\sigma_0^2}. \tag{5.41}$$

Based on $F_6$, the generalized $p$-value is given by

$$p_6 = P(F_6 \leqslant 0 | H_0) = 1 - E_{V_2} \left[ F_{\chi_{n_1}^2} \left( \frac{V_2 t_1}{t_2(b\delta_2^* + 1)} \right) \right]. \tag{5.42}$$

The null hypothesis $H_0$ will be rejected if $p_6$ is less than the nominal significance level of $\beta$.

To obtain the generalized confidence interval of $\sigma_1^2/\sigma_0^2$, we define

$$F_6^* = \frac{V_2 t_1}{b V_1 t_2} - \frac{1}{b},$$

where the observed value of $F_6^*$ is $\sigma_1^2/\sigma_0^2$. Therefore, we can utilize the percentile of $F_6^*$ to construct a generalized confidence interval for $\sigma_1^2/\sigma_0^2$.

**Remark 5.7.** *It is easily proven that (5.39) and (5.42) can be simplified to $P(T_{1B}/T_{2B} > t_1/t_2|H_0)$ and $P(T_1/T_2 > t_1/t_2|H_0)$, respectively. Hence, for hypothesis testing problem (5.35), the Bootstrap approach and generalized approach are nearly equivalent.*

## 5.5  Monte Carlo simulation

By the Monte Carlo Simulation, this section discusses the Type I error probability and power based on the above testing methods, especially whether the Type I error probability can maintain the nominal significance level.

For convenience, here we only provide the algorithm of the Bootstrap approach for hypothesis testing problem (5.19) as follows.

**Step 1:** For a given $(a, b, \sigma_0^2, \sigma_1^2, \delta_0^*)$, generate $t_1 \sim (\sigma_0^2 + b\sigma_1^2)\chi_{n_1}^2$ and $t_2 \sim \sigma_0^2 \chi_{n_2}^2$.

**Step 2:** By (5.21), $f_1$ is computed.

**Step 3:** Generate $T_{1B} \sim (t_2/n_2 + b\delta_0^*)\chi_{n_1}^2$ and $T_{2B} \sim (t_2/n_2)\chi_{n_2}^2$, then compute $F_{1B}$ by (5.22).

**Step 4:** Repeat Step 3 $k_1$ times and compute $p_1$ by (5.23). If $p_1 \leqslant \beta$, then $Q = 1$. Otherwise, $Q = 0$.

**Step 5:** Repeat Steps 1–4 $k_2$ times and get $Q_1, \cdots, Q_{k_2}$. Then the Type I error probability is $\sum_{i=1}^{k_2} Q_i/k_2$.

Based on the above algorithm, the power of hypothesis testing problem (5.19) under $H_1$ can be obtained similarly.

In this simulation, the parameters and sample sizes are set as follows. Firstly, let the nominal significance level $\beta$ be 0.025, 0.05, 0.075, 0.1, and the numbers of inner loops $k_1$ and outer loops $k_2$ both be 2500. For hypothesis testing problem (5.11), let $d = 0$, $a = 3, 4, 5$ and $b = 4, 8$. The random effect $\varepsilon_1$ is randomly generated from the skew-normal distribution with parameters $\sigma_1 = 1, 2, 4$, $\alpha = \alpha_* 1_a$ and $\alpha_* = 1/2, 1, 2$. The error term $\varepsilon_0$ is randomly generated from the normal distribution with parameters $\sigma_0 = 1, 2, 4$.

**Table 5.1:** Type I error probabilities for hypothesis testing problem (5.11).

| $a$ | $b$ | $\sigma_1$ | $\sigma_0$ | $\alpha_*$ | $\beta$ | | | |
|---|---|---|---|---|---|---|---|---|
| | | | | | 0.025 | 0.05 | 0.075 | 0.1 |
| 3 | 4 | 2 | 2 | 1/2 | 0.036 | 0.056 | 0.082 | 0.104 |
| | | | | 1 | 0.042 | 0.068 | 0.086 | 0.102 |
| | | | | 2 | 0.042 | 0.070 | 0.076 | 0.098 |
| 3 | 4 | 2 | 4 | 1/2 | 0.030 | 0.058 | 0.078 | 0.106 |
| | | | | 1 | 0.032 | 0.050 | 0.076 | 0.102 |
| | | | | 2 | 0.028 | 0.052 | 0.070 | 0.086 |
| 3 | 8 | 2 | 4 | 1/2 | 0.034 | 0.054 | 0.078 | 0.104 |
| | | | | 1 | 0.046 | 0.060 | 0.084 | 0.114 |
| | | | | 2 | 0.038 | 0.062 | 0.082 | 0.094 |
| 3 | 8 | 4 | 4 | 1/2 | 0.046 | 0.068 | 0.080 | 0.112 |
| | | | | 1 | 0.032 | 0.050 | 0.072 | 0.084 |
| | | | | 2 | 0.034 | 0.066 | 0.084 | 0.114 |
| 4 | 4 | 2 | 2 | 1/2 | 0.036 | 0.062 | 0.074 | 0.098 |
| | | | | 1 | 0.034 | 0.054 | 0.064 | 0.074 |
| | | | | 2 | 0.028 | 0.046 | 0.076 | 0.086 |
| 4 | 4 | 4 | 2 | 1/2 | 0.032 | 0.058 | 0.078 | 0.092 |
| | | | | 1 | 0.038 | 0.048 | 0.072 | 0.086 |
| | | | | 2 | 0.028 | 0.052 | 0.080 | 0.094 |
| 4 | 8 | 2 | 2 | 1/2 | 0.040 | 0.058 | 0.072 | 0.086 |
| | | | | 1 | 0.032 | 0.050 | 0.068 | 0.082 |
| | | | | 2 | 0.034 | 0.050 | 0.080 | 0.082 |
| 4 | 8 | 4 | 2 | 1/2 | 0.024 | 0.042 | 0.080 | 0.098 |
| | | | | 1 | 0.044 | 0.060 | 0.070 | 0.086 |
| | | | | 2 | 0.034 | 0.052 | 0.088 | 0.098 |
| 5 | 8 | 1 | 1 | 1/2 | 0.024 | 0.048 | 0.066 | 0.088 |
| | | | | 1 | 0.036 | 0.046 | 0.060 | 0.082 |
| | | | | 2 | 0.036 | 0.050 | 0.068 | 0.086 |
| 5 | 8 | 2 | 2 | 1/2 | 0.026 | 0.042 | 0.062 | 0.074 |
| | | | | 1 | 0.026 | 0.046 | 0.060 | 0.072 |
| | | | | 2 | 0.038 | 0.046 | 0.060 | 0.076 |
| 5 | 8 | 2 | 4 | 1/2 | 0.036 | 0.050 | 0.060 | 0.072 |
| | | | | 1 | 0.034 | 0.048 | 0.065 | 0.085 |
| | | | | 2 | 0.038 | 0.046 | 0.060 | 0.080 |
| 5 | 8 | 4 | 4 | 1/2 | 0.038 | 0.058 | 0.078 | 0.098 |
| | | | | 1 | 0.040 | 0.054 | 0.074 | 0.09 |
| | | | | 2 | 0.036 | 0.068 | 0.084 | 0.100 |
| 5 | 4 | 4 | 2 | 1/2 | 0.038 | 0.066 | 0.084 | 0.102 |
| | | | | 1 | 0.042 | 0.068 | 0.082 | 0.112 |
| | | | | 2 | 0.036 | 0.061 | 0.079 | 0.097 |

For hypothesis testing problem (5.19), $(a,b)$ are equal to (5,2), (6,3), (10,4), (15,5), (20,6). Let $\delta_0^* = 1$ and $\sigma_0^2 = 4, 4.5, 5.5, 6.5, 8$. For hypothesis testing problem (5.27), suppose $\delta_1^* = 5$, $\sigma_0^2 = 0.2, 0.4, 1, 1.5, 2.5$, and $(a,b) = (5,2)$, (6,3), (10,4), (15,5), (20,6). For hypothesis testing problem (5.35), let $\delta_2^* = 1$, $\sigma_0^2 = 4, 4.5, 5.5, 6.5, 8$, and $(a,b) = (5,2)$, (6,3), (10,4), (15,5), (20,6).

Under the null hypothesis $H_0$ in (5.11), the simulated Type I error probabilities for the above-mentioned testing methods are shown in Table 5.1. It can be observed from Table 5.1 that the simulated Type I error probabilities are close to the corresponding significance levels across different parameter settings. This indi-

**Table 5.2:** Powers for hypothesis testing problem (5.11) ($\sigma_0 = 2$).

| $a$ | $b$ | $\sigma_1$ | $\alpha_*$ | $\mu$ | $\beta$ | | | |
|---|---|---|---|---|---|---|---|---|
| | | | | | 0.025 | 0.05 | 0.075 | 0.1 |
| 3 | 4 | 1 | 1/3 | 1 | 0.252 | 0.316 | 0.376 | 0.428 |
| | | | | 2 | 0.634 | 0.728 | 0.786 | 0.826 |
| | | | | 3 | 0.912 | 0.946 | 0.960 | 0.984 |
| 3 | 4 | 2 | 1/2 | 1 | 0.248 | 0.304 | 0.338 | 0.394 |
| | | | | 2 | 0.478 | 0.534 | 0.614 | 0.678 |
| | | | | 3 | 0.692 | 0.758 | 0.826 | 0.848 |
| 3 | 4 | 2 | 1 | 1 | 0.236 | 0.286 | 0.352 | 0.384 |
| | | | | 2 | 0.518 | 0.614 | 0.666 | 0.696 |
| | | | | 3 | 0.748 | 0.812 | 0.856 | 0.908 |
| 3 | 8 | 1 | 1/3 | 1 | 0.386 | 0.472 | 0.526 | 0.588 |
| | | | | 2 | 0.794 | 0.858 | 0.912 | 0.932 |
| | | | | 3 | 0.976 | 0.988 | 0.994 | 0.996 |
| 3 | 8 | 2 | 1/2 | 1 | 0.258 | 0.318 | 0.370 | 0.396 |
| | | | | 2 | 0.478 | 0.540 | 0.610 | 0.652 |
| | | | | 3 | 0.764 | 0.826 | 0.862 | 0.888 |
| 3 | 8 | 2 | 1 | 1 | 0.226 | 0.308 | 0.380 | 0.410 |
| | | | | 2 | 0.618 | 0.696 | 0.750 | 0.790 |
| | | | | 3 | 0.832 | 0.886 | 0.936 | 0.958 |
| 4 | 4 | 1 | 1/3 | 1 | 0.256 | 0.342 | 0.400 | 0.450 |
| | | | | 2 | 0.730 | 0.802 | 0.854 | 0.880 |
| | | | | 3 | 0.940 | 0.960 | 0.976 | 0.994 |
| 4 | 4 | 2 | 1 | 1 | 0.172 | 0.220 | 0.292 | 0.336 |
| | | | | 2 | 0.506 | 0.608 | 0.670 | 0.732 |
| | | | | 3 | 0.804 | 0.886 | 0.914 | 0.934 |
| 4 | 8 | 1 | 1/3 | 1 | 0.358 | 0.432 | 0.480 | 0.532 |
| | | | | 2 | 0.854 | 0.904 | 0.932 | 0.954 |
| | | | | 3 | 0.994 | 0.998 | 0.998 | 0.998 |
| 4 | 8 | 2 | 1 | 1 | 0.214 | 0.270 | 0.312 | 0.344 |
| | | | | 2 | 0.546 | 0.634 | 0.736 | 0.794 |
| | | | | 3 | 0.870 | 0.926 | 0.96 | 0.970 |
| 5 | 4 | 2 | 1/2 | 1 | 0.170 | 0.226 | 0.292 | 0.328 |
| | | | | 2 | 0.466 | 0.574 | 0.628 | 0.680 |
| | | | | 3 | 0.792 | 0.856 | 0.906 | 0.924 |
| 5 | 4 | 2 | 1 | 1 | 0.180 | 0.238 | 0.292 | 0.334 |
| | | | | 2 | 0.496 | 0.598 | 0.692 | 0.740 |
| | | | | 3 | 0.852 | 0.914 | 0.948 | 0.968 |
| 5 | 8 | 2 | 1/2 | 1 | 0.192 | 0.262 | 0.324 | 0.364 |
| | | | | 2 | 0.526 | 0.61 | 0.682 | 0.744 |
| | | | | 3 | 0.850 | 0.918 | 0.946 | 0.964 |

cates that the parametric Bootstrap (PB) method can effectively control Type I error probability at various nominal significance levels. Furthermore, under the alternative hypothesis $H_1$ in (5.11), the corresponding powers are obtained through simulation and presented in Table 5.2. It can be observed from Table 5.2 that as the value of $\mu$ deviates from the null hypothesis $H_0$ in (5.11), the power increases rapidly. Meanwhile, when other parameters are the same, the parameter $\alpha_*$ does not significantly affect the power.

**Table 5.3:** Type I error probabilities for two testing methods in (5.19) ($\sigma_1^2 = \delta_0^* = 1$).

| | | | $\beta$ | | | | | | | |
|---|---|---|---|---|---|---|---|---|---|---|
| | | | 0.025 | | 0.05 | | 0.075 | | 0.1 | |
| $a$ | $b$ | $\sigma_0^2$ | PB | GA | PB | GA | PB | GA | PB | GA |
| 5 | 2 | 4 | 0.0420 | 0.0172 | 0.0692 | 0.0368 | 0.0880 | 0.0592 | 0.1128 | 0.0808 |
| | | 4.5 | 0.0448 | 0.0168 | 0.0696 | 0.0380 | 0.0876 | 0.0600 | 0.1172 | 0.0816 |
| | | 5.5 | 0.0468 | 0.0172 | 0.0708 | 0.0400 | 0.0920 | 0.0628 | 0.1176 | 0.0828 |
| | | 6.5 | 0.0472 | 0.0172 | 0.0720 | 0.0404 | 0.0936 | 0.0644 | 0.1232 | 0.0836 |
| | | 8 | 0.0496 | 0.0188 | 0.0732 | 0.0424 | 0.0936 | 0.0656 | 0.1236 | 0.0848 |
| 6 | 3 | 4 | 0.0288 | 0.0216 | 0.0544 | 0.0432 | 0.0792 | 0.0636 | 0.1016 | 0.0900 |
| | | 4.5 | 0.0296 | 0.0216 | 0.0548 | 0.0428 | 0.0800 | 0.0640 | 0.1032 | 0.0892 |
| | | 5.5 | 0.0312 | 0.0216 | 0.0556 | 0.0444 | 0.0816 | 0.0668 | 0.1028 | 0.0904 |
| | | 6.5 | 0.0332 | 0.0216 | 0.0560 | 0.0432 | 0.0824 | 0.0664 | 0.1032 | 0.0900 |
| | | 8 | 0.0340 | 0.0224 | 0.0556 | 0.0440 | 0.0824 | 0.0668 | 0.1036 | 0.0908 |
| 10 | 4 | 4 | 0.0268 | 0.0212 | 0.0504 | 0.0464 | 0.0760 | 0.0708 | 0.1004 | 0.0944 |
| | | 4.5 | 0.0276 | 0.0224 | 0.0500 | 0.0464 | 0.0760 | 0.0708 | 0.1008 | 0.0948 |
| | | 5.5 | 0.0272 | 0.0224 | 0.0500 | 0.0468 | 0.0784 | 0.0704 | 0.0992 | 0.0944 |
| | | 6.5 | 0.0252 | 0.0224 | 0.0508 | 0.0468 | 0.0768 | 0.0708 | 0.1008 | 0.0948 |
| | | 8 | 0.0260 | 0.0232 | 0.0512 | 0.0476 | 0.0772 | 0.0692 | 0.1000 | 0.0952 |
| 15 | 5 | 4 | 0.0256 | 0.0228 | 0.0508 | 0.0476 | 0.0756 | 0.0716 | 0.1016 | 0.0964 |
| | | 4.5 | 0.0260 | 0.0236 | 0.0512 | 0.0476 | 0.0752 | 0.0720 | 0.1016 | 0.0972 |
| | | 5.5 | 0.0252 | 0.0244 | 0.0508 | 0.0476 | 0.0752 | 0.0728 | 0.0996 | 0.0964 |
| | | 6.5 | 0.0252 | 0.0236 | 0.0508 | 0.0460 | 0.0772 | 0.0732 | 0.1000 | 0.0960 |
| | | 8 | 0.0256 | 0.0232 | 0.0504 | 0.0480 | 0.0776 | 0.0728 | 0.1008 | 0.0956 |
| 20 | 6 | 4 | 0.0248 | 0.0232 | 0.0512 | 0.0484 | 0.0752 | 0.0720 | 0.1000 | 0.0968 |
| | | 4.5 | 0.0252 | 0.0240 | 0.0500 | 0.0480 | 0.0752 | 0.0732 | 0.1000 | 0.0972 |
| | | 5.5 | 0.0252 | 0.0240 | 0.0496 | 0.0480 | 0.0748 | 0.0724 | 0.1016 | 0.0976 |
| | | 6.5 | 0.0256 | 0.0248 | 0.0500 | 0.0488 | 0.0752 | 0.0728 | 0.1004 | 0.0980 |
| | | 8 | 0.0260 | 0.0244 | 0.0496 | 0.0488 | 0.0752 | 0.0720 | 0.1004 | 0.0984 |

For hypothesis testing problem (5.19), Tables 5.3–5.4 provide the simulated Type I error probabilities and powers for the PB method and generalized (GA) method at different nominal significance levels. From Table 5.3, it is clear that when the sample size is small, the PB method tends to be slightly liberal, while the GA method is relatively conservative. As the sample size increases, both methods are closer to the nominal significance level $\beta$, but the PB method outperforms the GA method in most cases. Table 5.4 shows that for the specified parameters, sample size, and nominal significance level, the PB method is better than the GA method in the sense of power.

For hypothesis testing problem (5.27), Tables 5.5–5.6 present the simulated Type I error probabilities and powers for the PB method and GA method at different nominal significance levels. From Table 5.5, it can be observed that both PB and GA methods exhibit slightly conservative or liberal behavior for small sample sizes, which becomes more pronounced as $\sigma_0^2$ increases. However, as the sample size increases, both methods can effectively control the Type I error probability, but the PB method outperforms the GA method in most cases. Table 5.6 demonstrates that as $\sigma_0^2 + \sigma_1^2$ deviates from the null hypothesis $H_0$ in (5.11) and the

**Table 5.4:** Powers for two testing methods in (5.19) ($\sigma_0^2 = \delta_0^* = 1$).

| | | | | | | $\beta$ | | | | |
|---|---|---|---|---|---|---|---|---|---|---|
| $a$ | $b$ | $\sigma_1^2$ | 0.025 | | 0.05 | | 0.075 | | 0.1 | |
| | | | PB | GA | PB | GA | PB | GA | PB | GA |
| 5 | 2 | 1.2 | 0.0468 | 0.0228 | 0.0820 | 0.0492 | 0.1144 | 0.0736 | 0.1424 | 0.1032 |
| | | 1.5 | 0.0824 | 0.0404 | 0.1300 | 0.0820 | 0.1676 | 0.1228 | 0.1992 | 0.1552 |
| | | 2 | 0.1468 | 0.0816 | 0.2104 | 0.1516 | 0.2580 | 0.1952 | 0.3036 | 0.2412 |
| | | 2.5 | 0.2168 | 0.1364 | 0.2908 | 0.2156 | 0.3460 | 0.2768 | 0.3944 | 0.3316 |
| | | 5 | 0.5228 | 0.3984 | 0.6040 | 0.5160 | 0.6536 | 0.5844 | 0.6900 | 0.6344 |
| 6 | 3 | 1.2 | 0.0488 | 0.0412 | 0.0852 | 0.0728 | 0.1224 | 0.1092 | 0.1484 | 0.1372 |
| | | 1.5 | 0.1000 | 0.0844 | 0.1480 | 0.1336 | 0.1928 | 0.1724 | 0.2280 | 0.2064 |
| | | 2 | 0.1872 | 0.1688 | 0.2604 | 0.2372 | 0.3112 | 0.2908 | 0.3612 | 0.3404 |
| | | 2.5 | 0.2812 | 0.2624 | 0.3688 | 0.3436 | 0.4416 | 0.4136 | 0.4844 | 0.4684 |
| | | 5 | 0.6552 | 0.6312 | 0.7196 | 0.7032 | 0.7684 | 0.7504 | 0.7928 | 0.7796 |
| 10 | 4 | 1.2 | 0.0596 | 0.0572 | 0.0992 | 0.0976 | 0.1360 | 0.1324 | 0.1728 | 0.1676 |
| | | 1.5 | 0.1340 | 0.1304 | 0.1936 | 0.1908 | 0.2488 | 0.2416 | 0.2896 | 0.2836 |
| | | 2 | 0.2844 | 0.2784 | 0.3784 | 0.3724 | 0.4516 | 0.4440 | 0.5116 | 0.5020 |
| | | 2.5 | 0.4572 | 0.4508 | 0.5564 | 0.5512 | 0.6124 | 0.6056 | 0.6680 | 0.6580 |
| | | 5 | 0.8680 | 0.8628 | 0.9052 | 0.9032 | 0.9244 | 0.9236 | 0.9420 | 0.9384 |
| 15 | 5 | 1.2 | 0.0668 | 0.0656 | 0.1156 | 0.1120 | 0.1604 | 0.1584 | 0.1928 | 0.1896 |
| | | 1.5 | 0.1672 | 0.1672 | 0.2512 | 0.2472 | 0.3172 | 0.3140 | 0.3760 | 0.3708 |
| | | 2 | 0.4060 | 0.4036 | 0.5220 | 0.5172 | 0.5948 | 0.5940 | 0.6440 | 0.6376 |
| | | 2.5 | 0.6184 | 0.6172 | 0.7080 | 0.7040 | 0.7652 | 0.7624 | 0.8016 | 0.8000 |
| | | 5 | 0.9644 | 0.9640 | 0.9788 | 0.9784 | 0.9840 | 0.9840 | 0.9868 | 0.9868 |
| 20 | 6 | 1.2 | 0.0784 | 0.0772 | 0.1316 | 0.1304 | 0.1760 | 0.1748 | 0.2168 | 0.2152 |
| | | 1.5 | 0.2232 | 0.2212 | 0.3132 | 0.3096 | 0.3888 | 0.3860 | 0.4464 | 0.4444 |
| | | 2 | 0.5360 | 0.5328 | 0.6328 | 0.6316 | 0.6996 | 0.6956 | 0.7388 | 0.7388 |
| | | 2.5 | 0.7528 | 0.7512 | 0.8196 | 0.8176 | 0.8620 | 0.8608 | 0.8828 | 0.8824 |
| | | 5 | 0.9900 | 0.9900 | 0.9936 | 0.9936 | 0.9964 | 0.9964 | 0.9968 | 0.9968 |

sample size increases, both PB and GA methods exhibit significant increases in the power, since the latter is better than the former in most cases.

For hypothesis testing problem (5.35), Tables 5.7–5.8 present the simulated Type I error probabilities and powers for the PB and GA methods at different nominal significance levels. From Table 5.7, it can be observed that both PB and GA methods maintain the actual level close to the nominal significance level, regardless of small or large sample sizes. The simulated results of both methods are nearly consistent, which aligns with the conclusions in Remark 5.7. As $\sigma_1^2/\sigma_0^2$ deviates from the null hypothesis $H_0$ in (5.11) and the sample size increases, both methods exhibit significant increases in the power, with satisfactory performance.

**Table 5.5:** Type I error probabilities for two testing methods in (5.27) $(\sigma_1^2 + \sigma_0^2 = \delta_1^* = 5)$.

| | | | $\beta$ | | | | | | | |
|---|---|---|---|---|---|---|---|---|---|---|
| | | | 0.025 | | 0.05 | | 0.075 | | 0.1 | |
| $a$ | $b$ | $\sigma_0^2$ | PB | GA | PB | GA | PB | GA | PB | GA |
| 5 | 2 | 0.2 | 0.0252 | 0.0260 | 0.0496 | 0.0516 | 0.0736 | 0.0768 | 0.1004 | 0.1032 |
| | | 0.4 | 0.0248 | 0.0264 | 0.0504 | 0.0524 | 0.0752 | 0.0788 | 0.0992 | 0.1064 |
| | | 1 | 0.0228 | 0.0292 | 0.0480 | 0.0568 | 0.0724 | 0.0856 | 0.0964 | 0.1164 |
| | | 1.5 | 0.0188 | 0.0316 | 0.0436 | 0.0604 | 0.0676 | 0.0936 | 0.0924 | 0.1216 |
| | | 2.5 | 0.0136 | 0.0372 | 0.0360 | 0.0672 | 0.0632 | 0.1032 | 0.0928 | 0.1348 |
| 6 | 3 | 0.2 | 0.0244 | 0.0256 | 0.0492 | 0.0516 | 0.0748 | 0.0756 | 0.0996 | 0.1008 |
| | | 0.4 | 0.0248 | 0.0260 | 0.0496 | 0.0524 | 0.0740 | 0.0792 | 0.0992 | 0.1052 |
| | | 1 | 0.0232 | 0.0300 | 0.0488 | 0.0544 | 0.0736 | 0.0836 | 0.0984 | 0.1088 |
| | | 1.5 | 0.0212 | 0.0300 | 0.0464 | 0.0604 | 0.0688 | 0.0872 | 0.0940 | 0.1156 |
| | | 2.5 | 0.0108 | 0.0352 | 0.0288 | 0.0660 | 0.0600 | 0.0976 | 0.0828 | 0.1276 |
| 10 | 4 | 0.2 | 0.0248 | 0.0252 | 0.0496 | 0.0500 | 0.0748 | 0.0752 | 0.0996 | 0.1004 |
| | | 0.4 | 0.0248 | 0.0252 | 0.0496 | 0.0508 | 0.0748 | 0.0764 | 0.0992 | 0.1024 |
| | | 1 | 0.0248 | 0.0276 | 0.0492 | 0.0540 | 0.0732 | 0.0812 | 0.0984 | 0.1060 |
| | | 1.5 | 0.0240 | 0.0280 | 0.0456 | 0.0548 | 0.0736 | 0.0832 | 0.0980 | 0.1108 |
| | | 2.5 | 0.0128 | 0.0332 | 0.0336 | 0.0612 | 0.0548 | 0.0908 | 0.0844 | 0.1208 |
| 15 | 5 | 0.2 | 0.0248 | 0.0252 | 0.0496 | 0.0500 | 0.0748 | 0.0752 | 0.0996 | 0.0996 |
| | | 0.4 | 0.0248 | 0.0252 | 0.0496 | 0.0504 | 0.0748 | 0.0760 | 0.0996 | 0.1016 |
| | | 1 | 0.0248 | 0.0276 | 0.0500 | 0.0516 | 0.0760 | 0.0772 | 0.0988 | 0.1036 |
| | | 1.5 | 0.0244 | 0.0268 | 0.0484 | 0.0548 | 0.0736 | 0.0804 | 0.0996 | 0.1060 |
| | | 2.5 | 0.0184 | 0.0300 | 0.0408 | 0.0592 | 0.0632 | 0.0876 | 0.0904 | 0.1168 |
| 20 | 6 | 0.2 | 0.0248 | 0.0248 | 0.0496 | 0.0496 | 0.0748 | 0.0748 | 0.0996 | 0.1000 |
| | | 0.4 | 0.0248 | 0.0252 | 0.0496 | 0.0496 | 0.0748 | 0.0764 | 0.0996 | 0.1004 |
| | | 1 | 0.0252 | 0.0272 | 0.0496 | 0.0512 | 0.0748 | 0.0768 | 0.1000 | 0.1036 |
| | | 1.5 | 0.0248 | 0.0256 | 0.0500 | 0.0540 | 0.0744 | 0.0784 | 0.0992 | 0.1052 |
| | | 2.5 | 0.0188 | 0.0284 | 0.0460 | 0.0568 | 0.0676 | 0.0852 | 0.0948 | 0.1148 |

# 5.6 Illustrative examples

**Example 5.1** The data set used in this study is derived from the leaf area index of artificially planted Robinia pseudoacacia in Huaiping Forest Farm, Yongshou County, Shaanxi Province. The relevant data, including the leaf area index, can be found in Ye et al. (2019). From Figure 5.1, it is evident that the leaf area index data exhibits skewness. For testing the normality of the data, the p-values for Shapiro-Wilk test, Kolmogorov-Smirnov test and Cramer-von Mises are 0.0007, 0.0463 and 0.0098, respectively. Thus, at a 5% nominal significance level, the leaf area index does not follow a normal distribution. To further investigate its distribution, we assume $H_0$ as, leaf area index follows a skew-normal distribution. Through calculations, the chi-square goodness-of-fit test statistic is $\chi^2 = 5.0929 < \chi_2^2(0.95) = 5.9915$. Therefore, at a 5% nominal significance level, the null hypothesis $H_0$ cannot be rejected, indicating that the leaf area index follows a skew-normal distribution. Based on the method of moment estimation, the the leaf area index is approximately distributed as $SN(1.2730, 3.3060, 2.7411)$ and its density curve is given in Figure 5.1.

**Table 5.6:** Powers for two testing methods in (5.27) ($\sigma_0^2 = 2, \delta_1^* = 5$).

| $a$ | $b$ | $\sigma_1^2$ | $\beta$ | | | | | | | |
|---|---|---|---|---|---|---|---|---|---|---|
| | | | 0.025 | | 0.05 | | 0.075 | | 0.1 | |
| | | | PB | GA | PB | GA | PB | GA | PB | GA |
| 5 | 2 | 4.5 | 0.0552 | 0.0976 | 0.1104 | 0.1556 | 0.1652 | 0.2108 | 0.2048 | 0.2556 |
| | | 5 | 0.0724 | 0.1232 | 0.1396 | 0.1924 | 0.1952 | 0.2484 | 0.2384 | 0.2944 |
| | | 6 | 0.1204 | 0.1808 | 0.1960 | 0.2580 | 0.2704 | 0.3284 | 0.3156 | 0.3780 |
| | | 10 | 0.3056 | 0.3968 | 0.4216 | 0.4868 | 0.5028 | 0.5612 | 0.5584 | 0.6064 |
| | | 15 | 0.5160 | 0.5912 | 0.6176 | 0.6700 | 0.6848 | 0.7224 | 0.7188 | 0.7568 |
| 6 | 3 | 4.5 | 0.0676 | 0.1140 | 0.1284 | 0.1748 | 0.1828 | 0.2288 | 0.2276 | 0.2796 |
| | | 5 | 0.0952 | 0.1464 | 0.1652 | 0.2144 | 0.2240 | 0.2804 | 0.2812 | 0.3356 |
| | | 6 | 0.1568 | 0.2172 | 0.2428 | 0.3092 | 0.3184 | 0.3796 | 0.3708 | 0.4268 |
| | | 10 | 0.4092 | 0.4884 | 0.5176 | 0.5788 | 0.5948 | 0.6440 | 0.6448 | 0.6848 |
| | | 15 | 0.6328 | 0.6952 | 0.7204 | 0.7600 | 0.7748 | 0.8032 | 0.8060 | 0.8316 |
| 10 | 4 | 4.5 | 0.1280 | 0.1584 | 0.1896 | 0.2264 | 0.2528 | 0.2920 | 0.3052 | 0.3408 |
| | | 5 | 0.1776 | 0.2112 | 0.2556 | 0.2976 | 0.3256 | 0.3636 | 0.3772 | 0.4116 |
| | | 6 | 0.2920 | 0.3332 | 0.3816 | 0.4212 | 0.4528 | 0.4940 | 0.5076 | 0.5432 |
| | | 10 | 0.6668 | 0.6956 | 0.7436 | 0.7680 | 0.7912 | 0.8124 | 0.8220 | 0.8356 |
| | | 15 | 0.8660 | 0.8840 | 0.9040 | 0.9164 | 0.9272 | 0.9384 | 0.9452 | 0.9504 |
| 15 | 5 | 4.5 | 0.1736 | 0.1872 | 0.2608 | 0.2948 | 0.3304 | 0.3576 | 0.3800 | 0.4052 |
| | | 5 | 0.2504 | 0.2732 | 0.3512 | 0.3824 | 0.4192 | 0.4464 | 0.4800 | 0.5040 |
| | | 6 | 0.4096 | 0.4280 | 0.5228 | 0.5556 | 0.5932 | 0.6188 | 0.6472 | 0.6644 |
| | | 10 | 0.8312 | 0.8424 | 0.8848 | 0.8956 | 0.9124 | 0.9204 | 0.9316 | 0.9384 |
| | | 15 | 0.9640 | 0.9664 | 0.9804 | 0.9832 | 0.9856 | 0.9872 | 0.9892 | 0.9916 |
| 20 | 6 | 4.5 | 0.2328 | 0.2492 | 0.3348 | 0.3544 | 0.3948 | 0.4108 | 0.4480 | 0.4672 |
| | | 5 | 0.3384 | 0.3552 | 0.4404 | 0.4620 | 0.5140 | 0.5300 | 0.5640 | 0.5800 |
| | | 6 | 0.5336 | 0.5336 | 0.6436 | 0.6600 | 0.6984 | 0.7160 | 0.7444 | 0.7576 |
| | | 10 | 0.9260 | 0.9336 | 0.9560 | 0.9584 | 0.9644 | 0.9692 | 0.9748 | 0.9768 |
| | | 15 | 0.9912 | 0.9932 | 0.9964 | 0.9964 | 0.9976 | 0.9980 | 0.9980 | 0.9980 |

It is evident that the leaf area index belongs to longitudinal data. Next, we assume the model of the leaf area index to be,

$$y_j = \mu + 1_b \varepsilon_{1j} + \varepsilon_{0j}, j = 1, 2, 3, 4.$$

Using the ML estimation of Section 5.2, we can estimate $\hat{\mu} = 2.6358$. Under the null hypothesis $H_0 : \mu = 0$, the p-value of the proposed PB test is calculated as 0.000. Therefore, the null hypothesis $H_0 : \mu = 0$ is rejected at a 5% nominal significance level.

**Example 5.2** The data set used in this study is derived from the birth rate in China from 1986 to 2018. From Figure 5.2, it is evident that the birth rate data exhibits skewness. To verify this characteristic, we conduct a normality test on the data. The p-values for the Shapiro-Wilk test, Kolmogorov-Smirnov test, Anderson-Darling test and Cramer-von Mises test are 0.0001, 2.2e-16, 2.646e-05, and 6.41e-06, respectively. Therefore, the birth rate data in China does not follow a normal distribution. Furthermore, we perform a hypothesis test on the assumption $H_0$ that the birth rate data follows a skew-normal distribution. Through calculations, the test statistic is $\chi^2 = 5.3485 < \chi_3^2(0.95) = 7.8147$. Thus, at a 5%

**Table 5.7:** Type I error probabilities for two testing methods in (5.35) ($\sigma_1^2/\sigma_0^2 = \delta_2^* = 1$).

| $a$ | $b$ | $\sigma_0^2$ | $\beta$ 0.025 | | 0.05 | | 0.075 | | 0.1 | |
|---|---|---|---|---|---|---|---|---|---|---|
| | | | PB | GA | PB | GA | PB | GA | PB | GA |
| 5 | 2 | 4 | 0.0252 | 0.0252 | 0.0500 | 0.0496 | 0.0752 | 0.0748 | 0.0996 | 0.0996 |
| | | 4.5 | 0.0248 | 0.0248 | 0.0496 | 0.0496 | 0.0748 | 0.0752 | 0.0996 | 0.0996 |
| | | 5.5 | 0.0248 | 0.0248 | 0.0496 | 0.0496 | 0.0752 | 0.0748 | 0.0996 | 0.0996 |
| | | 6.5 | 0.0248 | 0.0248 | 0.0496 | 0.0496 | 0.0748 | 0.0752 | 0.0996 | 0.0996 |
| | | 8 | 0.0252 | 0.0252 | 0.0500 | 0.0496 | 0.0752 | 0.0748 | 0.0996 | 0.0996 |
| 6 | 3 | 4 | 0.0252 | 0.0248 | 0.0496 | 0.0500 | 0.0752 | 0.0748 | 0.0996 | 0.0996 |
| | | 4.5 | 0.0248 | 0.0248 | 0.0496 | 0.0496 | 0.0752 | 0.0752 | 0.1000 | 0.0996 |
| | | 5.5 | 0.0248 | 0.0248 | 0.0500 | 0.0500 | 0.0748 | 0.0748 | 0.0996 | 0.0996 |
| | | 6.5 | 0.0248 | 0.0248 | 0.0500 | 0.0496 | 0.0748 | 0.0752 | 0.0996 | 0.1000 |
| | | 8 | 0.0252 | 0.0248 | 0.0496 | 0.0500 | 0.0752 | 0.0748 | 0.0996 | 0.0996 |
| 10 | 4 | 4 | 0.0248 | 0.0248 | 0.0496 | 0.0496 | 0.0748 | 0.0748 | 0.1000 | 0.0996 |
| | | 4.5 | 0.0252 | 0.0248 | 0.0500 | 0.0500 | 0.0748 | 0.0748 | 0.0996 | 0.0996 |
| | | 5.5 | 0.0248 | 0.0248 | 0.0496 | 0.0496 | 0.0748 | 0.0748 | 0.1000 | 0.1000 |
| | | 6.5 | 0.0248 | 0.0248 | 0.0496 | 0.0500 | 0.0748 | 0.0748 | 0.1000 | 0.1000 |
| | | 8 | 0.0248 | 0.0248 | 0.0496 | 0.0496 | 0.0748 | 0.0748 | 0.1000 | 0.0996 |
| 15 | 5 | 4 | 0.0248 | 0.0248 | 0.0500 | 0.0500 | 0.0748 | 0.0748 | 0.1000 | 0.0996 |
| | | 4.5 | 0.0248 | 0.0248 | 0.0496 | 0.0500 | 0.0752 | 0.0748 | 0.0996 | 0.0996 |
| | | 5.5 | 0.0248 | 0.0252 | 0.0500 | 0.0496 | 0.0752 | 0.0748 | 0.0996 | 0.0996 |
| | | 6.5 | 0.0252 | 0.0252 | 0.0496 | 0.0496 | 0.0752 | 0.0748 | 0.0996 | 0.0996 |
| | | 8 | 0.0248 | 0.0248 | 0.0500 | 0.0500 | 0.0748 | 0.0748 | 0.1000 | 0.0996 |
| 20 | 6 | 4 | 0.0248 | 0.0248 | 0.0496 | 0.0496 | 0.0748 | 0.0748 | 0.0996 | 0.0996 |
| | | 4.5 | 0.0252 | 0.0252 | 0.0496 | 0.0496 | 0.0748 | 0.0748 | 0.0996 | 0.0996 |
| | | 5.5 | 0.0248 | 0.0252 | 0.0500 | 0.0496 | 0.0748 | 0.0748 | 0.0996 | 0.0996 |
| | | 6.5 | 0.0248 | 0.0248 | 0.0496 | 0.0496 | 0.0748 | 0.0748 | 0.1000 | 0.1000 |
| | | 8 | 0.0248 | 0.0248 | 0.0496 | 0.0496 | 0.0748 | 0.0748 | 0.0996 | 0.0996 |

nominal significance level, the null hypothesis $H_0$ cannot be rejected, indicating that the birth rate data from 1986 to 2018 in China follows a skew-normal distribution. Based on the method of moment estimation, the distribution of the data is determined as $SN(10.4314, 6.0171^2, 5.2324)$, and its density curve is shown in Figure 5.2.

In model (5.1), $Y$ represents the observed value of a $33 \times 1$ vector, $\varepsilon_1 \sim SN_3(0, \sigma_1^2 I_3, \alpha)$, $\varepsilon_0 \sim N_{33}(0, \sigma_0^2 I_{33})$, and $\varepsilon_1$ and $\varepsilon_0$ are mutually independent. Considering the one-sided hypothesis test for a single variance component

$$H_0 : \sigma_1^2 \leqslant 5 \quad versus \quad H_1 : \sigma_1^2 > 5. \tag{5.43}$$

**Table 5.8:** Powers for two testing methods in (5.35) ($\sigma_0^2 = 1, \delta_2^* = 1$).

| $a$ | $b$ | $\sigma_1^2$ | $\beta$ | | | | | | | |
|---|---|---|---|---|---|---|---|---|---|---|
| | | | \multicolumn{2}{c}{0.025} | | \multicolumn{2}{c}{0.05} | | \multicolumn{2}{c}{0.075} | | \multicolumn{2}{c}{0.1} | |
| | | | PB | GA | PB | GA | PB | GA | PB | GA |
| 5 | 2 | 1.2 | 0.0320 | 0.0320 | 0.0644 | 0.0644 | 0.0892 | 0.0892 | 0.1284 | 0.1284 |
| | | 1.5 | 0.0424 | 0.0424 | 0.0856 | 0.0856 | 0.1188 | 0.1188 | 0.1660 | 0.1660 |
| | | 2 | 0.0672 | 0.0672 | 0.1220 | 0.1220 | 0.1680 | 0.1680 | 0.2308 | 0.2308 |
| | | 4 | 0.1756 | 0.1756 | 0.2940 | 0.2940 | 0.3696 | 0.3696 | 0.4588 | 0.4588 |
| | | 6 | 0.2952 | 0.2952 | 0.4368 | 0.4368 | 0.5188 | 0.5188 | 0.5976 | 0.5976 |
| 6 | 3 | 1.2 | 0.0380 | 0.0380 | 0.0744 | 0.0744 | 0.1012 | 0.1012 | 0.1400 | 0.1400 |
| | | 1.5 | 0.0608 | 0.0608 | 0.1088 | 0.1088 | 0.1620 | 0.1620 | 0.2092 | 0.2092 |
| | | 2 | 0.1044 | 0.1044 | 0.1924 | 0.1924 | 0.2536 | 0.2536 | 0.3140 | 0.3140 |
| | | 4 | 0.3604 | 0.3604 | 0.4884 | 0.4884 | 0.5704 | 0.5704 | 0.6364 | 0.6364 |
| | | 6 | 0.5596 | 0.5596 | 0.6768 | 0.6768 | 0.7356 | 0.7356 | 0.7868 | 0.7868 |
| 10 | 4 | 1.2 | 0.0468 | 0.0468 | 0.0880 | 0.0880 | 0.1216 | 0.1216 | 0.1648 | 0.1648 |
| | | 1.5 | 0.0988 | 0.0988 | 0.1688 | 0.1688 | 0.2160 | 0.2160 | 0.2716 | 0.2716 |
| | | 2 | 0.2180 | 0.2180 | 0.3220 | 0.3220 | 0.3872 | 0.3872 | 0.4584 | 0.4584 |
| | | 4 | 0.6704 | 0.6704 | 0.7624 | 0.7624 | 0.8048 | 0.8048 | 0.8396 | 0.8396 |
| | | 6 | 0.8600 | 0.8600 | 0.9124 | 0.9124 | 0.9344 | 0.9344 | 0.9496 | 0.9496 |
| 15 | 5 | 1.2 | 0.0596 | 0.0596 | 0.1068 | 0.1068 | 0.1432 | 0.1432 | 0.1832 | 0.1832 |
| | | 1.5 | 0.1412 | 0.1412 | 0.2260 | 0.2260 | 0.2840 | 0.2840 | 0.3460 | 0.3460 |
| | | 2 | 0.3392 | 0.3392 | 0.4636 | 0.4636 | 0.5300 | 0.5300 | 0.5948 | 0.5948 |
| | | 4 | 0.8572 | 0.8572 | 0.9116 | 0.9116 | 0.9312 | 0.9312 | 0.9460 | 0.9460 |
| | | 6 | 0.9664 | 0.9664 | 0.9804 | 0.9804 | 0.9860 | 0.9860 | 0.9888 | 0.9888 |
| 20 | 6 | 1.2 | 0.0752 | 0.0752 | 0.1196 | 0.1196 | 0.1592 | 0.1592 | 0.2056 | 0.2056 |
| | | 1.5 | 0.1888 | 0.1888 | 0.2788 | 0.2788 | 0.3460 | 0.3460 | 0.4176 | 0.4176 |
| | | 2 | 0.4768 | 0.4768 | 0.5768 | 0.5768 | 0.6488 | 0.6488 | 0.7008 | 0.7008 |
| | | 4 | 0.9464 | 0.9464 | 0.9668 | 0.9668 | 0.9760 | 0.9760 | 0.9824 | 0.9824 |
| | | 6 | 0.9936 | 0.9936 | 0.9948 | 0.9948 | 0.9960 | 0.9960 | 0.9976 | 0.9976 |

Using (5.23) and (5.26), by $10^4$ simulation runs, the p-values for the Bootstrap test and generalized test are obtained as 0.0352 and 0.0358, respectively. Therefore, at 5% nominal significance level, both test methods reject the null hypothesis in (5.43).

Next, considering the one-sided hypothesis test for the sum of variance components

$$H_0 : \sigma_1^2 + \sigma_0^2 \leqslant 7 \quad versus \quad H_1 : \sigma_1^2 + \sigma_0^2 > 7. \tag{5.44}$$

Using (5.31) and (5.34), the p-values for the Bootstrap test and generalized test are obtained as 0.0240 and 0.0189, respectively. Hence, at a 5% nominal significance level, both test methods reject the null hypothesis in (5.44).

Finally, considering the one-sided hypothesis test for the ratio of variance components

$$H_0 : \sigma_1^2 / \sigma_0^2 \leqslant 1 \quad versus \quad H_1 : \sigma_1^2 / \sigma_0^2 > 1. \tag{5.45}$$

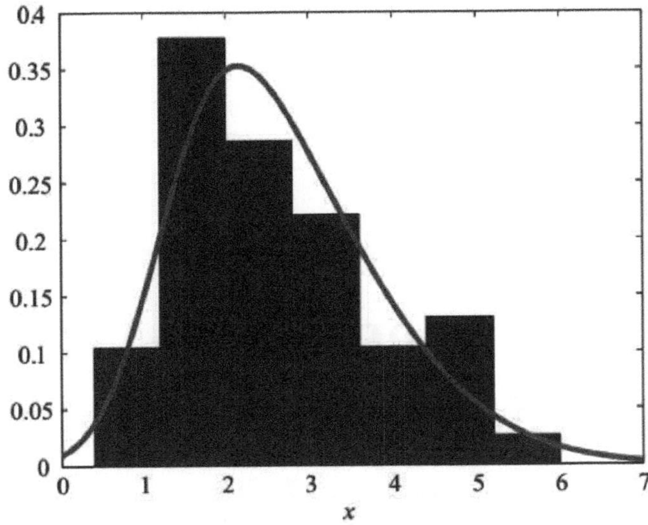

**Figure 5.1:** Histogram and probability density curve of the leaf index.

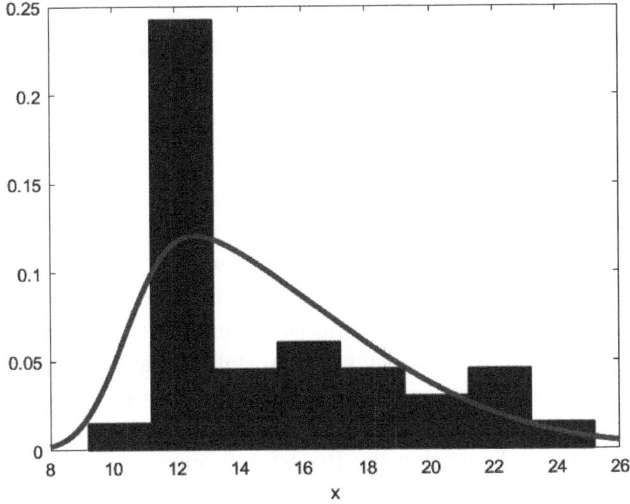

**Figure 5.2:** Histogram and probability density curve of the birth rate in China.

Using (5.39) and (5.42), the p-values for the Bootstrap test and generalized test are 0.0078. Therefore, at 5% nominal significance level, both methods reject the null hypothesis in (5.45).

# Chapter 6

# Unbalanced One-Way Classification Model with Skew-Normal Random Effects

This chapter addresses the one-sided hypothesis testing and interval estimation problems for fixed effect and variance component functions are considered in the unbalanced one-way classification model with skew-normal random effects. Firstly, the Bootstrap approach is used to establish test statistic for fixed effect. Secondly, utilizing the matrix decomposition technique, Bootstrap approach and generalized approach, we construct the test statistics and confidence intervals for the single variance component and sum of variance components. Next, the exact test statistic for the ratio of variance components is obtained. The Monte Carlo simulation results indicate that the Bootstrap approach performs better than the generalized approach in most cases. Finally, the above approaches are illustrated with a real example of carbon fibers' strength.

## 6.1   Model properties

Let $M_{n \times k}$ be the set of all $n \times k$ matrices over the real field. For any $A \in M_{n \times k}$, $A^{'}$ and $rk(A)$ denotes the transpose and rank of $A$ respectively. For any positive semidefinite matrix $B \in M_{n \times n}$, $tr(B)$ and $B^{1/2}$ denote the trace and square root of matrix $B$ respectively. Besides, $I_n$ is an identity matrix of order $n$, and $1_n$ is a $n \times 1$ vector with every element unity. $diag(\cdot)$, $\overset{asy}{\sim}$ and $\triangleq$ denote the diagonal matrix, "approximate distributed" and "defined as", respectively.

Given the prevalence of unbalanced data in application fields, we consider the unbalanced one-way classification model with skew-normal random effects given by

$$Y_{ij} = \mu + A_i + e_{ij}, i = 1, 2, \cdots, a, j = 1, 2, \cdots, n_i, \tag{6.1}$$

where $Y_{ij}$, $\mu$, $A_i$ and $e_{ij}$ represent the observation, fixed effect, $i$th treatment effect and random error respectively. The above model in matrix form is

$$Y = 1_n \mu + ZA + e, \tag{6.2}$$

where $Y = (Y_{11}, \cdots, Y_{1n_1}, \cdots, Y_{a1}, \cdots, Y_{an_a})'$, $A = (A_1, A_2, \cdots, A_a)'$, $Z = diag(1_{n_1}, 1_{n_2}, \cdots, 1_{n_a})$, $e = (e_{11}, \cdots, e_{1n_1}, \cdots, e_{a1}, \cdots, e_{an_a})'$, and $n = \sum_{i=1}^{a} n_i$. We assume that $A \sim SN_a(0, \sigma_A^2 I_a, \lambda_1)$, $e \sim N_n(0, \sigma_e^2 I_n)$, with $A$ and $e$ mutually independent, where $\sigma_A^2$ and $\sigma_e^2$ are the between-group variance component and within-group variance component respectively.

**Remark 6.1.** *If $n_1 = n_2 = \cdots = n_a = b$, the model (6.2) degenerates into the balanced model. In the balanced design, $T_1 = Y'\left(P_{(1_n:Z)} - P_{1_n}\right)Y$ and $T_2 = Y'\left(I_n - P_{(1_n:Z)}\right)Y$ in Ye and Qi (2022) are independent chi-square random variables with $a - 1$ and $n - a$ degrees of freedom respectively. However, design unbalancedness brings a problem concerning the distribution of $T_1$. Specifically, in the unbalanced case, $T_1$ and $T_2$ are independent, and $T_2$ still follows a chi-square distribution with $n - a$ degrees of freedom while $T_1$ does not. Hence, the results in Ye and Qi (2022) are not strictly valid. In other words, the main difficulty to establish the inference method in the unbalanced case is that the independent chi-square statistics are not readily available. Now we present alternative methods appropriate for this situation.*

**Theorem 6.1.** *For the model $Y$ given in (6.2), We have $Y \sim SN_n(\mu_Y, \Sigma_Y, \lambda_2)$, and the moment generating function (MGF) of $Y$ is*

$$M_Y(t) = 2\exp\left(t'\mu_Y + \frac{t'\Sigma_Y t}{2}\right)\Phi\left(\frac{\sigma_A \lambda_1' Z' t}{\left(1 + \lambda_1' \lambda_1\right)^{\frac{1}{2}}}\right), t \in R^n, \tag{6.3}$$

*where $\mu_Y = 1_n \mu$, $\Sigma_Y = \sigma_A^2 ZZ' + \sigma_e^2 I_n$ and $\lambda_2 = \dfrac{\sigma_A(\Sigma_Y)^{-1/2} Z\lambda_1}{\left[1 + \lambda_1'\left(I_a - \sigma_A^2 Z'\Sigma_Y^{-1}Z\right)\lambda_1\right]^{1/2}}.$*

Since the proof of Theorem 6.1 is similar to that given in Ye and Luo (2016), we omit it.

Let

$$
H = \begin{bmatrix}
\frac{1}{\sqrt{2}} & \frac{1}{\sqrt{6}} & \cdots & \frac{1}{\sqrt{n(n-1)}} \\[2mm]
\frac{-1}{\sqrt{2}} & \frac{1}{\sqrt{6}} & \cdots & \frac{1}{\sqrt{n(n-1)}} \\[2mm]
0 & \frac{-2}{\sqrt{6}} & \cdots & \frac{1}{\sqrt{n(n-1)}} \\[2mm]
0 & 0 & \cdots & \frac{1}{\sqrt{n(n-1)}} \\[2mm]
\vdots & \vdots & & \vdots \\[2mm]
0 & 0 & \cdots & \frac{-(n-1)}{\sqrt{n(n-1)}}
\end{bmatrix},
$$

satisfying that $H' 1_n = 0$ and $H' H = I_{n-1}$. We have

$$
H' Y \sim SN_{n-1}\left(0, \sigma_A^2 H' ZZ' H + \sigma_e^2 I_{n-1}, \lambda_3\right), \tag{6.4}
$$

where $\lambda_3 = \dfrac{\left(H' \Sigma_Y H\right)^{-1/2} H' \Sigma_Y^{1/2} \lambda_2}{\left\{1 + \lambda_2' \left[I_n - \Sigma_Y^{1/2} H \left(H' \Sigma_Y H\right)^{-1} H' \Sigma_Y^{1/2}\right] \lambda_2\right\}^{1/2}}.$

As $H' ZZ' H$ is a positive semidefinite matrix, there exists a $(n-1) \times (n-1)$ orthogonal matrix $P = [P_1, P_2, \cdots, P_d]$ such that $P' H' ZZ' HP$ is a diagonal matrix, that is

$$
P' H' ZZ' HP = diag\left(\Delta_1, \cdots, \Delta_1, \cdots, \Delta_d, \cdots, \Delta_d\right) \triangleq D, \tag{6.5}
$$

where $0 \le \Delta_1 < \Delta_2 < \cdots < \Delta_d$, each $\Delta_i$ is repeated $r_i$ times, $i = 1, 2, \cdots, d$, and $\sum_{i=1}^{d} r_i = n - 1$. Note that $rk\left(H' ZZ' H\right) = a - 1$, then $\Delta_1 = 0$ and $r_1 = n - a$. Accordingly,

$$
P' H' Y \sim SN_{n-1}\left(0, \sigma_A^2 D + \sigma_e^2 I_{n-1}, \lambda_4\right) \text{ and } P_i' H' Y \sim SN_{r_i}\left(0, \left(\Delta_i \sigma_A^2 + \sigma_e^2\right) I_{r_i}, \lambda_4^{(i)}\right),
$$

where $\lambda_4 = \dfrac{\left(P' \Sigma_H P\right)^{-1/2} P' \Sigma_H^{1/2} \lambda_3}{\left\{1 + \lambda_3' \left[I_{n-1} - \Sigma_H^{1/2} P \left(P' \Sigma_H P\right)^{-1} P' \Sigma_H^{1/2}\right] \lambda_3\right\}^{1/2}},$

$\lambda_4^{(i)} = \dfrac{\left(P_i' \Sigma_H P_i\right)^{-1/2} P_i' \Sigma_H^{1/2} \lambda_3}{\left\{1 + \lambda_3' \left[I_{n-1} - \Sigma_H^{1/2} P_i \left(P_i' \Sigma_H P_i\right)^{-1} P_i' \Sigma_H^{1/2}\right] \lambda_3\right\}^{1/2}}$ and $\Sigma_H = \sigma_A^2 H' ZZ' H + \sigma_e^2 I_{n-1}.$

**Theorem 6.2.** *For the model $Y$ given in (6.2), if $n_1 = n_2 = \cdots = n_a = b$, then $\Delta_1 = 0$, $\Delta_2 = b$, $r_1 = n - a$, $r_2 = a - 1$, and $d = 2$, where $\Delta_1$, $\Delta_2$, $r_1$, $r_2$, and $d$ are given in (6.5).*

*Proof.* Let $A = bI_n - ZZ'$. Clearly, the distinct eigenvalues of $A$ are $b$ and $0$, and $rk(A) = n - a$. Note that $\left[\frac{1}{\sqrt{n}} 1_n, H\right]$ is a $n \times n$ orthogonal matrix. It follows from

$$
\left[\frac{1}{\sqrt{n}} 1_n, H\right]' A \left[\frac{1}{\sqrt{n}} 1_n, H\right] = \begin{bmatrix} 0_{1 \times 1} & 0_{1 \times (n-1)} \\ 0_{(n-1) \times 1} & H' AH \end{bmatrix}
$$

that $rk\left(H'AH\right) = rk(A) = n - a$. As $bI_{n-1} - H'ZZ'H = H'AH$, we know that $bI_{n-1} - H'ZZ'H$ is a singular matrix. Thus, $b$ and 0 are the distinct eigenvalues of $H'ZZ'H$ with multiplicities $a - 1$ and $n - a$. Therefore, the proof of Theorem 6.1 is completed. $\qquad\square$

Wu et al. (2017a) and Ye and Wang (2015), propose Lemma 6.1 and Theorem 6.3 given below.

**Lemma 6.1.** *Suppose* $X \sim SN_n(0, \Sigma_0, \alpha_0)$, *and A is a symmetric matrix of order n, then* $X'AX$ *has the same distribution as* $V'AV$, *where* $V \sim N_n(0, \Sigma_0)$.

**Theorem 6.3.** *For the model Y given in* (6.2), *let* $Q_i^* = Y'B_iY/\sigma_{*i}^2$, $i = 1, 2, \cdots, l$, *where positive semidefinite matrix* $B_i \in M_{n\times n}$, $\sigma_{*i}^2 = \frac{1}{m_i}\left[\sigma_e^2 tr(B_i) + \sigma_A^2 tr\left(B_iZZ'\right)\right]$, *and* $m_i = rk(B_i)$. *If* $\lambda_2'\Omega_i^{1/2}B_i\mu_Y = 0$, *then* $\{Q_i^*\}_{i=1}^l$ *is a family of independent noncentral chi-square distributed random variables and each* $Q_i^* \sim \chi_{m_i}^2(\zeta_i)$ *if and only if for any distinct* $i, j \in \{1, 2, \cdots, l\}$:

*(i)* $\Omega_iB_i$ *is idempotent of rank* $m_i$,

*(ii)* $\zeta_i = \mu_Y'B_i\mu_Y/\sigma_{*i}^2$, *and*

*(iii)* $B_iB_j = 0$,

*where* $\mu_Y = 1_n\mu$ *and* $\Sigma_Y = \sigma_A^2ZZ' + \sigma_e^2I_n = \sigma_{*i}^2\Omega_i$.

**Theorem 6.4.** *For the model Y given in* (6.2), *let* $Q_i = Y'HP_iP_i'H'Y$, $i = 1, 2, \cdots, d$. *We have*

$$Q_i \sim \left(\sigma_e^2 + \Delta_i\sigma_A^2\right)\chi_{r_i}^2, \tag{6.6}$$

*and* $Q_1, Q_2, \cdots, Q_d$ *are independent to each other.*

*Proof.* Suppose $B_i = HP_iP_i'H'$, $i = 1, 2, \cdots, d$. To obtain Theorem 6.4, it suffices to show that $\lambda_2'\Omega_i^{1/2}B_i\mu_Y = 0$ and conditions (i)–(iii) hold in Theorem 6.3. Since $rk(B_i) = tr(B_i) = r_i$, and $tr\left(B_iZZ'\right) = \Delta_ir_i$, then $\sigma_{*i}^2 = \frac{1}{r_i}\left[\sigma_e^2 tr(B_i) + \sigma_A^2 tr\left(B_iZZ'\right)\right] = \sigma_e^2 + \sigma_A^2\Delta_i$. Let $Q_i^* = Q_i/\sigma_{*i}^2$. Obviously, $\Omega_i = \frac{1}{\sigma_e^2+\sigma_A^2\Delta_i}\sigma_e^2I_n + \frac{1}{\sigma_e^2+\sigma_A^2\Delta_i}\sigma_A^2ZZ'$, and it is easy to check that $\lambda_2'\Omega_i^{1/2}B_i\mu_Y = 0$. It follows from $B_i\Omega_iB_i = B_i$ that $rk(\Omega_iB_i) = tr(\Omega_iB_i) = r_i$, and hence Condition (i) is satisfied. By calculation, $\zeta_i = \mu_Y'B_i\mu_Y/\sigma_{*i}^2 = 0$, so Condition (ii) holds. Note that $B_kB_j = HP_kP_k'H'HP_jP_j'H' = 0$, where $k, j = 1, 2, \cdots, d, k \neq j$, Condition (iii) is established. By Theorem 6.3, $\{Q_i^*\}_{i=1}^d$ is a family of independent central chi-square distributed random variables and each $Q_i^* \sim \chi_{r_i}^2$. Therefore, the proof of Theorem 6.4 is complete. $\qquad\square$

**Remark 6.2.** *If $n_1 = n_2 = \cdots = n_a = b$, then $Q_1/\sigma_e^2 \sim \chi_{n-a}^2$ and $Q_2/(\sigma_e^2 + b\sigma_A^2) \sim \chi_{a-1}^2$. In fact, Theorem 6.4 is the generalization of the results in Ye and Qi (2022).*

**Theorem 6.5.** *For $Q_i$ in (6.6), then $\frac{1}{\sigma_e^2 + \sigma_A^2 \bar{\Delta}} \sum_{i=2}^{d} Q_i \overset{asy}{\sim} \chi_{a-1}^2$, where*

$$\bar{\Delta} = \sum_{i=2}^{d} r_i \Delta_i / \sum_{i=2}^{d} r_i.$$

*Proof.* By Lemma 6.1 and (6.4), there exists $V \sim N_{n-1}\left(0, \sigma_A^2 H' ZZ' H + \sigma_e^2 I_{n-1}\right)$ such that $Q_i = Y' HP_i P_i' H' Y$ has the same distribution as $V' P_i P_i' V$. It follows from Theorem 6.4 that $\sum_{i=2}^{d} \frac{1}{\sigma_e^2 + \sigma_A^2 \Delta_i} Q_i \sim \chi_{a-1}^2$, and hence $\sum_{i=2}^{d} \frac{1}{\sigma_e^2 + \sigma_A^2 \Delta_i} V' P_i P_i' V \sim \chi_{a-1}^2$. By Wimmer and Witkovsky (2003), the result of Theorem 6.5 is obtained immediately. Therefore, the proof of Theorem 6.5 is complete. $\square$

By Theorems 6.4–6.5, Corollary 6.1 is given as follows.

**Corollary 6.1.** *For $Q_i$ in (6.6), then the unbiased estimator of $\sigma_e^2$ and feasible estimator of $\sigma_A^2$ are given by $\hat{\sigma}_e^2 = Q_1/(n-a)$ and $\hat{\sigma}_A^2 = \frac{1}{(a-1)\bar{\Delta}} \sum_{i=2}^{d} Q_i - \frac{1}{(n-a)\bar{\Delta}} Q_1$ respectively.*

Let $R = \left(Z'Z\right)^{-1} Z'$. Premultiplying $R$ in (6.2), we get

$$RY = 1_a \mu + A + Re. \tag{6.7}$$

By the model (6.7), then $RY \sim SN_a\left(1_a\mu, \sigma_A^2 I_a + M, \lambda_5\right)$, where $M = diag\left\{\frac{\sigma_e^2}{n_i}\right\}$ and $\lambda_5 = \dfrac{\left(R\Sigma_Y R'\right)^{-1/2} R\Sigma_Y^{1/2} \lambda_2}{\left\{1 + \lambda_2'\left[I_n - \Sigma_Y^{1/2} R'\left(R\Sigma_Y R'\right)^{-1} R\Sigma_Y^{1/2}\right]\lambda_2\right\}^{1/2}}$.

Furthermore, we obtain

$$1_a' RY \sim SN\left(a\mu, a\sigma_s^2, \lambda_6\right), \tag{6.8}$$

where $\sigma_s^2 = \sigma_A^2 + \frac{1}{a}\sum_{i=1}^{a} \sigma_e^2/n_i$, $\lambda_6 = \dfrac{\left(1_a'\Sigma_R 1_a\right)^{-1/2} 1_a'\Sigma_R^{1/2} \lambda_5}{\left\{1 + \lambda_5'\left[I_a - \Sigma_R^{1/2} 1_a\left(1_a'\Sigma_R 1_a\right)^{-1} 1_a'\Sigma_R^{1/2}\right]\lambda_5\right\}^{1/2}}$ and $\Sigma_R = \sigma_A^2 I_a + M$.

**Theorem 6.6.** *Let $Q_0 = Y' R' 1_a 1_a' RY$. Then*

$$\frac{Q_0}{a\sigma_s^2} \sim S\chi_1^2\left(\frac{a\mu^2}{\sigma_s^2}, \frac{\sqrt{a}\mu}{\sigma_s}\lambda_6, \lambda_6^2\right). \tag{6.9}$$

By Definition 2.2 and (6.8), it is easy to get the result in (6.9), so the proof is omitted. In particular, if $\mu = 0$, then $Q_0/(a\sigma_s^2) \sim \chi_1^2$.

## 6.2 Inference on the fixed effect

In this section, we consider the one-sided hypothesis of the fixed effect in model (6.2) as

$$H_0 : \mu \le \mu_0 \quad \textit{versus} \quad H_1 : \mu > \mu_0, \tag{6.10}$$

where $\mu_0$ is a specified value. This hypothesis is equivalent to

$$H_0 : v \le 0 \quad \textit{versus} \quad H_1 : v > 0, \tag{6.11}$$

where $v = \mu - \mu_0$. Therefore, without loss of generality, we assume that $\mu_0 = 0$.

**Theorem 6.7.** *Let* $X \sim N_n(0, \Sigma_0)$, $L_{in} = B_{in}X$, *where* $B_{in}$ *is a* $m \times n$ *matrix,* $i = 1, 2$. *If* $B_{1n}\Sigma_0 B_{2n}' \overset{n \to \infty}{\longrightarrow} 0$ *and* $B_{in}\Sigma_0 B_{in}' \overset{n \to \infty}{\longrightarrow} M_i$, *then* $L_{1n}$ *and* $L_{2n}$ *are asymptotically independent.*

*Proof.* Obviously, the characteristic function of $L_n = \left[ L_{1n}', L_{2n}' \right]'$ is

$$\varphi_{L_n}(t_1, t_2) = \exp\left[ -\frac{1}{2}\left( t_1' B_{1n}\Sigma_0 B_{1n}' t_1 + 2t_1' B_{1n}\Sigma_0 B_{2n}' t_2 + t_2' B_{2n}\Sigma_0 B_{2n}' t_2 \right) \right], t_1, t_2 \in R^m,$$

thus $L_{1n}$ and $L_{2n}$ are mutually independent if and only if $B_{1n}\Sigma_0 B_{2n}' = 0$. If $B_{1n}\Sigma_0 B_{2n}' \overset{n \to \infty}{\longrightarrow} 0$ and $B_{in}\Sigma_0 B_{in}' \overset{n \to \infty}{\longrightarrow} M_i$, $i = 1, 2$, then

$$\varphi_{L_n}(t_1, t_2) \overset{n \to \infty}{\longrightarrow} \exp\left[ -\frac{1}{2}\left( t_1' M_1 t_1 + t_2' M_2 t_2 \right) \right].$$

Further, by Pan (1966), $L_{1n}$ and $L_{2n}$ are asymptotically independent, namely the result of Theorem 6.7. $\qquad\square$

Let $P_i = [p_{i1}, p_{i2}, \cdots, p_{ir_i}]$ in (6.5) and $w_{ij} = Y' H p_{ij} p_{ij}' H' Y$, where $p_{ij} \in R^{n-1}$, $i = 1, 2, \cdots, d$, $j = 1, 2, \cdots, r_i$. Then, $Q_i$ in (6.6) is rewritten as $Q_i = \sum_{j=1}^{r_i} w_{ij}$. For $l = 1, 2, \cdots, a$, suppose $n_l = m + k_l$, where $m$ is the minimum of $n_1, n_2, \cdots, n_a$, and $k_l$ is the given constant.

**Theorem 6.8.** *If* $\mu = 0$ *and* $\sigma_A^2 \overset{n \to \infty}{\longrightarrow} 0$, *then* $Q_i$ *and* $Q_0$ *are asymptotically independent, where* $Q_i$ *and* $Q_0$ *are given in (6.6) and (6.9) respectively,* $i = 1, 2, \cdots, d$.

*Proof.* For Theorem 6.8, it suffices to show that for any $i \in \{1, 2, \cdots, d\}$, $Q_0$ and $w_{ij}$ are asymptotically independent, $j = 1, 2, \cdots, r_i$. If $\mu = 0$, then $Y \sim SN_n(0, \Sigma_Y, \lambda_2)$. By Genton (2005), we rewrite $Y$ as

$$Y = \begin{cases} V, & U \le \Phi\left( \lambda_2' \Sigma_Y^{-1/2} V \right) \\ -V, & U > \Phi\left( \lambda_2' \Sigma_Y^{-1/2} V \right) \end{cases},$$

where $V \sim N_n(0, \Sigma_Y)$, $U \sim U[0,1]$, $U[0,1]$ denotes the uniform distribution on $[0,1]$. Thus, we obtain $Y'AY = V'AV$, where $A$ is any $n \times n$ matrix. Furthermore, $Q_0 = V'R'1_a1_a'RV$ and $w_{ij} = V'Hp_{ij}p_{ij}'H'V$, $j = 1, 2, \cdots, r_i$. For $n_l = m + k_l$, $l = 1, 2, \cdots, a$, we have $n = am + \sum\limits_{l=1}^{a} k_l$.

Denote $L_{0n} = 1_a'RV$ and $L_{ijn} = p_{ij}'H'V$. Obviously, $p_{ij}'H'\Sigma_Y R'1_a = \sigma_e^2 p_{ij}'H'R'1_a$, $p_{ij}'H'\Sigma_Y Hp_{ij} = \sigma_A^2 \Delta_i + \sigma_e^2$ and $1_a'R\Sigma_Y R'1_a = a\sigma_A^2 + \sigma_e^2 \sum\limits_{l=1}^{a} \frac{1}{n_l}$. For any $i \in \{1, 2, \cdots, d\}$, we have $p_{ij}'H'\Sigma_Y R'1_a \overset{n \to \infty}{\longrightarrow} 0$, $p_{ij}'H'\Sigma_Y Hp_{ij} \overset{n \to \infty}{\longrightarrow} \sigma_e^2$ and $1_a'R\Sigma_Y R'1_a \overset{n \to \infty}{\longrightarrow} 0$, $j = 1, 2, \cdots, r_i$. Further, $L_{0n}$ and $L_{ijn}$ are asymptotically independent by Theorem 6.7. Since $Q_0 = L_{0n}'L_{0n}$ and $w_{ij} = L_{ijn}'L_{ijn}$, $Q_0$ and $w_{ij}$ are asymptotically independent. Therefore, the proof of Theorem 6.8 is completed. $\square$

**Remark 6.3.** *If $\mu = 0$ and $n_1 = n_2 = \cdots = n_a = b$, then $Q_0$, $Q_1$ and $Q_2$ are mutually independent.*

For the hypothesis testing problem (6.10), we have

$$T_0 = \frac{Q_0}{a\sigma_s^2}. \tag{6.12}$$

If $\sigma_s^2$ is known, $T_0$ will be the test statistic for the hypothesis testing problem (6.10). However, $\sigma_s^2$ is often unknown in practical applications. In such cases, the parameter might be replaced by its estimator $\hat{\sigma}_s^2 = \hat{\sigma}_A^2 + \frac{1}{a}\sum\limits_{i=1}^{a} \hat{\sigma}_e^2 / n_i$ under the null hypothesis $H_0$ in (6.10). Then the test statistic is expressed as

$$T_0^* = \frac{Q_0}{a\left[\dfrac{\sum\limits_{i=2}^{d} Q_i}{(a-1)\Delta} + \left(\dfrac{1}{a}\sum\limits_{i=1}^{a}\dfrac{1}{n_i} - \dfrac{1}{\Delta}\right)\dfrac{Q_1}{n-a}\right]}. \tag{6.13}$$

It is difficult to obtain the exact distribution of $T_0^*$, so the Bootstrap approach is used to construct the test statistic. Thus, based on (6.13), the Bootstrap test statistic for hypothesis testing problem (6.10) is defined as

$$T_{0B}^* = \frac{Q_{0B}}{a\left[\dfrac{\sum\limits_{i=2}^{d} Q_{iB}}{(a-1)\Delta} + \left(\dfrac{1}{a}\sum\limits_{i=1}^{a}\dfrac{1}{n_i} - \dfrac{1}{\Delta}\right)\dfrac{Q_{1B}}{n-a}\right]}, \tag{6.14}$$

where $Q_{0B} \sim \left\{ a \left[ \frac{1}{(a-1)\bar{\Delta}} \sum_{i=2}^{d} q_i + \left( \frac{1}{a} \sum_{i=1}^{a} \frac{1}{n_i} - \frac{1}{\Delta} \right) q_1 / (n-a) \right] \right\} \chi_1^2, Q_{1B} \sim (q_1/(n-a))$

$\chi_{n-a}^2, \sum_{i=2}^{d} Q_{iB} \overset{asy}{\sim} \left( \frac{1}{a-1} \sum_{i=2}^{d} q_i \right) \chi_{a-1}^2$, and $q_1, q_2, \cdots, q_d$ denote the observed values of $Q_1, Q_2, \cdots, Q_d$ respectively. Further, the Bootstrap $p$-value is computed by $T_{0B}^*$ in (6.14) as

$$p_{T_0} = P\left( T_{0B}^* > t_0^* | H_0 \right), \tag{6.15}$$

where $t_0^*$ denotes the observed value of $T_0^*$. Let $\beta$ be the nominal significance level. The null hypothesis $H_0$ in (6.10) is rejected whenever the above $p$-value is less than the nominal significance level of $\beta$.

## 6.3 Inference on variance component functions

### 6.3.1 Inference on the single variance component

In this section, we consider the one-sided hypothesis of the single variance component in model (6.2) as

$$H_0 : \sigma_A^2 \leq c_1 \quad versus \quad H_1 : \sigma_A^2 > c_1, \tag{6.16}$$

where $c_1$ is a specified value.

#### 6.3.1.1 Bootstrap approach

For hypothesis testing problem (6.16), we get

$$T_1 = \sum_{i=2}^{d} \frac{Q_i}{\sigma_e^2 + c_1 \Delta_i}. \tag{6.17}$$

Since $\sigma_e^2$ is often unknown in the applications, the parameter can be replaced by its estimator $\hat{\sigma}_e^2 = Q_1/(n-a)$ under the null hypothesis $H_0$ in (6.16). Then the test statistic is constructed as

$$T_1^* = \sum_{i=2}^{d} \frac{Q_i}{\frac{Q_1}{n-a} + c_1 \Delta_i}. \tag{6.18}$$

Similar to (6.13), the exact distribution of $T_1^*$ is difficult to obtain, so the Bootstrap approach is used to construct the test statistic. Therefore, the Bootstrap test statistic for hypothesis testing problem (6.16) has the form of

$$T_{1B}^* = \sum_{i=2}^{d} \frac{Q_{iB}}{\frac{Q_{1B}}{n-a} + c_1 \Delta_i}, \tag{6.19}$$

where $Q_{1B} \sim (q_1/(n-a)) \chi^2_{n-a}$ and $Q_{iB} \sim (c_1\Delta_i + q_1/(n-a)) \chi^2_{r_i}, i = 2, 3, \cdots, d$. Then, the Bootstrap $p$-value is computed by $T^*_{1B}$ in (6.19) as

$$p_{T_1} = P\left(T^*_{1B} > t^*_1 | H_0\right), \tag{6.20}$$

where $t^*_1$ denotes the observed value of $T^*_1$. The null hypothesis $H_0$ in (6.16) is rejected whenever $p_{T_1}$ is less than the nominal significance level of $\beta$.

**Remark 6.4.** *If $n_1 = n_2 = \cdots = n_a = b$, then $T^*_{1B}$ in (6.19) degenerates into the result given by Ye and Qi (2022).*

**Remark 6.5.** *If $\lambda_1 = 0$ and $n_1 = n_2 = \cdots = n_a = b$, then $T^*_{1B}$ in (6.19) degenerates into the result given by Yang et al. (2012).*

**Remark 6.6.** *Based on $T^*_{1B}$ in (6.19), the Bootstrap pivot quantity of $\sigma^2_A$ can be constructed as*

$$\tilde{T}^*_{1B} = \sum_{i=2}^{d} \frac{\tilde{Q}_{iB}}{\frac{\tilde{Q}_{1B}}{n-a} + \tilde{\sigma}^2_A \Delta_i}, \tag{6.21}$$

*where $\tilde{\sigma}^2_A = \frac{1}{(a-1)\bar{\Delta}} \sum_{i=2}^{d} q_i - \frac{1}{(n-a)\bar{\Delta}} q_1$ and $\tilde{Q}_{iB} \sim (q_i/r_i) \chi^2_{r_i}, i = 1, 2, \cdots, d$. $\tilde{T}^*_{1B}(\gamma)$*

*denotes the $100\gamma$ empirical percentile of $\tilde{T}^*_{1B}$. Let $\bar{\Delta} = \sum_{i=2}^{d} r_i \Delta_i / \sum_{i=2}^{d} r_i$. By Burch (2011), $\Delta_2, \Delta_3, \cdots, \Delta_d$ in (6.21) are replaced with $\bar{\Delta}$. Then, the approximate $1 - \beta$ Bootstrap confidence interval for $\sigma^2_A$ is*

$$\left[ \frac{\sum_{i=2}^{d} q_i}{\bar{\Delta}\tilde{T}^*_{1B}(1-\beta/2)} - \frac{q_1}{\bar{\Delta}(n-a)}, \frac{\sum_{i=2}^{d} q_i}{\bar{\Delta}\tilde{T}^*_{1B}(\beta/2)} - \frac{q_1}{\bar{\Delta}(n-a)} \right].$$

### 6.3.1.2 Generalized approach

Let $R_1 = Q_1/\sigma^2_e$ and $R_i = Q_i/(\sigma^2_e + \sigma^2_A \Delta_i), i = 2, 3, \cdots, d$. For the hypothesis testing problem (6.16), the generalized test variable is

$$F_1 = \sum_{i=2}^{d} R_i \left( \frac{1}{R_1} + \frac{\sigma^2_A \Delta_i}{q_1} \right) \sim \sum_{i=2}^{d} \chi^2_{r_i} \left( \frac{1}{\chi^2_{n-a}} + \frac{\sigma^2_A \Delta_i}{q_1} \right). \tag{6.22}$$

It is apparent that the observed value of $F_1$ is $f_1 = \sum_{i=2}^{d} q_i/q_1$. From the second expression in (6.22), we know that the distribution of $F_1$ is free of nuisance parameters. By (6.22), $F_1$ is stochastically increasing in $\sigma^2_A$. Namely, $F_1$ is a generalized test variable for hypothesis testing problem (6.16). Based on $F_1$ in (6.22), the generalized *p*-value is given by

$$
\begin{aligned}
p_{F_1} &= P\left(F_1 \geq f_1 | H_0\right) = P\left(\frac{1}{R_1} \geq \frac{f_1 - \sum_{i=2}^{d} \frac{c_1 \Delta_i R_i}{q_1}}{\sum_{i=2}^{d} R_i}\right) \\
&= 1 - E_{R_2, R_3, \cdots, R_d}\left[ F_{I\Gamma(\frac{n-a}{2}, \frac{1}{2})}\left(\frac{f_1 - \sum_{i=2}^{d} \frac{c_1 \Delta_i R_i}{q_1}}{\sum_{i=2}^{d} R_i}\right) \right],
\end{aligned}
\tag{6.23}
$$

where $F_{I\Gamma(\frac{n-a}{2}, \frac{1}{2})}$ denotes the cumulative distribution function of the inverse gamma distribution with parameters $(n-a)/2$ and $1/2$, and the expectation $E_{R_2, R_3, \cdots, R_d}$ is taken with respect to $R_2, R_3, \cdots, R_d$. The null hypothesis $H_0$ in (6.16) will be rejected if $p_{F_1}$ is less than the nominal significance level of $\beta$.

A testing approach is supposed to stay invariant with the change of the observation unit, so we consider the p-invariance of the generalized testing approach. Under the scale transformations

$$
\begin{aligned}
\left(\sigma_e^2, \sigma_A^2\right) &\rightarrow \left(k\sigma_e^2, k\sigma_A^2\right), \\
(Q_1, Q_2, \cdots, Q_d) &\rightarrow (kQ_1, kQ_2, \cdots, kQ_d), k > 0,
\end{aligned}
\tag{6.24}
$$

although the generalized test variable $F_1$ is invariant, the hypothesis testing problem (6.16) is not. Hence, consider the equivalent hypothesis

$$
H_0 : \theta \leq \theta_1 \quad versus \quad H_1 : \theta > \theta_1,
\tag{6.25}
$$

where $\theta = \sigma_A^2 / q_1$ and $\theta_1 = c_1 / q_1$. By the following scale transformations

$$
\begin{aligned}
\left(\sigma_e^2, \theta\right) &\rightarrow \left(k\sigma_e^2, \theta\right), \\
(Q_1, Q_2, \cdots, Q_d) &\rightarrow (kQ_1, kQ_2, \cdots, kQ_d), k > 0,
\end{aligned}
\tag{6.26}
$$

the hypothesis testing problem (6.25) is invariant. Then, the generalized *p*-value can be computed as

$$
\tilde{p}_{F_1} = 1 - E_{R_2, R_3, \cdots, R_d}\left[ F_{I\Gamma(\frac{n-a}{2}, \frac{1}{2})}\left(\frac{f_1 - \sum_{i=2}^{d} \theta_1 \Delta_i R_i}{\sum_{i=2}^{d} R_i}\right) \right].
\tag{6.27}
$$

Therefore, for the hypothesis testing problem (6.25), the test based on $\tilde{p}_{F_1}$ in (6.27) is p-invariant under the scale transformations (6.26).

**Remark 6.7.** *If $n_1 = n_2 = \cdots = n_a = b$, then $F_1$ in (6.22) degenerates into the result given by Ye and Qi (2022).*

**Remark 6.8.** *If $\lambda_1 = 0$ and $n_1 = n_2 = \cdots = n_a = b$, then $F_1$ in (6.22) degenerates into the result given by Weerahandi (1991).*

Next, to obtain the generalized confidence interval of $\sigma_A^2$, we define

$$F_1^* = \frac{1}{d-1}\sum_{i=2}^{d}\frac{1}{\Delta_i}\left[\frac{q_i\left(\sigma_e^2 + \sigma_A^2\Delta_i\right)}{Q_i} - \frac{q_1\sigma_e^2}{Q_1}\right]. \tag{6.28}$$

Apparently, the observed value of $F_1^*$ is $\sigma_A^2$, and the distribution of $F_1^*$ is free of any unknown parameters. Thus, $F_1^*$ is a generalized pivot quantity. By the quantile of $F_1^*$, the generalized lower confidence limit and upper confidence limit of $\sigma_A^2$ are obtained at the confidence level of $1 - \beta$, which are written as $F_1^*\left(\beta/2\right)$ and $F_1^*\left(1 - \beta/2\right)$, respectively.

The generalized confidence interval is not based on the frequency theory, so it is necessary to study the coverage probability of $[F_1^*\left(\beta/2\right), F_1^*\left(1 - \beta/2\right)]$.

**Theorem 6.9.** *If $n_1 = n_2 = \cdots = n_a = b$, then*

$$\lim_{\sigma_e^2 \to 0} P\left(F_1^*\left(\frac{\beta}{2}\right) \leq \sigma_A^2 \leq F_1^*\left(1 - \frac{\beta}{2}\right)\right) = 1 - \beta,$$

$$\lim_{\sigma_A^2 \to 0} P\left(F_1^*\left(\frac{\beta}{2}\right) \leq \sigma_A^2 \leq F_1^*\left(1 - \frac{\beta}{2}\right)\right) = 1 - \beta,$$

$$\lim_{b \to \infty} P\left(F_1^*\left(\frac{\beta}{2}\right) \leq \sigma_A^2 \leq F_1^*\left(1 - \frac{\beta}{2}\right)\right) = 1 - \beta,$$

$$\lim_{\sigma_e^2 \to 0, b \to \infty} P\left(F_1^*\left(\frac{\beta}{2}\right) \leq \sigma_A^2 \leq F_1^*\left(1 - \frac{\beta}{2}\right)\right) = 1 - \beta.$$

*Proof.* Firstly, we should prove the first equation. Clearly, to obtain the result, it suffices to show that

$$\lim_{\sigma_e^2 \to 0} P\left(\sigma_A^2 \geq F_1^*\left(\frac{\beta}{2}\right)\right) = 1 - \frac{\beta}{2},$$

$$\lim_{\sigma_e^2 \to 0} P\left(\sigma_A^2 \leq F_1^*\left(1 - \frac{\beta}{2}\right)\right) = 1 - \frac{\beta}{2}.$$

By Theorem 6.2, since $n_1 = n_2 = \cdots = n_a = b$, then $\Delta_2 = b$ and $d = 2$. By Theorem 6.4, $Q_1 \sim \sigma_e^2 \chi_{n-a}^2$ and $Q_2 \sim \left(\sigma_e^2 + b\sigma_A^2\right)\chi_{a-1}^2$. Suppose that $(R_1^*, R_2^*)$ and

$(R_1, R_2)$ are independently and identically distributed. Further,

$$
\begin{aligned}
P\left(\sigma_A^2 \geq F_1^*\left(\frac{\beta}{2}\right)\right) &= P\left(P\left(F_1^* \leq \sigma_A^2\right) \geq \frac{\beta}{2}\right)\\
&= P\left(P\left(\frac{1}{b}\left(\frac{Q_2}{R_2} - \frac{Q_1}{R_1}\right) \leq \sigma_A^2 \mid Q_1, Q_2\right) \geq \frac{\beta}{2}\right)\\
&= \tilde{P}\left(P\left(\frac{1}{b}\left(\frac{\left(\sigma_e^2 + b\sigma_A^2\right)R_2^*}{R_2} - \frac{\sigma_e^2 R_1^*}{R_1}\right) \leq \sigma_A^2 \mid R_1^*, R_2^*\right) \geq \frac{\beta}{2}\right),
\end{aligned}
$$

where $\tilde{P}$ denotes the joint distribution of $(R_1^*, R_2^*)$. Then,

$$
\begin{aligned}
\lim_{\sigma_e^2 \to 0} P\left(\sigma_A^2 \geq F_1^*\left(\frac{\beta}{2}\right)\right) &= \tilde{P}\left(P\left(R_2^* \leq R_2 \mid R_1^*, R_2^*\right) \geq \frac{\beta}{2}\right)\\
&= \tilde{P}\left(F_{\chi_{a-1}^2}\left(R_2^*\right) \leq 1 - \frac{\beta}{2}\right)\\
&= 1 - \frac{\beta}{2},
\end{aligned}
$$

where $F_{\chi_{a-1}^2}$ denotes the cumulative distribution function of $\chi^2$ distribution with degrees of freedom $a - 1$. Furthermore, we get $\lim_{\sigma_e^2 \to 0} P\left(\sigma_A^2 \leq F_1^*\left(1 - \beta/2\right)\right) = 1 - \beta/2$. So, the first equation is satisfied. Similarly, the other three equations can be obtained. Therefore, the proof of Theorem 6.9 is completed. □

**Remark 6.9.** *If $n_1 = n_2 = \cdots = n_a = b$, then the generalized confidence interval $\left[F_1^*\left(\beta/2\right), F_1^*\left(1 - \beta/2\right)\right]$ degenerates into the result given by Ye and Qi (2022).*

**Remark 6.10.** *If $\lambda_1 = 0$ and $n_1 = n_2 = \cdots = n_a = b$, then the generalized confidence interval $\left[F_1^*\left(\beta/2\right), F_1^*\left(1 - \beta/2\right)\right]$ degenerates into the result given by Weerahandi (1993).*

### 6.3.2 *Inference on the sum of variance components*

In this section, we consider the one-sided hypothesis of the sum of variance components in model (6.2) as

$$
H_0: \sigma_A^2 + \sigma_e^2 \leq c_2 \quad versus \quad H_1: \sigma_A^2 + \sigma_e^2 > c_2 \tag{6.29}
$$

where $c_2$ is a specified value.

### 6.3.2.1 *Bootstrap approach*

For hypothesis testing problem (6.29), we obtain

$$
T_2 = \sum_{i=2}^{d} \frac{Q_i}{c_2 \Delta_i + \left(1 - \Delta_i\right)\sigma_e^2}. \tag{6.30}
$$

Similar to (6.18), the test statistic is defined as

$$T_2^* = \sum_{i=2}^{d} \frac{Q_i}{c_2 \Delta_i + (1 - \Delta_i) \frac{Q_1}{n-a}}. \tag{6.31}$$

Then, the Bootstrap test statistic for hypothesis testing problem (6.29) is

$$T_{2B}^* = \sum_{i=2}^{d} \frac{Q_{iB}}{c_2 \Delta_i + (1 - \Delta_i) \frac{Q_{1B}}{n-a}}. \tag{6.32}$$

where $Q_{1B} \sim (q_1/(n-a)) \chi_{n-a}^2$ and $Q_{iB} \sim (c_2 \Delta_i + (1 - \Delta_i) q_1/(n-a)) \chi_{r_i}^2$, $i = 2, 3, \cdots, d$. Then, the Bootstrap $p$-value is computed by $T_{2B}^*$ in (6.32) as

$$p_{T_2} = P\left(T_{2B}^* > t_2^* | H_0\right), \tag{6.33}$$

where $t_2^*$ denotes the observed value of $T_2^*$. The null hypothesis $H_0$ in (6.29) is rejected whenever $p_{T_2}$ is less than the nominal significance level of $\beta$.

**Remark 6.11.** *If $n_1 = n_2 = \cdots = n_a = b$, then $T_{2B}^*$ in (6.32) degenerates into the result given by Ye and Qi (2022).*

**Remark 6.12.** *Based on $T_{2B}^*$ in (6.32), the Bootstrap pivot quantity of $\sigma_A^2 + \sigma_e^2$ can be constructed as*

$$\tilde{T}_{2B}^* = \sum_{i=2}^{d} \frac{\tilde{Q}_{iB}}{\left(\tilde{\sigma}_A^2 + \tilde{\sigma}_e^2\right) \Delta_i + (1 - \Delta_i) \frac{\tilde{Q}_{1B}}{n-a}}, \tag{6.34}$$

*where $\tilde{\sigma}_e^2 = q_1/(n-a)$. Let $\tilde{T}_{2B}^*(\gamma)$ be the $100\gamma$ empirical percentile of $\tilde{T}_{2B}^*$. Similar to Remark 6.6, the approximate $1 - \beta$ Bootstrap confidence interval for $\sigma_A^2 + \sigma_e^2$ is given by*

$$\left[ \frac{\sum_{i=2}^{d} q_i}{\tilde{T}_{2B}^*\left(1 - \frac{\beta}{2}\right)\bar{\Delta}} - \frac{(1 - \bar{\Delta}) q_1}{(n-a)\bar{\Delta}}, \frac{\sum_{i=2}^{d} q_i}{\tilde{T}_{2B}^*\left(\frac{\beta}{2}\right)\bar{\Delta}} - \frac{(1 - \bar{\Delta}) q_1}{(n-a)\bar{\Delta}} \right].$$

### 6.3.2.2  *Generalized approach*

Let $R_* = \dfrac{1}{\sigma_e^2 + \bar{\Delta}\sigma_A^2} \sum\limits_{i=2}^{d} Q_i$. For the hypothesis testing problem (6.29), we define

$$
\begin{aligned}
F_2 &= \left( \frac{\sum\limits_{i=2}^{d} q_i}{\bar{\Delta}} \frac{1}{R_*} + \frac{q_1}{\bar{\Delta}} \frac{\bar{\Delta}-1}{R_1} \right) - \left( \sigma_A^2 + \sigma_e^2 \right) \\[2ex]
&\overset{asy}{\sim} \left( \frac{\sum\limits_{i=2}^{d} q_i}{\bar{\Delta}} \frac{1}{\chi_{a-1}^2} + \frac{q_1}{\bar{\Delta}} \frac{\bar{\Delta}-1}{\chi_{n-a}^2} \right) - \left( \sigma_A^2 + \sigma_e^2 \right).
\end{aligned}
\tag{6.35}
$$

Obviously, the observed value of $F_2$ is $f_2 = 0$. From the second expression in (6.35), the approximate distribution of $F_2$ is free of nuisance parameters. By (6.35), $F_2$ is stochastically decreasing in $\sigma_A^2 + \sigma_e^2$. Therefore, $F_2$ is an approximate generalized test variable for hypothesis testing problem (6.29). Based on $F_2$ in (6.35), the generalized $p$-value is given by

$$
\begin{aligned}
p_{F_2} = P\left(F_2 \le f_2 | H_0\right) &= P\left( \frac{1}{R_*} \le \frac{c_2\bar{\Delta} - \dfrac{q_1\left(\bar{\Delta}-1\right)}{R_1}}{\sum\limits_{i=2}^{d} q_i} \right) \\[2ex]
&= E_{R_1}\left[ F_{I\Gamma\left(\frac{a-1}{2},\frac{1}{2}\right)}\left( \frac{c_2\bar{\Delta} - \dfrac{q_1\left(\bar{\Delta}-1\right)}{R_1}}{\sum\limits_{i=2}^{d} q_i} \right) \right].
\end{aligned}
\tag{6.36}
$$

The null hypothesis $H_0$ in (6.29) will be rejected if $p_{F_2}$ is less than the nominal significance level of $\beta$.

Apparently, under the scale transformations

$$
\begin{aligned}
\left( \sigma_e^2, \sigma_A^2 \right) &\to \left( k\sigma_e^2, k\sigma_A^2 \right), \\
\left( Q_1, Q_2, \cdots, Q_d \right) &\to \left( kQ_1, kQ_2, \cdots, kQ_d \right), k > 0,
\end{aligned}
\tag{6.37}
$$

both the approximate generalized test variable $F_2$ and hypothesis testing problem (6.29) are not invariant. Therefore, consider the equivalent hypothesis

$$
H_0 : \xi \le \xi_2 \quad versus \quad H_1 : \xi > \xi_2,
\tag{6.38}
$$

where $\xi = (\sigma_A^2 + \sigma_e^2)/q_1$ and $\xi_2 = c_2/q_1$. Then, we obtain

$$F_{2G} = \left( \frac{\sum\limits_{i=2}^{d} q_i}{\bar{\Delta} q_1} \frac{1}{R_*} + \frac{\bar{\Delta}-1}{\bar{\Delta}} \frac{1}{R_1} \right) - \xi. \tag{6.39}$$

It is easy to check that $F_{2G}$ is an approximate generalized test variable for the hypothesis testing problem (6.38). The corresponding generalized $p$-value is

$$\tilde{p}_{F_{2G}} = E_{R_1} \left[ F_{I\Gamma(\frac{a-1}{2}, \frac{1}{2})} \left( \frac{\xi_2 \bar{\Delta} - \frac{\bar{\Delta}-1}{R_1}}{\sum\limits_{i=2}^{d} \frac{q_i}{q_1}} \right) \right]. \tag{6.40}$$

By the following scale transformations

$$
\begin{aligned}
\left( \sigma_e^2, \xi \right) &\rightarrow \left( k\sigma_e^2, \xi \right), \\
(Q_1, Q_2, \cdots, Q_d) &\rightarrow (kQ_1, kQ_2, \cdots, kQ_d), k > 0,
\end{aligned} \tag{6.41}
$$

the approximate generalized test variable $F_{2G}$ and hypothesis testing problem (6.38) are both invariant. Accordingly, for hypothesis testing problem (6.38), the test based on $\tilde{p}_{F_{2G}}$ is $p$-invariant under the scale transformations (6.41).

**Remark 6.13.** *If $n_1 = n_2 = \cdots = n_a = b$, then $F_2$ in (6.35) degenerates into the result given by Ye and Qi (2022).*

To obtain the generalized confidence interval of $\sigma_A^2 + \sigma_e^2$, we define

$$F_2^* = \frac{\sum\limits_{i=2}^{d} q_i}{\bar{\Delta}} \frac{\sigma_e^2 + \bar{\Delta}\sigma_A^2}{\sum\limits_{i=2}^{d} Q_i} + \frac{q_1}{\bar{\Delta}} \frac{(\bar{\Delta}-1)\sigma_e^2}{Q_1}. \tag{6.42}$$

Apparently, the observed value of $F_2^*$ is $\sigma_A^2 + \sigma_e^2$, and the approximate distribution of $F_2^*$ is free of any unknown parameters. Thus, $F_2^*$ is an approximate generalized pivot quantity. Then, at the confidence level of $1 - \beta$, the approximate generalized lower confidence limit and upper confidence limit of $\sigma_A^2 + \sigma_e^2$ are constructed as $F_2^* (\beta/2)$ and $F_2^* (1 - \beta/2)$, respectively.

**Theorem 6.10.** *If $n_1 = n_2 = \cdots = n_a = b$, then*

$$\lim_{\sigma_e^2 \to 0} P\left( F_2^*\left(\frac{\beta}{2}\right) \leq \sigma_A^2 + \sigma_e^2 \leq F_2^*\left(1 - \frac{\beta}{2}\right) \right) = 1 - \beta,$$

$$\lim_{\sigma_A^2 \to 0, b \to \infty} P\left( F_2^*\left(\frac{\beta}{2}\right) \leq \sigma_A^2 + \sigma_e^2 \leq F_2^*\left(1 - \frac{\beta}{2}\right) \right) = 1 - \beta,$$

$$\lim_{\sigma_e^2 \to 0, b \to \infty} P\left( F_2^*\left(\frac{\beta}{2}\right) \leq \sigma_A^2 + \sigma_e^2 \leq F_2^*\left(1 - \frac{\beta}{2}\right) \right) = 1 - \beta.$$

Similar to Theorem 6.9, it is easy to get the above results, so the proof is omitted.

**Remark 6.14.** *If $n_1 = n_2 = \cdots = n_a = b$, then the generalized confidence interval $[F_2^*(\beta/2), F_2^*(1 - \beta/2)]$ degenerates into the result given by Ye and Qi (2022).*

### 6.3.3 Inference on the ratio of variance components

We consider the one-sided hypothesis of the ratio of variance components in model (6.2) as

$$H_0 : \frac{\sigma_A^2}{\sigma_e^2} \leq c_3 \quad versus \quad H_1 : \frac{\sigma_A^2}{\sigma_e^2} > c_3, \tag{6.43}$$

where $c_3$ is a specified value.

For hypothesis testing problem (6.43), the test statistic is defined as

$$T_3 = \frac{\dfrac{\sum\limits_{i=2}^{d} \frac{Q_i}{1 + c_3 \Delta_i}}{a - 1}}{\dfrac{Q_1}{n - a}} \sim F_{a-1, n-a}, \tag{6.44}$$

where $F_{a-1, n-a}$ denotes the $F$ distribution with degrees of freedom $a - 1$ and $n - a$. Then, the $p$-value is computed by $T_3$ in (6.44) as

$$p_{T_3} = P\left(T_3 > t_3 \,|\, H_0\right), \tag{6.45}$$

where $t_3$ denotes the observed value of $T_3$. The null hypothesis $H_0$ in (6.43) is rejected whenever $p_{T_3}$ is less than the nominal significance level of $\beta$.

**Remark 6.15.** *The pivot quantity $\sigma_A^2/\sigma_e^2$ can be constructed based on $T_3$ in (6.44). Similar to Remark 6.6, the approximate $1 - \beta$ confidence interval for $\sigma_A^2/\sigma_e^2$ is*

$$\left[ \frac{\sum\limits_{i=2}^{d} q_i}{\frac{a-1}{n-a} \bar{\Delta} q_1 F_{a-1, n-a}\left(1 - \frac{\beta}{2}\right)} - \frac{1}{\bar{\Delta}}, \; \frac{\sum\limits_{i=2}^{d} q_i}{\frac{a-1}{n-a} \bar{\Delta} q_1 F_{a-1, n-a}\left(\frac{\beta}{2}\right)} - \frac{1}{\bar{\Delta}} \right]. \tag{6.46}$$

## 6.4 Monte Carlo simulation

In this section, the sizes and powers of the above testing approaches are studied from the numerical perspective by the Monte Carlo simulation. For convenience, we only provide the steps of the Bootstrap approach for hypothesis testing problem (6.10) as follows.

**Step 1:** For a given $\left((n_1, n_2, \ldots, n_a), \sigma_A^2, \sigma_e^2, \lambda_1\right)$, generate $y \sim SN_n\left(0, \Sigma_Y, \lambda_2\right)$, then $q_0 = y' R' 1_a 1_a' R y$ and $q_i = y' H P_i P_i' H' y$, $i = 1, 2, \cdots, d$.

**Step 2:** Compute $T_0^*$ in (6.13) and denote it as $t_0^*$.

**Step 3:** Generate $Q_{0B} \sim \left\{ a \left[ \frac{1}{(a-1)\bar{\Delta}} \sum_{i=2}^{d} q_i + \left( \frac{1}{a}\sum_{i=1}^{a} \frac{1}{n_i} - \frac{1}{\Delta} \right) q_1 / (n-a) \right] \right\} \chi_1^2$, $Q_{1B} \sim (q_1 / (n-a)) \chi_{n-a}^2$, and $\sum_{i=2}^{d} Q_{iB} \overset{asy}{\sim} \left( \frac{1}{a-1} \sum_{i=2}^{d} q_i \right) \chi_{a-1}^2$. Further, $T_{0B}^*$ is computed by (6.14).

**Step 4:** Repeat Step 3 $k_1$ times and compute $p_{T_0}$ by (6.15). If $p_{T_0} \le \beta$, then $l = 1$. Otherwise, $l = 0$.

**Step 5:** Repeat Steps 1–4 $k_2$ times and get $l_1, l_2, \cdots, l_{k_2}$. Then the size is $\sum_{i=1}^{k_2} l_i / k_2$.

Based on the above steps, the power of the hypothesis testing problem (6.10) under $H_1$ can be obtained similarly.

In simulation, let the nominal significance levels $\beta = 0.025, 0.05, 0.075, 0.1$, and the number of inner loops $k_1$ and outer loops $k_2$ both be 2500. Then, we give five settings of sample size: $N_1 = (n_1, n_2) = (5, 6)$, $N_2 = (n_1, n_2, n_3) = (6, 8, 10)$, $N_3 = (n_1, n_2, n_3, n_4) = (9, 12, 15, 18)$, $N_4 = (n_1, n_2, n_3, n_4, n_5) = (16, 20, 24, 28, 32)$, and $N_5 = (n_1, n_2, n_3, n_4, n_5, n_6) = (30, 35, 40, 45, 50, 55)$. The parameters are set in Table 6.1.

**Table 6.1:** Settings of parameters.

| Testing problem | Size | Power |
|---|---|---|
| (6.10) | $\sigma_e^2 = 0.5, \lambda_1 = 1_a,$ $\sigma_A^2 = 0.6, 0.8, 1, 1.5, 2$ | $\sigma_e^2 = 0.5, \sigma_A^2 = 0.6, \lambda_1 = 1_a,$ $\mu = 0.2, 0.4, 0.6, 0.8, 1$ |
| (6.16) | $c_1 = 3, \lambda_1 = 1_a, \mu = 1,$ $\sigma_e^2 = 0.5, 1, 2, 3, 4$ | $c_1 = 3, \sigma_e^2 = 1, \lambda_1 = 1_a, \mu = 1,$ $\sigma_A^2 = 5, 10, 15, 20, 25$ |
| (6.29) | $c_2 = 5, \lambda_1 = 1_a, \mu = 1,$ $\sigma_e^2 = 0.3, 0.5, 1, 1.5, 2$ | $c_2 = 5, \sigma_e^2 = 2, \lambda_1 = 1_a, \mu = 1,$ $\sigma_A^2 = 5, 10, 15, 20, 25$ |
| (6.43) | $c_3 = \sigma_A^2 / \sigma_e^2, \sigma_e^2 = 0.5, \lambda_1 = 1_a, \mu = 1,$ $\sigma_A^2 = 1, 2, 3, 4, 5$ | $c_3 = 3, \sigma_e^2 = 0.5, \lambda_1 = 1_a, \mu = 1,$ $\sigma_A^2 = 3, 5, 7, 10, 15$ |

**Table 6.2:** Sizes for testing problem (6.10) ($\sigma_e^2 = 0.5$).

| Sample size | $\sigma_A^2$ | $\beta$ | | | |
|---|---|---|---|---|---|
| | | 0.025 | 0.05 | 0.075 | 0.1 |
| | | BA | BA | BA | BA |
| $N_1$ | 0.6 | 0.0232 | 0.0460 | 0.0716 | 0.0988 |
| | 0.8 | 0.0244 | 0.0484 | 0.0748 | 0.0980 |
| | 1.0 | 0.0248 | 0.0512 | 0.0772 | 0.0976 |
| | 1.5 | 0.0268 | 0.0552 | 0.0792 | 0.1016 |
| | 2.0 | 0.0324 | 0.0568 | 0.0816 | 0.1012 |
| $N_2$ | 0.6 | 0.0368 | 0.0592 | 0.0860 | 0.1084 |
| | 0.8 | 0.0376 | 0.0580 | 0.0824 | 0.1052 |
| | 1.0 | 0.0368 | 0.0592 | 0.0824 | 0.1044 |
| | 1.5 | 0.0336 | 0.0580 | 0.0796 | 0.1008 |
| | 2.0 | 0.0344 | 0.0572 | 0.0808 | 0.1024 |
| $N_3$ | 0.6 | 0.0312 | 0.0536 | 0.0760 | 0.1020 |
| | 0.8 | 0.0292 | 0.0532 | 0.0736 | 0.1000 |
| | 1.0 | 0.0280 | 0.0504 | 0.0748 | 0.1000 |
| | 1.5 | 0.0244 | 0.0472 | 0.0712 | 0.0952 |
| | 2.0 | 0.0240 | 0.0460 | 0.0708 | 0.0948 |
| $N_4$ | 0.6 | 0.0244 | 0.0508 | 0.0784 | 0.1016 |
| | 0.8 | 0.0224 | 0.0492 | 0.0772 | 0.1040 |
| | 1.0 | 0.0220 | 0.0508 | 0.0764 | 0.1004 |
| | 1.5 | 0.0256 | 0.0496 | 0.0752 | 0.1012 |
| | 2.0 | 0.0284 | 0.0524 | 0.0756 | 0.0964 |
| $N_5$ | 0.6 | 0.0224 | 0.0476 | 0.0752 | 0.0952 |
| | 0.8 | 0.0224 | 0.0496 | 0.0728 | 0.0952 |
| | 1.0 | 0.0236 | 0.0484 | 0.0708 | 0.0980 |
| | 1.5 | 0.0232 | 0.0456 | 0.0716 | 0.0968 |
| | 2.0 | 0.0232 | 0.0440 | 0.0720 | 0.0944 |

*Note:* $N_1 = (n_1, n_2) = (5, 6)$, $N_2 = (n_1, n_2, n_3) = (6, 8, 10)$, $N_3 = (n_1, n_2, n_3, n_4) = (9, 12, 15, 18)$, $N_4 = (n_1, n_2, n_3, n_4, n_5) = (16, 20, 24, 28, 32)$, $N_5 = (n_1, n_2, n_3, n_4, n_5, n_6) = (30, 35, 40, 45, 50, 55)$.

For hypothesis testing problem (6.10), Tables 6.2–6.3 present the simulated sizes and powers of the Bootstrap approach (BA) under the various nominal significance levels. As in Table 6.2, the empirical sizes are close to the various nominal significance levels, but they are slightly liberal for the small samples. From Table 6.3, in cases where $\mu$ departs from the null hypothesis, the powers of the BAs increase significantly with the sample size enlarging.

For the hypothesis testing problem (6.16), Tables 6.4–6.5 present the simulated sizes and powers of the BA and generalized approach (GA) under various nominal significance levels. By Table 6.4, both approaches are satisfactory in controlling the sizes in most cases. The results of Table 6.5 indicate that the BA is uniformly better than the GA for the above parameter configurations, sample size and nominal significance levels in terms of the power.

**Table 6.3:** Powers for testing problem (6.10) ($\sigma_A^2 = 0.6, \sigma_e^2 = 0.5$).

| | | $\beta$ | | | |
| | | 0.025 | 0.05 | 0.075 | 0.1 |
| Sample size | $\mu$ | BA | BA | BA | BA |
|---|---|---|---|---|---|
| $N_1$ | 0.2 | 0.0312 | 0.0640 | 0.0972 | 0.1348 |
| | 0.4 | 0.0416 | 0.0868 | 0.1304 | 0.1760 |
| | 0.6 | 0.0536 | 0.1056 | 0.1624 | 0.2140 |
| | 0.8 | 0.0624 | 0.1264 | 0.1956 | 0.2528 |
| | 1.0 | 0.0732 | 0.1464 | 0.2256 | 0.2964 |
| $N_2$ | 0.2 | 0.0660 | 0.1040 | 0.1420 | 0.1832 |
| | 0.4 | 0.0988 | 0.1604 | 0.2208 | 0.2800 |
| | 0.6 | 0.1372 | 0.2292 | 0.3132 | 0.3868 |
| | 0.8 | 0.1860 | 0.3048 | 0.4048 | 0.4948 |
| | 1.0 | 0.2392 | 0.3748 | 0.4936 | 0.6000 |
| $N_3$ | 0.2 | 0.0652 | 0.1104 | 0.1688 | 0.2168 |
| | 0.4 | 0.1212 | 0.2120 | 0.2988 | 0.3732 |
| | 0.6 | 0.2028 | 0.3348 | 0.4560 | 0.5448 |
| | 0.8 | 0.2988 | 0.4752 | 0.6124 | 0.7072 |
| | 1.0 | 0.4044 | 0.6164 | 0.7432 | 0.8380 |
| $N_4$ | 0.2 | 0.0732 | 0.1344 | 0.1916 | 0.2468 |
| | 0.4 | 0.1600 | 0.2752 | 0.3764 | 0.4644 |
| | 0.6 | 0.2912 | 0.4700 | 0.6008 | 0.6932 |
| | 0.8 | 0.4580 | 0.6572 | 0.7856 | 0.8648 |
| | 1.0 | 0.6128 | 0.8160 | 0.9072 | 0.9484 |
| $N_5$ | 0.2 | 0.0816 | 0.1468 | 0.2064 | 0.2644 |
| | 0.4 | 0.1992 | 0.3368 | 0.4484 | 0.5372 |
| | 0.6 | 0.3900 | 0.5804 | 0.7076 | 0.7956 |
| | 0.8 | 0.5972 | 0.7924 | 0.8960 | 0.9432 |
| | 1.0 | 0.7740 | 0.9256 | 0.9728 | 0.9912 |

*Note:* $N_1 = (n_1, n_2) = (5, 6)$, $N_2 = (n_1, n_2, n_3) = (6, 8, 10)$, $N_3 = (n_1, n_2, n_3, n_4) = (9, 12, 15, 18)$, $N_4 = (n_1, n_2, n_3, n_4, n_5) = (16, 20, 24, 28, 32)$, $N_5 = (n_1, n_2, n_3, n_4, n_5, n_6) = (30, 35, 40, 45, 50, 55)$.

For hypothesis testing problem (6.29), Tables 6.6–6.7 present the simulated sizes and powers of the BA and GA under the different nominal significance levels. As in Table 6.6, it is clear that the actual levels of the BA are close to the nominal significance level regardless of the sample size. The GA appears to be slightly liberal, but its performance improves with the sample size increasing. Accordingly, the BA performs better than the GA in terms of the size. From Table 6.7, as $\sigma_A^2 + \sigma_e^2$ departs from the null hypothesis, the powers of two approaches are both significantly raised, but the GA is slightly better than the BA across the wide array of scenarios.

For the hypothesis testing problem (6.43), Tables 6.8–6.9 present the simulated sizes and powers of the exact testing approach under the different nominal significance levels. The results show that the exact testing approach maintains the nominal sizes quite well in all sample size settings. As $\sigma_A^2 / \sigma_e^2$ departs from the null hypothesis, the powers apparently improve with the sample size increasing.

**Table 6.4:** Sizes for testing problem (6.16) ($\sigma_A^2 = c_1 = 3$).

| | | \multicolumn{2}{c}{0.025} | | 0.05 | | 0.075 | | 0.1 | |
|---|---|---|---|---|---|---|---|---|---|
| Sample size | $\sigma_e^2$ | BA | GA | BA | GA | BA | GA | BA | GA |
| | 0.5 | 0.0304 | 0.0300 | 0.0540 | 0.0532 | 0.0732 | 0.0720 | 0.0936 | 0.0920 |
| | 1.0 | 0.0268 | 0.0260 | 0.0536 | 0.0516 | 0.0744 | 0.0732 | 0.0956 | 0.0940 |
| $N_1$ | 2.0 | 0.0256 | 0.0232 | 0.0532 | 0.0504 | 0.0732 | 0.0712 | 0.0980 | 0.0944 |
| | 3.0 | 0.0264 | 0.0224 | 0.0552 | 0.0504 | 0.0744 | 0.0692 | 0.0992 | 0.0932 |
| | 4.0 | 0.0260 | 0.0232 | 0.0528 | 0.0488 | 0.0736 | 0.0700 | 0.0972 | 0.0924 |
| | 0.5 | 0.0252 | 0.0264 | 0.0536 | 0.0476 | 0.0756 | 0.0768 | 0.0984 | 0.1004 |
| | 1.0 | 0.0276 | 0.0264 | 0.0496 | 0.0476 | 0.0744 | 0.0764 | 0.1032 | 0.1024 |
| $N_2$ | 2.0 | 0.0268 | 0.0260 | 0.0512 | 0.0484 | 0.0772 | 0.0744 | 0.1012 | 0.1060 |
| | 3.0 | 0.0260 | 0.0248 | 0.0548 | 0.0504 | 0.0768 | 0.0732 | 0.1048 | 0.1040 |
| | 4.0 | 0.0252 | 0.0240 | 0.0552 | 0.0512 | 0.0796 | 0.0732 | 0.1052 | 0.1036 |
| | 0.5 | 0.0276 | 0.0312 | 0.0556 | 0.0548 | 0.0832 | 0.0796 | 0.1092 | 0.1072 |
| | 1.0 | 0.0276 | 0.0276 | 0.0568 | 0.0572 | 0.0872 | 0.0800 | 0.1116 | 0.1060 |
| $N_3$ | 2.0 | 0.0280 | 0.0312 | 0.0572 | 0.0560 | 0.0844 | 0.0756 | 0.1060 | 0.1032 |
| | 3.0 | 0.0312 | 0.0288 | 0.0556 | 0.0544 | 0.0844 | 0.0776 | 0.1052 | 0.0996 |
| | 4.0 | 0.0292 | 0.0292 | 0.0564 | 0.0540 | 0.0804 | 0.0740 | 0.1068 | 0.1016 |
| | 0.5 | 0.0280 | 0.0264 | 0.0512 | 0.0524 | 0.0772 | 0.0744 | 0.1016 | 0.0968 |
| | 1.0 | 0.0272 | 0.0260 | 0.0528 | 0.0540 | 0.0784 | 0.0772 | 0.1012 | 0.0956 |
| $N_4$ | 2.0 | 0.0280 | 0.0288 | 0.0508 | 0.0508 | 0.0764 | 0.0736 | 0.1016 | 0.0980 |
| | 3.0 | 0.0292 | 0.0276 | 0.0492 | 0.0496 | 0.0736 | 0.0712 | 0.0992 | 0.0944 |
| | 4.0 | 0.0296 | 0.0280 | 0.0496 | 0.0500 | 0.0708 | 0.0724 | 0.0960 | 0.0968 |
| | 0.5 | 0.0216 | 0.0228 | 0.0492 | 0.0472 | 0.0776 | 0.0748 | 0.0992 | 0.1000 |
| | 1.0 | 0.0208 | 0.0240 | 0.0508 | 0.0488 | 0.0796 | 0.0772 | 0.1028 | 0.1012 |
| $N_5$ | 2.0 | 0.0216 | 0.0216 | 0.0480 | 0.0472 | 0.0784 | 0.0776 | 0.1064 | 0.1040 |
| | 3.0 | 0.0236 | 0.0256 | 0.0476 | 0.0520 | 0.0760 | 0.0768 | 0.1096 | 0.1028 |
| | 4.0 | 0.0240 | 0.0256 | 0.0448 | 0.0504 | 0.0784 | 0.0772 | 0.1084 | 0.1052 |

*Note:* $N_1 = (n_1, n_2) = (5, 6)$, $N_2 = (n_1, n_2, n_3) = (6, 8, 10)$, $N_3 = (n_1, n_2, n_3, n_4) = (9, 12, 15, 18)$, $N_4 = (n_1, n_2, n_3, n_4, n_5) = (16, 20, 24, 28, 32)$, $N_5 = (n_1, n_2, n_3, n_4, n_5, n_6) = (30, 35, 40, 45, 50, 55)$.

## 6.5   Illustrative example

To verify the reasonableness and effectiveness of the proposed approaches, an example of carbon fibers' strength is presented in this section.

Kundu and Gupta (2006) presented a data set possessing the strength of a single carbon fiber. The histogram of the data is given in Figure 6.1. It can be seen from Figure 6.1 that the data clearly exhibit skew distribution characteristics. To verify the conclusion, we first conduct the normality test for the data. It turns out that the $p$-value of Shapiro-Wilk test for the data is 0.0127. Therefore, the carbon fibers' strength data are not normally distributed at the nominal significance level of 5%.

**Table 6.5:** Powers for testing problem (6.16) ($\sigma_e^2 = 1, c_1 = 3$).

| | | | $\beta$ | | | | | | |
| | | 0.025 | | 0.05 | | 0.075 | | 0.1 | |
| Sample size | $\sigma_A^2$ | BA | GA | BA | GA | BA | GA | BA | GA |
|---|---|---|---|---|---|---|---|---|---|
| | 5.0 | 0.0752 | 0.0736 | 0.1164 | 0.1148 | 0.1496 | 0.1468 | 0.1872 | 0.1840 |
| | 10.0 | 0.2012 | 0.1968 | 0.2672 | 0.2652 | 0.3152 | 0.3108 | 0.3580 | 0.3516 |
| $N_1$ | 15.0 | 0.3040 | 0.2996 | 0.3716 | 0.3688 | 0.4220 | 0.4200 | 0.4556 | 0.4532 |
| | 20.0 | 0.3796 | 0.3756 | 0.4404 | 0.4384 | 0.4844 | 0.4832 | 0.5176 | 0.5140 |
| | 25.0 | 0.4284 | 0.4244 | 0.4868 | 0.4864 | 0.5332 | 0.5304 | 0.5656 | 0.5624 |
| | 5.0 | 0.1052 | 0.1028 | 0.1596 | 0.1572 | 0.2024 | 0.1980 | 0.2444 | 0.2404 |
| | 10.0 | 0.3140 | 0.3096 | 0.3972 | 0.3872 | 0.4532 | 0.4448 | 0.4904 | 0.4912 |
| $N_2$ | 15.0 | 0.4696 | 0.4604 | 0.5364 | 0.5328 | 0.5856 | 0.5852 | 0.6200 | 0.6196 |
| | 20.0 | 0.5640 | 0.5580 | 0.6276 | 0.6228 | 0.6688 | 0.6644 | 0.6976 | 0.6940 |
| | 25.0 | 0.6316 | 0.6268 | 0.6876 | 0.6816 | 0.7240 | 0.7188 | 0.7528 | 0.7480 |
| | 5.0 | 0.1372 | 0.1284 | 0.2016 | 0.1932 | 0.2524 | 0.2452 | 0.2944 | 0.2868 |
| | 10.0 | 0.4252 | 0.4180 | 0.5136 | 0.5008 | 0.5660 | 0.5588 | 0.6016 | 0.5960 |
| $N_3$ | 15.0 | 0.6064 | 0.5948 | 0.6624 | 0.6580 | 0.7020 | 0.6968 | 0.7368 | 0.7284 |
| | 20.0 | 0.6968 | 0.6864 | 0.7488 | 0.7420 | 0.7848 | 0.7732 | 0.8112 | 0.8012 |
| | 25.0 | 0.7624 | 0.7520 | 0.8088 | 0.7968 | 0.8436 | 0.8328 | 0.8632 | 0.8552 |
| | 5.0 | 0.1500 | 0.1412 | 0.2160 | 0.2096 | 0.2744 | 0.2680 | 0.3168 | 0.3140 |
| | 10.0 | 0.4924 | 0.4764 | 0.5772 | 0.5612 | 0.6244 | 0.6168 | 0.6632 | 0.6560 |
| $N_4$ | 15.0 | 0.6812 | 0.6700 | 0.7420 | 0.7368 | 0.7812 | 0.7744 | 0.8068 | 0.8016 |
| | 20.0 | 0.7800 | 0.7744 | 0.8312 | 0.8208 | 0.8584 | 0.8492 | 0.8720 | 0.8692 |
| | 25.0 | 0.8460 | 0.8364 | 0.8764 | 0.8732 | 0.8992 | 0.8960 | 0.9128 | 0.9092 |
| | 5.0 | 0.1804 | 0.1784 | 0.2500 | 0.2428 | 0.3124 | 0.3028 | 0.3604 | 0.3512 |
| | 10.0 | 0.5756 | 0.5596 | 0.6452 | 0.6440 | 0.7056 | 0.6912 | 0.7420 | 0.7276 |
| $N_5$ | 15.0 | 0.7676 | 0.7568 | 0.8192 | 0.8144 | 0.8564 | 0.8496 | 0.8768 | 0.8700 |
| | 20.0 | 0.8640 | 0.8580 | 0.8976 | 0.8952 | 0.9168 | 0.9148 | 0.9268 | 0.9232 |
| | 25.0 | 0.9140 | 0.9060 | 0.9340 | 0.9304 | 0.9452 | 0.9444 | 0.9524 | 0.9532 |

*Note:* $N_1 = (n_1, n_2) = (5, 6)$, $N_2 = (n_1, n_2, n_3) = (6, 8, 10)$, $N_3 = (n_1, n_2, n_3, n_4) = (9, 12, 15, 18)$, $N_4 = (n_1, n_2, n_3, n_4, n_5) = (16, 20, 24, 28, 32)$, $N_5 = (n_1, n_2, n_3, n_4, n_5, n_6) = (30, 35, 40, 45, 50, 55)$.

In addition, we should prove whether the distribution of the data is skew-normal by the chi-square goodness-of-fit test. Namely, set $H_0$: the carbon fibers' strength data are skew-normally distributed. By calculation, the fitted value of the data is $\chi^2 = 1.7521 < \chi_3^2(0.95) = 7.8147$ with $p$-value 0.6254. Consequently, the null hypothesis $H_0$ is not rejected at the nominal significance level of 5%. That is, the carbon fibers' strength data can be considered to follow the skew-normal distribution. Based on the method of moment estimation, the data are distributed as $SN\left(2.1180, 0.9140^2, 2.8797\right)$ whose density curve is given in Figure 6.1.

**Table 6.6:** Sizes for testing problem (6.29) ($\sigma_A^2 + \sigma_e^2 = c_2 = 5$).

| | | $\beta$ | | | | | | | |
| | | 0.025 | | 0.05 | | 0.075 | | 0.1 | |
| Sample size | $\sigma_e^2$ | BA | GA | BA | GA | BA | GA | BA | GA |
|---|---|---|---|---|---|---|---|---|---|
| | 0.3 | 0.0292 | 0.0288 | 0.0500 | 0.0536 | 0.0736 | 0.0760 | 0.0956 | 0.0976 |
| | 0.5 | 0.0300 | 0.0300 | 0.0524 | 0.0544 | 0.0752 | 0.0784 | 0.0960 | 0.1024 |
| $N_1$ | 1.0 | 0.0284 | 0.0348 | 0.0540 | 0.0600 | 0.0752 | 0.0824 | 0.0940 | 0.1052 |
| | 1.5 | 0.0220 | 0.0360 | 0.0512 | 0.0628 | 0.0740 | 0.0896 | 0.0928 | 0.1108 |
| | 2.0 | 0.0176 | 0.0364 | 0.0516 | 0.0700 | 0.0780 | 0.0944 | 0.1004 | 0.1224 |
| | 0.3 | 0.0264 | 0.0260 | 0.0508 | 0.0504 | 0.0752 | 0.0780 | 0.0984 | 0.0988 |
| | 0.5 | 0.0248 | 0.0264 | 0.0504 | 0.0528 | 0.0764 | 0.0808 | 0.0976 | 0.1004 |
| $N_2$ | 1.0 | 0.0256 | 0.0284 | 0.0488 | 0.0520 | 0.0740 | 0.0848 | 0.1004 | 0.1088 |
| | 1.5 | 0.0244 | 0.0276 | 0.0456 | 0.0568 | 0.0732 | 0.0844 | 0.0964 | 0.1152 |
| | 2.0 | 0.0184 | 0.0284 | 0.0436 | 0.0620 | 0.0676 | 0.0864 | 0.0912 | 0.1220 |
| | 0.3 | 0.0308 | 0.0340 | 0.0580 | 0.0576 | 0.0824 | 0.0808 | 0.1088 | 0.1112 |
| | 0.5 | 0.0288 | 0.0328 | 0.0564 | 0.0584 | 0.0828 | 0.0824 | 0.1084 | 0.1112 |
| $N_3$ | 1.0 | 0.0276 | 0.0316 | 0.0540 | 0.0632 | 0.0840 | 0.0852 | 0.1076 | 0.1108 |
| | 1.5 | 0.0284 | 0.0324 | 0.0548 | 0.0604 | 0.0828 | 0.0852 | 0.1056 | 0.1120 |
| | 2.0 | 0.0260 | 0.0352 | 0.0516 | 0.0616 | 0.0796 | 0.0872 | 0.0996 | 0.1172 |
| | 0.3 | 0.0240 | 0.0304 | 0.0532 | 0.0512 | 0.0748 | 0.0780 | 0.0984 | 0.1004 |
| | 0.5 | 0.0248 | 0.0300 | 0.0524 | 0.0556 | 0.0760 | 0.0772 | 0.1008 | 0.0996 |
| $N_4$ | 1.0 | 0.0272 | 0.0300 | 0.0504 | 0.0588 | 0.0768 | 0.0816 | 0.0996 | 0.0980 |
| | 1.5 | 0.0256 | 0.0308 | 0.0500 | 0.0564 | 0.0760 | 0.0816 | 0.0988 | 0.1028 |
| | 2.0 | 0.0268 | 0.0312 | 0.0476 | 0.0548 | 0.0756 | 0.0812 | 0.0968 | 0.1072 |
| | 0.3 | 0.0220 | 0.0264 | 0.0516 | 0.0480 | 0.0736 | 0.0748 | 0.1032 | 0.0976 |
| | 0.5 | 0.0232 | 0.0260 | 0.0504 | 0.0492 | 0.0728 | 0.0740 | 0.1004 | 0.1024 |
| $N_5$ | 1.0 | 0.0212 | 0.0248 | 0.0480 | 0.0508 | 0.0768 | 0.0804 | 0.1052 | 0.1072 |
| | 1.5 | 0.0220 | 0.0260 | 0.0496 | 0.0512 | 0.0808 | 0.0800 | 0.1036 | 0.1100 |
| | 2.0 | 0.0232 | 0.0260 | 0.0464 | 0.0532 | 0.0796 | 0.0844 | 0.1084 | 0.1124 |

*Note:* $N_1 = (n_1, n_2) = (5, 6)$, $N_2 = (n_1, n_2, n_3) = (6, 8, 10)$, $N_3 = (n_1, n_2, n_3, n_4) = (9, 12, 15, 18)$, $N_4 = (n_1, n_2, n_3, n_4, n_5) = (16, 20, 24, 28, 32)$, $N_5 = (n_1, n_2, n_3, n_4, n_5, n_6) = (30, 35, 40, 45, 50, 55)$.

Then, the model for the carbon fibers' strength data is written as (6.2), where $Y$ is the 123-vector of all measurements, $A \sim SN_2\left(0, \sigma_A^2 I_2, \lambda_1\right)$, $e \sim N_{123}\left(0, \sigma_e^2 I_{123}\right)$, and $A$ and $e$ are mutually independent.

First, consider the hypothesis testing problem for the fixed effect

$$H_0 : \mu \leq 2.5 \quad versus \quad H_1 : \mu > 2.5. \tag{6.47}$$

Based on (6.15), the Bootstrap $p$-value is 0.4839 by $10^4$ loops. Thus, at the nominal significance level of 5%, this approach cannot reject the null hypothesis $H_0$ in (6.47).

**Table 6.7:** Powers for testing problem (6.29) ($\sigma_e^2 = 2, c_2 = 5$).

| Sample size | $\sigma_A^2$ | $\beta$ 0.025 BA | GA | 0.05 BA | GA | 0.075 BA | GA | 0.1 BA | GA |
|---|---|---|---|---|---|---|---|---|---|
| $N_1$ | 5.0 | 0.0608 | 0.0880 | 0.1064 | 0.1312 | 0.1432 | 0.1824 | 0.1848 | 0.2164 |
|  | 10.0 | 0.1616 | 0.2048 | 0.2408 | 0.2788 | 0.2944 | 0.3324 | 0.3384 | 0.3772 |
|  | 15.0 | 0.2528 | 0.3024 | 0.3392 | 0.3772 | 0.3952 | 0.4332 | 0.4428 | 0.4780 |
|  | 20.0 | 0.3256 | 0.3768 | 0.4128 | 0.4512 | 0.4676 | 0.4980 | 0.5072 | 0.5388 |
|  | 25.0 | 0.3868 | 0.4328 | 0.4676 | 0.4964 | 0.5144 | 0.5464 | 0.5520 | 0.5776 |
| $N_2$ | 5.0 | 0.0836 | 0.1172 | 0.1440 | 0.1740 | 0.1908 | 0.2252 | 0.2384 | 0.2648 |
|  | 10.0 | 0.2728 | 0.3224 | 0.3608 | 0.4000 | 0.4184 | 0.4516 | 0.4712 | 0.4968 |
|  | 15.0 | 0.4196 | 0.4616 | 0.5124 | 0.5364 | 0.5640 | 0.5880 | 0.5976 | 0.6260 |
|  | 20.0 | 0.5228 | 0.5616 | 0.5984 | 0.6272 | 0.6440 | 0.6716 | 0.6796 | 0.7012 |
|  | 25.0 | 0.5920 | 0.6232 | 0.6608 | 0.6892 | 0.7060 | 0.7244 | 0.7380 | 0.7508 |
| $N_3$ | 5.0 | 0.1272 | 0.1408 | 0.1884 | 0.2072 | 0.2444 | 0.2548 | 0.2940 | 0.3028 |
|  | 10.0 | 0.4012 | 0.4184 | 0.4872 | 0.5096 | 0.5424 | 0.5620 | 0.5896 | 0.6016 |
|  | 15.0 | 0.5824 | 0.5944 | 0.6524 | 0.6588 | 0.6948 | 0.6984 | 0.7264 | 0.7344 |
|  | 20.0 | 0.6836 | 0.6900 | 0.7380 | 0.7484 | 0.7772 | 0.7808 | 0.8028 | 0.8084 |
|  | 25.0 | 0.7460 | 0.7560 | 0.7988 | 0.8060 | 0.8328 | 0.8356 | 0.8544 | 0.8544 |
| $N_4$ | 5.0 | 0.1376 | 0.1492 | 0.2072 | 0.2148 | 0.2636 | 0.2780 | 0.3128 | 0.3216 |
|  | 10.0 | 0.4804 | 0.4860 | 0.5680 | 0.5680 | 0.6168 | 0.6248 | 0.6604 | 0.6644 |
|  | 15.0 | 0.6784 | 0.6776 | 0.7384 | 0.7420 | 0.7736 | 0.7764 | 0.7976 | 0.7996 |
|  | 20.0 | 0.7772 | 0.7760 | 0.8228 | 0.8228 | 0.8540 | 0.8496 | 0.8692 | 0.8692 |
|  | 25.0 | 0.8376 | 0.8392 | 0.8716 | 0.8712 | 0.8944 | 0.8956 | 0.9100 | 0.9100 |
| $N_5$ | 5.0 | 0.1740 | 0.1860 | 0.2452 | 0.2496 | 0.3104 | 0.3116 | 0.3544 | 0.3564 |
|  | 10.0 | 0.5688 | 0.5704 | 0.6464 | 0.6516 | 0.6980 | 0.6980 | 0.7360 | 0.7332 |
|  | 15.0 | 0.7644 | 0.7600 | 0.8160 | 0.8152 | 0.8468 | 0.8468 | 0.8708 | 0.8660 |
|  | 20.0 | 0.8624 | 0.8568 | 0.8948 | 0.8904 | 0.9104 | 0.9096 | 0.9228 | 0.9224 |
|  | 25.0 | 0.9064 | 0.9064 | 0.9312 | 0.9312 | 0.9436 | 0.9424 | 0.9496 | 0.9500 |

*Note:* $N_1 = (n_1, n_2) = (5, 6)$, $N_2 = (n_1, n_2, n_3) = (6, 8, 10)$, $N_3 = (n_1, n_2, n_3, n_4) = (9, 12, 15, 18)$, $N_4 = (n_1, n_2, n_3, n_4, n_5) = (16, 20, 24, 28, 32)$, $N_5 = (n_1, n_2, n_3, n_4, n_5, n_6) = (30, 35, 40, 45, 50, 55)$.

Secondly, consider the hypothesis testing problem for the single variance component

$$H_0 : \sigma_A^2 \leq 0.03 \quad versus \quad H_1 : \sigma_A^2 > 0.03 \tag{6.48}$$

The Bootstrap $p$-value based on (6.20) is 0.0274, and the generalized $p$-value based on (6.23) is 0.0276. Consequently, the null hypothesis $H_0$ in (6.48) is rejected by the two approaches at the nominal significance level of 5%.

Next, consider the hypothesis testing problem for the sum of variance components

$$H_0 : \sigma_A^2 + \sigma_e^2 \leq 0.5 \quad versus \quad H_1 : \sigma_A^2 + \sigma_e^2 > 0.5 \tag{6.49}$$

The Bootstrap $p$-value based on (6.33) is 0.3895, and the generalized $p$-value based on (6.36) is 0.3641. Therefore, at the nominal significance level of 5%, these two approaches cannot reject the null hypothesis $H_0$ in (6.49).

**Table 6.8:** Sizes for testing problem (6.43) ($\sigma_e^2 = 0.5, c_3 = \sigma_A^2/\sigma_e^2$).

| | | $\beta$ | | | |
|---|---|---|---|---|---|
| Sample size | $\sigma_A^2$ | 0.025 | 0.05 | 0.075 | 0.1 |
| | 1.0 | 0.0244 | 0.0564 | 0.0760 | 0.1020 |
| | 2.0 | 0.0252 | 0.0536 | 0.0768 | 0.0984 |
| $N_1$ | 3.0 | 0.0252 | 0.0484 | 0.0752 | 0.1012 |
| | 4.0 | 0.0224 | 0.0460 | 0.0780 | 0.0988 |
| | 5.0 | 0.0220 | 0.0464 | 0.0764 | 0.0984 |
| | 1.0 | 0.0250 | 0.0480 | 0.0740 | 0.1000 |
| | 2.0 | 0.0190 | 0.0540 | 0.0780 | 0.0980 |
| $N_2$ | 3.0 | 0.0210 | 0.0510 | 0.0710 | 0.1010 |
| | 4.0 | 0.0210 | 0.0500 | 0.0700 | 0.1010 |
| | 5.0 | 0.0210 | 0.0470 | 0.0700 | 0.1060 |
| | 1.0 | 0.0284 | 0.0596 | 0.0836 | 0.1124 |
| | 2.0 | 0.0304 | 0.0580 | 0.0848 | 0.1092 |
| $N_3$ | 3.0 | 0.0296 | 0.0604 | 0.0832 | 0.1080 |
| | 4.0 | 0.0304 | 0.0596 | 0.0828 | 0.1064 |
| | 5.0 | 0.0304 | 0.0608 | 0.0812 | 0.1064 |
| | 1.0 | 0.0272 | 0.0528 | 0.0772 | 0.1016 |
| | 2.0 | 0.0268 | 0.0480 | 0.0828 | 0.1024 |
| $N_4$ | 3.0 | 0.0268 | 0.0500 | 0.0808 | 0.1028 |
| | 4.0 | 0.0244 | 0.0496 | 0.0776 | 0.1016 |
| | 5.0 | 0.0240 | 0.0496 | 0.0776 | 0.1020 |
| | 1.0 | 0.0208 | 0.0500 | 0.0748 | 0.1036 |
| | 2.0 | 0.0220 | 0.0468 | 0.0756 | 0.0992 |
| $N_5$ | 3.0 | 0.0220 | 0.0492 | 0.0752 | 0.0996 |
| | 4.0 | 0.0224 | 0.0508 | 0.0732 | 0.0980 |
| | 5.0 | 0.0228 | 0.0512 | 0.0736 | 0.0976 |

*Note:* $N_1 = (n_1, n_2) = (5, 6)$, $N_2 = (n_1, n_2, n_3) = (6, 8, 10)$, $N_3 = (n_1, n_2, n_3, n_4) = (9, 12, 15, 18)$, $N_4 = (n_1, n_2, n_3, n_4, n_5) = (16, 20, 24, 28, 32)$, $N_5 = (n_1, n_2, n_3, n_4, n_5, n_6) = (30, 35, 40, 45, 50, 55)$.

At last, consider the hypothesis testing problem for the ratio of variance components

$$H_0 : \frac{\sigma_A^2}{\sigma_e^2} \leq 0.2 \quad versus \quad H_1 : \frac{\sigma_A^2}{\sigma_e^2} > 0.2 \tag{6.50}$$

Based on (6.44) and (6.45), $t_3 = 2.8729 < F_{1,121}(0.95) = 3.9195$ with $p$-value 0.0927. Thus, at the nominal significance level of 5%, this approach cannot reject the null hypothesis $H_0$ in (6.50).

**Table 6.9:** Powers for testing problem (6.43) ($\sigma_e^2 = 0.5, c_3 = 3$).

| Sample size | $\sigma_A^2$ | $\beta$ | | | |
| | | 0.025 | 0.05 | 0.075 | 0.1 |
|---|---|---|---|---|---|
| $N_1$ | 3.0 | 0.0876 | 0.1376 | 0.1824 | 0.2240 |
|  | 5.0 | 0.1644 | 0.2404 | 0.2940 | 0.3312 |
|  | 7.0 | 0.2376 | 0.3124 | 0.3660 | 0.4132 |
|  | 10.0 | 0.3184 | 0.3972 | 0.4540 | 0.4932 |
|  | 15.0 | 0.4124 | 0.4900 | 0.5408 | 0.5804 |
| $N_2$ | 3.0 | 0.1280 | 0.1932 | 0.2432 | 0.2880 |
|  | 5.0 | 0.2708 | 0.3504 | 0.4132 | 0.4624 |
|  | 7.0 | 0.3872 | 0.4772 | 0.5324 | 0.5760 |
|  | 10.0 | 0.5176 | 0.5948 | 0.6424 | 0.6800 |
|  | 15.0 | 0.6432 | 0.7048 | 0.7432 | 0.7696 |
| $N_3$ | 3.0 | 0.1844 | 0.2588 | 0.3180 | 0.3596 |
|  | 5.0 | 0.3908 | 0.4832 | 0.5416 | 0.5784 |
|  | 7.0 | 0.5436 | 0.6188 | 0.6628 | 0.6984 |
|  | 10.0 | 0.6728 | 0.7324 | 0.7728 | 0.8008 |
|  | 15.0 | 0.7944 | 0.8404 | 0.8640 | 0.8808 |
| $N_4$ | 3.0 | 0.2152 | 0.2988 | 0.3624 | 0.4068 |
|  | 5.0 | 0.4792 | 0.5568 | 0.6100 | 0.6520 |
|  | 7.0 | 0.6372 | 0.7024 | 0.7476 | 0.7764 |
|  | 10.0 | 0.7692 | 0.8232 | 0.8500 | 0.8720 |
|  | 15.0 | 0.8752 | 0.9040 | 0.9208 | 0.9304 |
| $N_5$ | 3.0 | 0.2600 | 0.3560 | 0.4248 | 0.4748 |
|  | 5.0 | 0.5632 | 0.6440 | 0.6948 | 0.7336 |
|  | 7.0 | 0.7308 | 0.7892 | 0.8244 | 0.8540 |
|  | 10.0 | 0.8588 | 0.8936 | 0.9148 | 0.9268 |
|  | 15.0 | 0.9384 | 0.9512 | 0.9596 | 0.9676 |

*Note:* $N_1 = (n_1, n_2) = (5, 6)$, $N_2 = (n_1, n_2, n_3) = (6, 8, 10)$, $N_3 = (n_1, n_2, n_3, n_4) = (9, 12, 15, 18)$, $N_4 = (n_1, n_2, n_3, n_4, n_5) = (16, 20, 24, 28, 32)$, $N_5 = (n_1, n_2, n_3, n_4, n_5, n_6) = (30, 35, 40, 45, 50, 55)$.

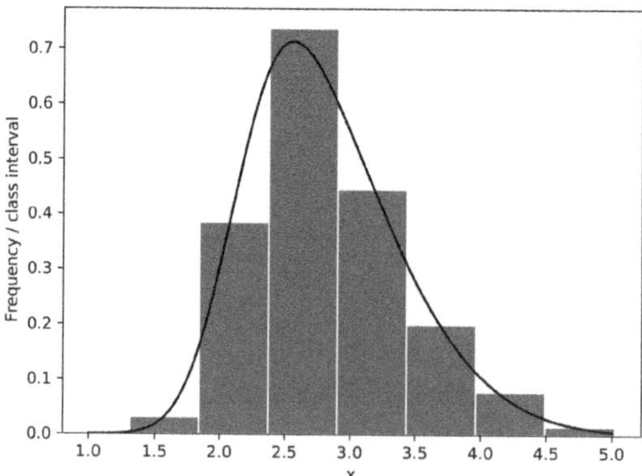


**Figure 6.1:** Histogram of the carbon fibers' strength data with superimposed skew-normal density curve.

# Chapter 7

# Skew-Normal Unbalanced Heteroscedastic One-Way Classification Random Effects Model

This chapter addresses the one-sided hypothesis testing and interval estimation problems for the fixed effect and variance component functions in the skew-normal unbalanced heteroscedastic one-way classification random effects model. Firstly, the Bootstrap approach is used to establish the test statistic for the fixed effect. Secondly, the test statistics and confidence intervals for variance component functions are constructed by the Bootstrap approach and generalized approach, and their theoretical properties are discussed. The Monte Carlo simulation results indicate that the Bootstrap approach performs better than the generalized approach in most cases. Finally, the above approaches are illustrated with two real examples of the annual average concentrations of fine particulate matter and nitrogen dioxide.

## 7.1 Model properties

Let $M_{n \times k}$ be the set of all $n \times k$ matrices over the real field. For any matrix $A \in M_{n \times k}$ and positive semidefinite matrix $B \in M_{n \times n}$, $rk(A)$ and $A'$ denote the rank and transpose of $A$ respectively, and $tr(B)$ and $B^{1/2}$ denote the trace and square root matrix of $B$ respectively. Let $I_n$, $diag(\cdot)$, $1_n$, and $R^n$ be diagonal identity matrix of order $n$, $n \times 1$ vector with each element $= 1$ and $n$-dimensional real vector space, respectively. The symbols $\rightarrow$, $\overset{asy}{\sim}$, $\overset{d}{=}$, and $\overset{\triangle}{=}$ respectively denote "approach", "approximately distributed", "identically distributed", and "defined as".

In this chapter, we consider the skew-normal unbalanced heteroscedastic one-way classification random effects model given by

$$Y_{ij} = \mu + A_i + e_{ij}, i = 1, 2, \cdots, a, j = 1, 2, \cdots, n_i, \tag{7.1}$$

where $Y_{ij}$, $\mu$, $A_i$, and $e_{ij}$ respectively represent the observation, fixed effect, $i$th treatment effect, and error term. The above model in matrix form is expressed as

$$Y = 1_n \mu + ZA + e, \tag{7.2}$$

where $Y = [Y_{11}, \cdots, Y_{1n_1}, \cdots, Y_{a1}, \cdots, Y_{an_a}]'$, $A = [A_1, A_2, \cdots, A_a]'$, $Z = diag\{1_{n_1}, 1_{n_2}, \cdots, 1_{n_a}\}$, $e = [e_{11}, \cdots, e_{1n_1}, \cdots, e_{a1}, \cdots, e_{an_a}]'$, and $n = \sum_{i=1}^{a} n_i$. We assume that $A \sim SN_a(0, \sigma_A^2 I_a, \lambda_1)$, $e \sim N_n(0, diag\{\sigma_i^2 I_{n_i}\})$, and $A$ and $e$ are mutually independent. By Wu et al. (2017b), Lemma 7.1 is as follows.

**Lemma 7.1.** *Suppose $X \sim SN_n(0, \Sigma_0, \alpha_0)$, and $A$ and $B$ are $n \times n$ symmetric matrices, then*

*(i) $X'AX \sim \chi_r^2$ if and only if $A\Sigma_0 A = A$ and $rk(A) = r$,*

*(ii) $X'AX$ and $X'BX$ are mutually independent if and only if $A\Sigma_0 B = 0$.*

**Theorem 7.1.** *For the model $Y$ given in (7.2), We have $Y \sim SN_n(\mu_Y, \Sigma_Y, \lambda_2)$, and the moment generating function of $Y$ is*

$$M_Y(t) = 2 \exp\left(t'\mu_Y + \frac{t'\Sigma_Y t}{2}\right) \Phi\left(\frac{\sigma_A \lambda_1' Z' t}{\left(1 + \lambda_1'\lambda_1\right)^{1/2}}\right), t \in R^n, \tag{7.3}$$

*where $\mu_Y = 1_n \mu$, $\Sigma_Y = \sigma_A^2 ZZ' + diag\{\sigma_i^2 I_{n_i}\}$ and $\lambda_2 = \dfrac{\sigma_A \Sigma_Y^{-1/2} Z \lambda_1}{\left[1 + \lambda_1'\left(I_a - \sigma_A^2 Z' \Sigma_Y^{-1} Z\right)\lambda_1\right]^{1/2}}$.*

The proof of Theorem 7.1 is similar to that given in Ye and Luo (2016) and thus is omitted.

Let partitioned matrix $C_i = [0_{1i}, I_{n_i}, 0_{2i}]$, $i = 1, 2, \cdots, a$, where $0_{1i}$ and $0_{2i}$ are $n_i \times \sum_{j=1}^{i-1} n_j$ zero matrix and $n_i \times \sum_{j=i+1}^{a} n_j$ zero matrix respectively. Premultiplying $C_i$ in (7.2), we get

$$Y_i = 1_{n_i}\mu + 1_{n_i}A_i + e_i, \tag{7.4}$$

where $Y_i = [Y_{i1}, Y_{i2}, \cdots, Y_{in_i}]'$ and $e_i = [e_{i1}, e_{i2}, \cdots, e_{in_i}]'$. Let

$$H_i = \begin{bmatrix} \frac{1}{\sqrt{2}} & \frac{1}{\sqrt{6}} & \cdots & \frac{1}{\sqrt{n_i(n_i-1)}} \\ \frac{-1}{\sqrt{2}} & \frac{1}{\sqrt{6}} & \cdots & \frac{1}{\sqrt{n_i(n_i-1)}} \\ 0 & \frac{-2}{\sqrt{6}} & \cdots & \frac{1}{\sqrt{n_i(n_i-1)}} \\ 0 & 0 & \cdots & \frac{1}{\sqrt{n_i(n_i-1)}} \\ \vdots & \vdots & & \vdots \\ 0 & 0 & \cdots & \frac{-(n_i-1)}{\sqrt{n_i(n_i-1)}} \end{bmatrix},$$

satisfying that $H_i' 1_{n_i} = 0$ and $H_i' H_i = I_{n_i-1}$. Then premultiplying $H_i'$ in (7.4), we obtain

$$H_i' Y_i = H_i' e_i. \tag{7.5}$$

**Theorem 7.2.** *For the model $Y_i$ given in (7.4), let $W_i = Y_i' H_i H_i' Y_i$, $i = 1, 2, \cdots, a$, then*

*(i) $W_i \sim \sigma_i^2 \chi_{n_i-1}^2$,*

*(ii) $W_1, W_2, \cdots, W_a$ are independent to each other,*

*(iii) $W_i = (n_i - 1) S_i$, where $S_i = \frac{1}{n_i-1} \sum_{j=1}^{n_i} (Y_{ij} - \bar{Y}_i)^2$ and $\bar{Y}_i = \frac{1}{n_i} \sum_{j=1}^{n_i} Y_{ij}$.*

*Proof.* By (7.5), $H_i' Y_i \sim N_{n_i-1}(0, \sigma_i^2 I_{n_i-1})$. It is easy to show that $W_i \sim \sigma_i^2 \chi_{n_i-1}^2$, so the result (i) holds. Let $D_i = H_i' C_i Y$. By calculation, $H_k' C_k \Sigma_Y C_q' H_q = 0$ and $H_k' C_k \Sigma_Y^{1/2} \lambda_2 = 0$, where $k, q = 1, 2, \cdots, a, k \neq q$. From Theorem 2.3, $D_1, D_2, \cdots, D_a$ are mutually independent. Since $W_i = Y' C_i' H_i H_i' C_i Y = D_i' D_i$, $W_1, W_2, \cdots, W_a$ are independent of each other, namely the result (ii).

Obviously, $H_i H_i' Y_i = \left(I_{n_i} - \frac{1}{n_i} 1_{n_i} 1_{n_i}'\right) Y_i = [Y_{i1} - \bar{Y}_i, Y_{i2} - \bar{Y}_i, \cdots, Y_{in_i} - \bar{Y}_i]'$, then $W_i = \sum_{j=1}^{n_i} (Y_{ij} - \bar{Y}_i)^2$, namely the result (iii). Therefore, the proof of Theorem 7.2 is completed. $\qquad \square$

Let $R = \left(Z'Z\right)^{-1} Z'$. Premultiplying $R$ in (7.2), we get

$$RY = 1_a\mu + A + Re, \tag{7.6}$$

and

$$RY \sim SN_a\left(1_a\mu, \sigma_A^2 I_a + M, \lambda_3\right), \tag{7.7}$$

where $M = diag\left\{\sigma_i^2/n_i\right\}$ and $\lambda_3 = \dfrac{\left(R\Sigma_Y R'\right)^{-1/2} R\Sigma_Y^{1/2}\lambda_2}{\left\{1+\lambda_2'\left[I_n - \Sigma_Y^{1/2}R'\left(R\Sigma_Y R'\right)^{-1}R\Sigma_Y^{1/2}\right]\lambda_2\right\}^{1/2}}$. Similar to $H_i$, let $H_0 \in M_{a\times(a-1)}$, satisfying $H_0'1_a = 0$ and $H_0'H_0 = I_{a-1}$. Further, premultiplying $H_0'$ in (7.6), we have

$$H_0'RY = H_0'A + H_0'Re,$$

and

$$H_0'RY \sim SN_{a-1}\left(0, \sigma_A^2 I_{a-1} + H_0'MH_0, \lambda_4\right), \tag{7.8}$$

where $\lambda_4 = \dfrac{\left(H_0'\Sigma_R H_0\right)^{-1/2}H_0'\Sigma_R^{1/2}\lambda_3}{\left\{1+\lambda_3'\left[I_a - \Sigma_R^{1/2}H_0\left(H_0'\Sigma_R H_0\right)^{-1}H_0'\Sigma_R^{1/2}\right]\lambda_3\right\}^{1/2}}$ and $\Sigma_R = \sigma_A^2 I_a + M$.

As $H_0'MH_0$ is a positive definite matrix, there exists a $(a-1)\times(a-1)$ orthogonal matrix $P = [P_1, \cdots, P_d]$ so that $P'H_0'MH_0 P$ is a diagonal matrix, that is

$$P'H_0'MH_0 P = diag\left\{\Delta_1, \cdots, \Delta_1, \cdots, \Delta_d, \cdots, \Delta_d\right\} \triangleq D, \tag{7.9}$$

where $0 < \Delta_1 < \Delta_2 < \cdots < \Delta_d$, each $\Delta_i$ is repeated $r_i$ times, $i = 1, 2, \cdots, d$, and $\sum_{i=1}^{d} r_i = a - 1$. By (7.8) and (7.9), $P_i'H_0'RY \sim SN_{r_i}\left(0, \left(\sigma_A^2 + \Delta_i\right)I_{r_i}, \lambda_5^{(i)}\right)$, where

$$\lambda_5^{(i)} = \dfrac{\left(P_i'\Sigma_H P_i\right)^{-1/2}P_i'\Sigma_H^{1/2}\lambda_4}{\left\{1+\lambda_4'\left[I_{a-1} - \Sigma_H^{1/2}P_i\left(P_i'\Sigma_H P_i\right)^{-1}P_i'\Sigma_H^{1/2}\right]\lambda_4\right\}^{1/2}}$$ and $\Sigma_H = \sigma_A^2 I_{a-1} + H_0'MH_0$. Clearly,

$$\bar{\Delta} = \frac{\sum_{i=1}^{d} r_i\Delta_i}{\sum_{i=1}^{d} r_i} = \frac{1}{a}\sum_{i=1}^{a}\frac{\sigma_i^2}{n_i}.$$

**Theorem 7.3.** *For the model $Y$ given in (7.2), let $Q_i = Y'R'H_0 P_i P_i' H_0'RY$, $i = 1, 2, \cdots, d$, then*

*(i) $Q_i \sim \left(\sigma_A^2 + \Delta_i\right)\chi_{r_i}^2$,*

*(ii) $Q_1, Q_2, \cdots, Q_d$ are independent to each other,*

*(iii) $\sum_{i=1}^{d} Q_i = (a-1)S_0$, where $S_0 = \frac{1}{a-1}\sum_{i=1}^{a}\left(\bar{Y}_i - \bar{Y}_.\right)^2$, $\bar{Y}_i = \frac{1}{n_i}\sum_{j=1}^{n_i}Y_{ij}$ and $\bar{Y}_. = \frac{1}{a}\sum_{i=1}^{a}\bar{Y}_i.$*

*Proof.* Suppose $Q_i^* = Q_i/\sigma_A^2 + \Delta_i$. Obviously, $\frac{P_i P_i'}{\sigma_A^2 + \Delta_i}\left(\sigma_A^2 I_{a-1} + H_0' M H_0\right)\frac{P_i P_i'}{\sigma_A^2 + \Delta_i} = (P_i P_i')/(\sigma_A^2 + \Delta_i)$ and $rk\left(P_i P_i'\right) = r_i$. It follows from Lemma 7.1 and (7.8) that $Q_i^* \sim \chi_{r_i}^2$, so the result (i) is true. It is easy to show that $P_k P_k'\left(\sigma_A^2 I_{a-1} + H_0' M H_0\right) P_q P_q' = 0$, where $k, q = 1, 2, \cdots, d, k \neq q$. By Lemma 7.1, $Q_1, Q_2, \cdots, Q_d$ are mutually independent, namely the result (ii). Note that $H_0 H_0' R Y = \left(I_a - \frac{1}{a}1_a 1_a'\right) R Y = [\bar{Y}_1 - \bar{Y}_., \bar{Y}_2 - \bar{Y}_., \cdots, \bar{Y}_a - \bar{Y}_.]'$, then the result (iii) holds. Hence, the proof of Theorem 7.3 is completed. $\square$

**Theorem 7.4.** *For the model* $Y$ *given in (7.2), let* $U_0 = \frac{(a-1)S_0}{\sigma_s^2}$, *then* $U_0 \overset{asy}{\sim} \chi_{a-1}^2$, *where* $S_0 = \frac{1}{a-1}\sum_{j=1}^{d} Q_j$, $Q_j = Y' R' H_0 P_j P_j' H_0' R Y$ *and* $\sigma_s^2 = \sigma_A^2 + \frac{1}{a}\sum_{k=1}^{a}\frac{\sigma_k^2}{n_k}$.

*Proof.* Without loss of generality, we assume that $d = a - 1$, $P = [P_1, \cdots, P_{a-1}]$ and $D = diag\{\delta_1, \delta_2, \cdots, \delta_{a-1}\}$ in (7.9), where $0 < \delta_1 \leq \delta_2 \leq \cdots \leq \delta_{a-1}$. Let $\varphi_x(\cdot)$ denote the characteristic function of random variable $x$. By Theorem 7.3, it is easy to show that $\xi_j = Q_j/(\sigma_A^2 + \delta_j) \sim \chi_1^2$, $j = 1, 2, \cdots, a - 1$, and the characteristic function of $\xi_j$ is

$$\varphi_{\xi_j}(t) = E\left[\exp\left(it\frac{Q_j}{\sigma_A^2 + \delta_j}\right)\right] = \varphi_{Q_j}\left(\frac{t}{\sigma_A^2 + \delta_j}\right) = (1 - 2it)^{-1/2}, t \in R,$$

so $\varphi_{Q_j}(t) = \left[1 - 2it\left(\sigma_A^2 + \delta_j\right)\right]^{-1/2}$. Let $\Gamma_j = \frac{\sigma_A^2 + \delta_j}{\sigma_A^2 + \frac{1}{a}\sum_{k=1}^{a}\frac{\sigma_k^2}{n_k}}$, we have

$$U_0 = \frac{\sum_{j=1}^{a-1} Q_j}{\sigma_A^2 + \frac{1}{a}\sum_{k=1}^{a}\frac{\sigma_k^2}{n_k}} = \sum_{j=1}^{a-1}\Gamma_j \xi_j.$$ It follows from

$$\varphi_{\Gamma_j \xi_j}(t) = E\left[\exp\left(it\Gamma_j\frac{Q_j}{\sigma_A^2 + \delta_j}\right)\right] = \varphi_{Q_j}\left(\frac{\Gamma_j}{\sigma_A^2 + \delta_j}t\right) = (1 - 2i\Gamma_j t)^{-1/2}$$

that $\varphi_{U_0}(t) = \prod_{j=1}^{a-1}(1 - 2i\Gamma_j t)^{-1/2}$.

Furthermore, the Taylor expansion of $\varphi_{U_0}(t)$ at $\Gamma_{j0} = 1$ is

$$\varphi_{U_0}(t) = (1 - 2it)^{-(a-1)/2} - (1 - 2it)^{-(a+3)/2}t^2\sum_{j=1}^{a-1}(\Gamma_j - 1)^2 + R^*,$$

where $R^*$ is the remainder term. Let $\tilde{U}_0 = \sum_{j=1}^{a-1} Q_j/(\sigma_A^2 + \delta_j)$. From Theorem 7.3, we obtain that $\tilde{U}_0 \sim \chi_{a-1}^2$ and $\varphi_{\tilde{U}_0}(t) = (1-2it)^{-(a-1)/2}$. By the characteristic function of $\tilde{U}_0$ and Taylor expansion of $\varphi_{U_0}(t)$, we have $U_0 \overset{asy}{\sim} \chi_{a-1}^2$. So the proof of Theorem 7.4 is complete. $\qquad\square$

**Theorem 7.5.** *For the models $Y$ in (7.2) and $Y_i$ in (7.4), let $W_i = Y_i^{'} H_i H_i^{'} Y_i$ and $Q_j = Y^{'} R^{'} H_0 P_j P_j^{'} H_0^{'} RY$, $i = 1, 2, \cdots, a$, $j = 1, 2, \cdots, d$, then $W_i$ and $\sum_{j=1}^{d} Q_j$ are independent to each other.*

*Proof.* Obviously, $Y \sim SN_n(\mu_Y, \Sigma_Y, \lambda_2)$, $W_i = Y^{'} C_i^{'} H_i H_i^{'} C_i Y$ and $\sum_{j=1}^{d} Q_j = Y^{'} R^{'} H_0 H_0^{'} RY$. It is easy to check that $H_i^{'} C_i \Sigma_Y R^{'} H_0 = 0$ and $H_i^{'} C_i \Sigma_Y^{1/2} \lambda_2 = 0$. By Theorem 2.3, $W_i$ and $\sum_{j=1}^{d} Q_j$ are mutually independent. Therefore, the proof of Theorem 7.5 is complete. $\qquad\square$

**Corollary 7.1.** *For the model $Y$ given in (7.2), the unbiased estimator of $\sigma_i^2$ is $\hat{\sigma}_i^2 = S_i$, $i = 1, 2, \cdots, a$, and the feasible estimators of $\sigma_s^2$ and $\sigma_A^2$ are $\hat{\sigma}_s^2 = S_0$ and $\hat{\sigma}_A^2 = S_0 - \frac{1}{a} \sum_{i=1}^{a} \frac{S_i}{n_i}$ respectively.*

## 7.2 Inference on the fixed effect

In this section, we consider the one-sided hypothesis for fixed effect in model (7.2) as

$$H_0 : \mu \leq \mu_0 \quad versus \quad H_1 : \mu > \mu_0, \tag{7.10}$$

where $\mu_0$ is a specified value. This hypothesis is equivalent to

$$H_0 : v \leq 0 \quad versus \quad H_1 : v > 0,$$

where $v = \mu - \mu_0$. So, without loss of generality, we assume that $\mu_0 = 0$.

Denote

$$\lambda_6 = \frac{\left(1_a^{'} \Sigma_R 1_a\right)^{-1/2} 1_a^{'} \Sigma_R^{1/2} \lambda_3}{\left\{1 + \lambda_3^{'} \left[I_a - \Sigma_R^{1/2} 1_a \left(1_a^{'} \Sigma_R 1_a\right)^{-1} 1_a^{'} \Sigma_R^{1/2}\right] \lambda_3\right\}^{1/2}}. \tag{7.11}$$

**Theorem 7.6.** *For the model Y given in (7.2), let* $Q_0 = Y' R' 1_a 1'_a RY$, *then*

$$Q_0 \sim a\sigma_s^2 S\chi_1^2 \left( \frac{a\mu^2}{\sigma_s^2}, \frac{\sqrt{a}\mu}{\sigma_s} \lambda_6, \lambda_6^2 \right).$$

*Particularly, if* $\mu = 0$, *then* $Q_0/(a\sigma_s^2) \sim \chi_1^2$.

*Proof.* It follows from Lemma 7.1 and (7.7) that $1'_a RY = a\bar{Y}. \sim SN\left(a\mu, a\sigma_s^2, \lambda_6\right)$, where $\lambda_6$ is given by (7.11). Let $X = \frac{1'_a RY}{\sqrt{a}\sigma_s} \sim SN\left(\frac{\sqrt{a}\mu}{\sigma_s}, 1, \lambda_6\right)$. By Definition 2.2, we have $X'X \sim S\chi_1^2\left(\frac{a\mu^2}{\sigma_s^2}, \frac{\sqrt{a}\mu}{\sigma_s}\lambda_6, \lambda_6^2\right)$. Thus the result of Theorem 7.6 is obtained. Obviously, if $\mu = 0$, then $Q_0/(a\sigma_s^2) \sim \chi_1^2$. Therefore, the proof of Theorem 7.6 is complete. $\square$

For hypothesis testing problem (7.10), we have

$$T_0 = \frac{Q_0}{a\sigma_s^2}. \tag{7.12}$$

By Theorem 7.6, if $\sigma_s^2$ is known, $T_0$ would be the test statistic. However, $\sigma_s^2$ is often unknown in practical applications. In such cases, the parameter $\sigma_s^2$ might be replaced by its estimator $\hat{\sigma}_s^2 = S_0$ under the null hypothesis $H_0$ in (7.10). Then the test statistic is expressed as

$$T_0 = \frac{Q_0}{aS_0}. \tag{7.13}$$

It is difficult to obtain the exact distribution of $T_0$, so the Bootstrap approach is used to construct the test statistic. Let $s_0$ and $s_i$ be the observed values of $S_0$ and $S_i$ respectively, $i = 1, 2, \cdots, a$. By (7.13), the Bootstrap test statistic is defined as

$$T_{0B} = \frac{Q_{0B}}{aS_{0B_1}}, \tag{7.14}$$

where $Q_{0B} = Y'_B R' 1_a 1'_a RY_B$, $S_{0B_1} = \frac{1}{a-1} Y'_B R' H_0 H'_0 RY_B$, $Y_B \sim SN_n(0, \tilde{\Sigma}_Y, \tilde{\lambda}_2)$, $\tilde{\Sigma}_Y = \left( s_0 - \frac{1}{a} \sum_{i=1}^{a} \frac{s_i}{n_i} \right) ZZ' + diag\{s_i I_{n_i}\}$, and $\tilde{\lambda}_2$ is the ML estimator of $\lambda_2$.

Since $Y_B \sim SN_n(0, \tilde{\Sigma}_Y, \tilde{\lambda}_2)$, the density function of $Y_B$ is $f(y) = 2 \phi_n\left(y; 0, \tilde{\Sigma}_Y\right) \Phi\left(\tilde{\lambda}'_2 \tilde{\Sigma}_Y^{-1/2} y\right)$. According to Genton (2005), we rewrite $Y_B$ as

$$Y_B = \begin{cases} V_B, & U \leq \Phi\left(\tilde{\lambda}'_2 \tilde{\Sigma}_Y^{-1/2} V_B\right) \\ -V_B, & U > \Phi\left(\tilde{\lambda}'_2 \tilde{\Sigma}_Y^{-1/2} V_B\right) \end{cases}, \tag{7.15}$$

where $V_B \sim N_n(0, \tilde{\Sigma}_Y)$, $U \sim U[0,1]$, and $U[0,1]$ denotes the uniform distribution on $[0,1]$. By (7.15), $Y_B' A Y_B = V_B' A V_B$, where $A$ is any $n \times n$ matrix. Therefore, $T_{0B}$ in (7.14) can be redefined as

$$T_{0B} = \frac{(a-1)V_B' R' 1_a 1_a' R V_B}{a V_B' R' H_0 H_0' R V_B}.$$
(7.16)

Further, the Bootstrap $p$-value is computed by $T_{0B}$ in (7.16) as

$$p_{T_0} = P\left(T_{0B} > t_0 | H_0\right),$$
(7.17)

where $t_0$ denotes the observed value of $T_0$ in (7.13). Let $\beta$ be the nominal significance level. The null hypothesis $H_0$ in (7.10) is rejected whenever the above $p$-value is less than the nominal significance level of $\beta$.

**Theorem 7.7.** *For the model Y given in (7.2), under the transformation*

$$\left(Y_{11}, \cdots, Y_{1n_1}, \cdots, Y_{a1}, \cdots, Y_{an_a}\right) \mapsto \left(Y_{1(1)}, \cdots, Y_{1(n_1)}, \cdots, Y_{a(1)}, \cdots, Y_{a(n_a)}\right),$$
(7.18)

*the distribution of $T_{0B}$ in (7.16) and $t_0$ in (7.17) are invariant, where $i(1), \cdots, i(n_i)$ represent all permutations of $i1, \cdots, in_i$, $i = 1, 2, \cdots, a$.*

*Proof.* Let $\bar{y}_i$, $\bar{y}_.$, $s_0$, and $s_i$ respectively denote the observed values of $\bar{Y}_i$, $\bar{Y}_.$, $S_0$, and $S_i$. Clearly, $\bar{Y}_i$, $\bar{Y}_.$, $S_0$, $S_i$, $\bar{y}_i$, $\bar{y}_.$, $s_0$, $s_i$, and $t_0$ are all invariant under the transformation (7.18). From the distribution of $V_B$ in (7.15), the invariance of the distribution of $T_{0B}$ in (7.16) is easily obtained. Therefore, the proof of Theorem 7.7 is complete. $\qquad\square$

## 7.3 Inference on the single variance component

In this section, we consider the one-sided hypothesis for single variance component in model (7.2) as

$$H_0 : \sigma_A^2 \leq c_1 \quad versus \quad H_1 : \sigma_A^2 > c_1,$$
(7.19)

where $c_1$ is a specified value.

### 7.3.1 Bootstrap approach

For hypothesis testing problem (7.19), we get

$$T_1 = \frac{(a-1)S_0}{c_1 + \frac{1}{a}\sum_{i=1}^{a} \sigma_i^2/n_i}.$$

By Theorem 7.4, if $\sigma_i^2$ is known, $T_1$ could be the test statistic for hypothesis testing problem (7.19). Note that $\sigma_i^2$ is often unknown, then $\sigma_i^2$ can be substituted by its estimator $\hat{\sigma}_i^2 = S_i$ under the null hypothesis $H_0$ in (7.19). The test statistic is constructed as

$$T_1 = \frac{(a-1)S_0}{c_1 + \frac{1}{a}\sum_{i=1}^{a} S_i/n_i}. \tag{7.20}$$

Similar to (7.14), the Bootstrap test statistic is given by

$$T_{1B} = \frac{(a-1)S_{0B_2}}{c_1 + \frac{1}{a}\sum_{i=1}^{a} S_{iB}/n_i}, \tag{7.21}$$

where $S_{0B_2} \overset{asy}{\sim} \frac{1}{a-1}\left(c_1 + \frac{1}{a}\sum_{i=1}^{a}\frac{s_i}{n_i}\right)\chi_{a-1}^2$ and $S_{iB} \sim \frac{s_i}{n_i-1}\chi_{n_i-1}^2$, $i = 1,2,\cdots,a$. Then the Bootstrap $p$-value is computed by $T_{1B}$ as

$$p_{T_1} = P(T_{1B} > t_1 | H_0), \tag{7.22}$$

where $t_1$ denotes the observed value of $T_1$. The null hypothesis $H_0$ in (7.19) is rejected whenever $p_{T_1}$ is less than the nominal significance level of $\beta$.

**Theorem 7.8.** *Under the transformation (7.18), the distribution of $T_{1B}$ in (7.21) and $t_1$ in (7.22) are both invariant.*

The proof is similar to that of Theorem 7.7, so it is omitted.

Let $\zeta = \sigma_A^2/s_0$, $\zeta_1 = c_1/s_0$, $\tilde{T}_1 = \frac{(a-1)S_0/s_0}{\zeta_1 + \frac{1}{a}\sum_{i=1}^{a} S_i/(n_i s_0)}$, $\tilde{T}_{1B} = \frac{(a-1)S_{0B_2}/s_0}{\zeta_1 + \frac{1}{a}\sum_{i=1}^{a} S_{iB}/(n_i s_0)}$, and $p_{\tilde{T}_1} = P(\tilde{T}_{1B} > \tilde{t}_1 | H_0)$, where $\tilde{t}_1$ is the observed value of $\tilde{T}_1$.

**Theorem 7.9.** *For hypothesis testing problem (7.19), consider the equivalent hypothesis*

$$H_0 : \zeta \leq \zeta_1 \quad versus \quad H_1 : \zeta > \zeta_1, \tag{7.23}$$

*then the test based on $p_{\tilde{T}_1}$ is affine-invariant under the affine transformation*

$$Y_{ij}^* = dY_{ij} + \xi, i = 1,2,\cdots,a, j = 1,2,\cdots,n_i, \tag{7.24}$$

*where $\xi$ and $d$ respectively are any given constant and non-zero constant.*

*Proof.* By (7.24), $Y_{ij}^*$ can be rewritten as

$$Y^* = 1_n \mu^* + ZA^* + e^*,$$

where $\mu^* = d\mu + \xi$, $A^* = dA \sim SN_a\left(0, d^2\sigma_A^2 I_a, \lambda_1\right)$, and $e^* = de \sim N_n(0, diag\{d^2\sigma_i^2 I_{n_i}\})$.

Denote $\bar{Y}_i^* = \frac{1}{n_i}\sum_{j=1}^{n_i} Y_{ij}^*$, $\bar{Y}_.^* = \frac{1}{a}\sum_{i=1}^{a}\bar{Y}_i^*$, $S_0^* = \frac{1}{a-1}\sum_{i=1}^{a}(\bar{Y}_i^* - \bar{Y}_.^*)^2$, $S_i^* = \frac{1}{n_i-1}\sum_{j=1}^{n_i}(Y_{ij}^*$

$- \bar{Y}_i^*)^2$, $S_{0B_2}^* \overset{asy}{\sim} \frac{1}{a-1}(s_0^*\zeta_1 + \frac{1}{a}\sum_{i=1}^{a}\frac{s_i^*}{n_i})\chi_{a-1}^2$, and $S_{iB}^* \sim \frac{s_i^*}{n_i-1}\chi_{n_i-1}^2$, $i = 1, 2, \cdots, a$,

where $s_0^*$ and $s_i^*$ are the observed values of $S_0^*$ and $S_i^*$ respectively. We can easily check that $S_0^* = d^2 S_0$, $S_i^* = d^2 S_i$, $s_0^* = d^2 s_0$, and $s_i^* = d^2 s_i$. Based on the above facts, it follows that $S_{0B_2}^* \overset{d}{=} d^2 S_{0B_2}$ and $S_{iB}^* \overset{d}{=} d^2 S_{iB}$. Similar to Theorems 7.2 and 7.5, we obtain $S_{0B_2}^*, S_{1B}^*, \cdots, S_{aB}^*$ that are independent of each other. By calculation, the affine-transformed Bootstrap test statistic is given by

$$\tilde{T}_{1B}^* = \frac{(a-1)S_{0B_2}^*/s_0^*}{\zeta_1 + \frac{1}{a}\sum_{i=1}^{a}S_{iB}^*/(n_i s_0^*)} \overset{d}{=} \frac{(a-1)S_{0B_2}/s_0}{\zeta_1 + \frac{1}{a}\sum_{i=1}^{a}S_{iB}/(n_i s_0)} = \tilde{T}_{1B}.$$

Hence, the distribution of $\tilde{T}_{1B}$ remains invariant.

Let $\tilde{T}_1^* = \frac{(a-1)S_0^*/s_0^*}{\zeta_1 + \frac{1}{a}\sum_{i=1}^{a}S_i^*/(n_i s_0^*)}$, and $\tilde{t}_1^*$ be the observed value of $\tilde{T}_1^*$. It is easy to show that $\tilde{t}_1^* = \tilde{t}_1$, and thus the affine-invariance of $\tilde{t}_1$ is satisfied. Obviously, the hypothesis testing problem (7.23) is invariant under the affine transformation (7.24). Then the Bootstrap test based on $p_{\tilde{T}_1}$ is affine-invariant for hypothesis testing problem (7.23). Therefore, the proof of Theorem 7.9 is complete. $\square$

Further, by Theorem 7.4, we define

$$T_2 = \frac{(a-1)S_0}{\sigma_A^2 + \frac{1}{a}\sum_{i=1}^{a}\sigma_i^2/n_i}.$$

In general, the parameter $\sigma_i^2$ is replaced by its estimator $\hat{\sigma}_i^2 = S_i$, then $T_2$ is given by

$$T_2 = \frac{(a-1)S_0}{\sigma_A^2 + \frac{1}{a}\sum_{i=1}^{a}S_i/n_i}.$$

Thus, the Bootstrap pivot quantity is expressed as

$$T_{2B} = \frac{(a-1)S_{0B_3}}{\tilde{\sigma}_A^2 + \frac{1}{a}\sum_{i=1}^{a}S_{iB}/n_i}, \tag{7.25}$$

where $S_{0B_3} \overset{asy}{\sim} \frac{s_0}{a-1}\chi_{a-1}^2$ and $\tilde{\sigma}_A^2 = s_0 - \frac{1}{a}\sum_{i=1}^{a}\frac{s_i}{n_i}$. For the given $s_0$ and $s_i$, the distribution of $T_{2B}$ does not depend on any unknown parameters. Let $T_{2B}(\beta)$ denote the

$100\beta$ empirical percentile of $T_{2B}$, then the $1 - \beta$ Bootstrap confidence interval for $\sigma_A^2$ is

$$\left[ \frac{(a-1)s_0}{T_{2B}(1-\beta/2)} - \frac{1}{a}\sum_{i=1}^{a}\frac{s_i}{n_i}, \frac{(a-1)s_0}{T_{2B}(\beta/2)} - \frac{1}{a}\sum_{i=1}^{a}\frac{s_i}{n_i} \right].$$

**Remark 7.1.** *Under the affine transformation (7.24), the Bootstrap pivot quantity for affine-invariant parameter $\zeta$ can be constructed as*

$$\tilde{T}_{2B} = \frac{(a-1)S_{0B_3}/s_0}{\tilde{\zeta} + \frac{1}{a}\sum_{i=1}^{a}S_{iB}/(n_i s_0)},$$

*where $\tilde{\zeta} = 1 - \frac{1}{a}\sum_{i=1}^{a}\frac{s_i}{n_i s_0}$. Then the $1 - \beta$ invariant Bootstrap confidence interval for $\zeta$ is*

$$\left[ \frac{a-1}{\tilde{T}_{2B}(1-\beta/2)} - \frac{1}{a}\sum_{i=1}^{a}\frac{s_i}{n_i s_0}, \frac{a-1}{\tilde{T}_{2B}(\beta/2)} - \frac{1}{a}\sum_{i=1}^{a}\frac{s_i}{n_i s_0} \right].$$

### 7.3.2  Generalized approach

Let $U_i = \frac{(n_i-1)S_i}{\sigma_i^2}, i = 1, 2, \cdots, a$. For hypothesis testing problem (7.19), we define

$$F_1 = U_0 \left[ \sigma_A^2 + \frac{1}{a}\sum_{i=1}^{a}\frac{(n_i-1)s_i}{n_i U_i} \right] \overset{asy}{\sim} \chi_{a-1}^2 \left[ \sigma_A^2 + \frac{1}{a}\sum_{i=1}^{a}\frac{(n_i-1)s_i}{n_i \chi_{n_i-1}^2} \right]. \qquad (7.26)$$

It is apparent that the observed value of $F_1$ is $f_1 = (a-1)s_0$, and $F_1$ is stochastically increasing in $\sigma_A^2$. From the last expression in (7.26), we know that its distribution is free of nuisance parameters. Hence, $F_1$ is an approximate generalized test variable. Based on $F_1$, the generalized $p$-value is given by

$$p_{F_1} = P(F_1 > f_1 | H_0) = P\left( U_0 > \frac{f_1}{c_1 + \frac{1}{a}\sum_{i=1}^{a}(n_i-1)s_i/(n_i U_i)} \right)$$

$$= 1 - E_{U_1, U_2, \cdots, U_a}\left[ F_{\chi_{a-1}^2}\left( \frac{f_1}{c_1 + \frac{1}{a}\sum_{i=1}^{a}(n_i-1)s_i/(n_i U_i)} \right) \right], \qquad (7.27)$$

where $F_{\chi_{a-1}^2}$ denotes the cumulative distribution function of the chi-square distribution with degrees of freedom $a - 1$, and the expectation $E_{U_1, U_2, \cdots, U_a}$ is taken with respect to $U_1, U_2, \cdots, U_a$. The null hypothesis $H_0$ in (7.19) will be rejected if $p_{F_1}$ is less than the nominal significance level of $\beta$.

Under the scale transformation

$$\left(\sigma_A^2, \sigma_i^2\right) \mapsto \left(l\sigma_A^2, l\sigma_i^2\right),$$
$$(S_0, S_i) \mapsto (lS_0, lS_i), l > 0, i = 1, 2, \cdots, a, \tag{7.28}$$

both the hypothesis testing problem (7.19) and approximate generalized test variable $F_1$ are not invariant. To establish a $p$-invariant test for (7.19), we consider the equivalent hypothesis (7.23). Further, the approximate generalized test variable is defined as

$$F_{1G} = U_0 \left[ \zeta + \frac{1}{a} \sum_{i=1}^{a} \frac{(n_i - 1) s_i}{n_i U_i s_0} \right].$$

The corresponding generalized $p$-value is

$$p_{F_{1G}} = 1 - E_{U_1, U_2, \ldots, U_a} \left[ F_{\chi_{a-1}^2} \left( \frac{a-1}{\zeta_1 + \frac{1}{a} \sum_{i=1}^{a} (n_i - 1) s_i / (n_i U_i s_0)} \right) \right]. \tag{7.29}$$

Under the scale transformation

$$\left(\zeta, \sigma_i^2\right) \mapsto \left(\zeta, l\sigma_i^2\right),$$
$$(S_0, S_i) \mapsto (lS_0, lS_i), l > 0, i = 1, 2, \cdots, a, \tag{7.30}$$

the hypothesis testing problem (7.23) and approximate generalized test variable $F_{1G}$ are both invariant. Accordingly, for hypothesis testing problem (7.23), the test based on $p_{F_{1G}}$ is $p$-invariant under the scale transformation (7.30).

To obtain the approximate generalized confidence interval for $\sigma_A^2$, we get

$$F_2 = \frac{(a-1) s_0}{U_0} - \frac{1}{a} \sum_{i=1}^{a} \frac{(n_i - 1) s_i}{n_i U_i} \overset{asy}{\sim} \frac{(a-1) s_0}{\chi_{a-1}^2} - \frac{1}{a} \sum_{i=1}^{a} \frac{(n_i - 1) s_i}{n_i \chi_{n_i - 1}^2}. \tag{7.31}$$

Note that the observed value of $F_2$ is $\sigma_A^2$. From the last expression in (7.31), its distribution is free of any unknown parameters. Thus, $F_2$ is an approximate generalized pivot quantity. Then, at the confidence level of $1 - \beta$, the approximate generalized lower confidence limit and upper confidence limit for $\sigma_A^2$ are constructed as $F_2(\beta/2)$ and $F_2(1 - \beta/2)$ respectively.

The approximate generalized confidence interval is not based on the frequency theory and may not be the confidence interval in the frequentist sense, so we consider it necessary to explore the coverage probability of the approximate generalized confidence interval from the analytical perspective.

**Theorem 7.10.** *For $F_2$ in (7.31), we have*

$$\lim_{\sigma_1^2,\cdots,\sigma_a^2\to 0} P\left(F_2\left(\frac{\beta}{2}\right)\le\sigma_A^2\le F_2\left(1-\frac{\beta}{2}\right)\right)=1-\beta,$$

$$\lim_{n_1,\cdots,n_a\to\infty} P\left(F_2\left(\frac{\beta}{2}\right)\le\sigma_A^2\le F_2\left(1-\frac{\beta}{2}\right)\right)=1-\beta,$$

$$\lim_{\substack{\sigma_1^2,\cdots,\sigma_a^2\to 0\\ n_1,\cdots,n_a\to\infty}} P\left(F_2\left(\frac{\beta}{2}\right)\le\sigma_A^2\le F_2\left(1-\frac{\beta}{2}\right)\right)=1-\beta,$$

$$\lim_{\substack{\sigma_A^2\to 0\\ \sigma_1^2,\cdots,\sigma_{j-1}^2,\sigma_{j+1}^2,\cdots,\sigma_a^2\to 0}} P\left(F_2\left(\frac{\beta}{2}\right)\le\sigma_A^2\le F_2\left(1-\frac{\beta}{2}\right)\right)=1-\beta, \qquad (7.32)$$

$$\lim_{\substack{\sigma_A^2\to 0\\ n_1,\cdots,n_{j-1},n_{j+1},\cdots,n_a\to\infty}} P\left(F_2\left(\frac{\beta}{2}\right)\le\sigma_A^2\le F_2\left(1-\frac{\beta}{2}\right)\right)=1-\beta,$$

$$\lim_{\substack{\sigma_A^2\to 0,\sigma_1^2,\cdots,\sigma_{j-1}^2,\sigma_{j+1}^2,\cdots,\sigma_a^2\to 0\\ n_1,\cdots,n_{j-1},n_{j+1},\cdots,n_a\to\infty}} P\left(F_2\left(\frac{\beta}{2}\right)\le\sigma_A^2\le F_2\left(1-\frac{\beta}{2}\right)\right)=1-\beta,$$

*where $\sigma_1^2,\cdots,\sigma_a^2\to 0$ and $n_1,\cdots,n_a\to\infty$ denote $\sigma_1^2\to 0,\cdots,\sigma_a^2\to 0$ and $n_1\to\infty,\cdots,n_a\to\infty$ respectively, meanwhile $\sigma_1^2,\cdots,\sigma_{j-1}^2,\sigma_{j+1}^2,\cdots,\sigma_a^2\to 0$ and $n_1,\cdots,n_{j-1},n_{j+1},\cdots,n_a\to\infty$ denote $\sigma_1^2\to 0,\cdots,\sigma_{j-1}^2\to 0,\sigma_{j+1}^2\to 0,\cdots,\sigma_a^2\to 0$ and $n_1\to\infty,\cdots,n_{j-1}\to\infty,n_{j+1}\to\infty,\cdots,n_a\to\infty$ respectively.*

*Proof.* Firstly, we should prove the first equation in (7.32). Obviously, to obtain this conclusion, it suffices to show that

$$\lim_{\sigma_1^2,\cdots,\sigma_a^2\to 0} P\left(\sigma_A^2\ge F_2\left(\frac{\beta}{2}\right)\right)=1-\frac{\beta}{2},$$

$$\lim_{\sigma_1^2,\cdots,\sigma_a^2\to 0} P\left(\sigma_A^2\le F_2\left(1-\frac{\beta}{2}\right)\right)=1-\frac{\beta}{2}.$$

Suppose that $(U_0^*,U_1^*,\cdots,U_a^*)$ and $(U_0,U_1,\cdots,U_a)$ are independent and identically distributed, we have

$$P\left(\sigma_A^2\ge F_2\left(\frac{\beta}{2}\right)\right)$$

$$=P\left(P\left(F_2\le\sigma_A^2\right)\ge\frac{\beta}{2}\right)$$

$$=P\left(P\left(\frac{(a-1)S_0}{U_0}-\frac{1}{a}\sum_{i=1}^{a}\frac{(n_i-1)S_i}{n_iU_i}\le\sigma_A^2\,\bigg|\,S_0,S_i\right)\ge\frac{\beta}{2}\right)$$

$$=\tilde{P}\left(P\left(\left(\sigma_A^2+\frac{1}{a}\sum_{i=1}^{a}\frac{\sigma_i^2}{n_i}\right)\frac{U_0^*}{U_0}-\frac{1}{a}\sum_{i=1}^{a}\frac{\sigma_i^2U_i^*}{n_iU_i}\le\sigma_A^2\,\bigg|\,U_0^*,U_i^*\right)\ge\frac{\beta}{2}\right),$$

where $\tilde{P}$ denotes the joint distribution of $(U_0^*, U_1^*, \cdots, U_a^*)$. Then,

$$\lim_{\sigma_1^2, \cdots, \sigma_a^2 \to 0} P\left(\sigma_A^2 \geq F_2\left(\frac{\beta}{2}\right)\right) = \tilde{P}\left(P(U_0^* \leq U_0 \mid U_0^*, U_i^*) \geq \frac{\beta}{2}\right)$$

$$= \tilde{P}\left(F_{\chi_{a-1}^2}(U_0^*) \leq 1 - \frac{\beta}{2}\right) = 1 - \frac{\beta}{2}.$$

Furthermore, we get $\displaystyle\lim_{\sigma_1^2, \cdots, \sigma_a^2 \to 0} P\left(\sigma_A^2 \leq F_2\left(1 - \frac{\beta}{2}\right)\right) = 1 - \frac{\beta}{2}$, thus the first equation holds. Similarly, the other five equations in (7.32) can be obtained. Therefore, the proof of Theorem 7.10 is completed. $\qquad\square$

**Remark 7.2.** *Under the scale transformation (7.30), the approximate generalized pivot quantity for scale-invariant parameter $\zeta$ is given by*

$$\tilde{F}_2 = \frac{a-1}{U_0} - \frac{1}{a}\sum_{i=1}^{a} \frac{(n_i - 1)s_i}{n_i s_0 U_i}.$$

*Then the $1 - \beta$ invariant generalized confidence interval for $\zeta$ is $\left[\tilde{F}_2(\beta/2), \tilde{F}_2(1 - \beta/2)\right]$.*

## 7.4 Inference on the sum of variance components

For $k = 1, 2, \cdots, a$, we consider the one-sided hypothesis for the sum of the variance components in model (7.2) as

$$H_0 : \sigma_A^2 + \sigma_k^2 \leq c_{2k} \quad versus \quad H_1 : \sigma_A^2 + \sigma_k^2 > c_{2k}, \tag{7.33}$$

where $c_{2k}$ is a specified value.

### 7.4.1 Bootstrap approach

For hypothesis testing problem (7.33), we obtain

$$T_{3k} = \frac{(a-1)S_0}{c_{2k} - \sigma_k^2 + \frac{1}{a}\sum_{i=1}^{a}\sigma_i^2/n_i}.$$

Similar to (7.20), the test statistic is defined as

$$T_{3k} = \frac{(a-1)S_0}{c_{2k} - S_k + \frac{1}{a}\sum_{i=1}^{a}S_i/n_i}. \tag{7.34}$$

Then the Bootstrap test statistic for hypothesis testing problem (7.33) can be constructed as

$$T_{3kB} = \frac{(a-1)S_{0B_4}}{c_{2k} - S_{kB} + \frac{1}{a}\sum_{i=1}^{a} S_{iB}/n_i},\qquad(7.35)$$

where $S_{0B_4} \overset{asy}{\sim} \frac{1}{a-1}\left(c_{2k} - S_k + \frac{1}{a}\sum_{i=1}^{a}\frac{S_i}{n_i}\right)\chi^2_{a-1}$. The Bootstrap $p$-value is computed by $T_{3kB}$ as

$$p_{T_{3k}} = P\left(T_{3kB} > t_{3k}|H_0\right),\qquad(7.36)$$

where $t_{3k}$ is the observed value of $T_{3k}$ in (7.34). The null hypothesis $H_0$ in (7.33) is rejected whenever $p_{T_{3k}}$ is less than the nominal significance level of $\beta$.

**Theorem 7.11.** *Under the transformation (7.18), the distribution of $T_{3kB}$ in (7.35) and $t_{3k}$ in (7.36) are both invariant.*

Similar to Theorem 7.7, it is easy to obtain the above results, so the proof is omitted.

Let

$$\Theta_k = \left(\sigma_A^2 + \sigma_k^2\right)/s_0,\ \theta_{2k} = c_{2k}/s_0,\ \tilde{T}_{3k} = \frac{(a-1)S_0/s_0}{\theta_{2k} - S_k/s_0 + \frac{1}{a}\sum_{i=1}^{a} S_i/(n_i s_0)},$$

$$\tilde{T}_{3kB} = \frac{(a-1)S_{0B_4}/s_0}{\theta_{2k} - S_{kB}/s_0 + \frac{1}{a}\sum_{i=1}^{a} S_{iB}/(n_i s_0)},\ p_{\tilde{T}_{3k}} = P\left(\tilde{T}_{3kB} > \tilde{t}_{3k}|H_0\right),$$

where $\tilde{t}_{3k}$ is the observed value of $\tilde{T}_{3k}$.

**Theorem 7.12.** *For hypothesis testing problem (7.33), consider the equivalent hypothesis*

$$H_0 : \Theta_k \leq \theta_{2k} \quad versus \quad H_1 : \Theta_k > \theta_{2k},\qquad(7.37)$$

*then the test based on $p_{\tilde{T}_{3k}}$ is affine-invariant under the affine transformation (7.24).*

The proof is similar to that given in Theorem 7.9 and thus is omitted.

Next, to construct the Bootstrap confidence interval for $\sigma_A^2 + \sigma_k^2$, we define

$$T_{4k} = \frac{(a-1)S_0}{\sigma_A^2 + \sigma_k^2 - S_k + \frac{1}{a}\sum_{i=1}^{a} S_i/n_i}.$$

Similar to (7.25), the Bootstrap pivot quantity is given by

$$T_{4kB} = \frac{(a-1)S_{0B_3}}{\tilde{\sigma}_A^2 + \tilde{\sigma}_k^2 - S_{kB} + \frac{1}{a}\sum_{i=1}^{a} S_{iB}/n_i},\qquad(7.38)$$

where $\tilde{\sigma}_k^2 = s_k$. Let $T_{4kB}(\beta)$ denote the $100\beta$ empirical percentile of $T_{4kB}$, then the $1 - \beta$ Bootstrap confidence interval for $\sigma_A^2 + \sigma_k^2$ is

$$\left[ \frac{(a-1)s_0}{T_{4kB}(1-\beta/2)} + s_k - \frac{1}{a}\sum_{i=1}^{a}\frac{s_i}{n_i}, \frac{(a-1)s_0}{T_{4kB}(\beta/2)} + s_k - \frac{1}{a}\sum_{i=1}^{a}\frac{s_i}{n_i} \right].$$

**Remark 7.3.** *Under the affine transformation (7.24), the Bootstrap pivot quantity for affine-invariant parameter $\Theta_k$ can be expressed as*

$$\tilde{T}_{4kB} = \frac{(a-1)S_{0B_3}/s_0}{\tilde{\Theta}_k - S_{kB}/s_0 + \frac{1}{a}\sum_{i=1}^{a}S_{iB}/(n_i s_0)},$$

*where $\tilde{\Theta}_k = 1 + \frac{s_k}{s_0} - \frac{1}{a}\sum_{i=1}^{a}\frac{s_i}{n_i s_0}$. Then the $1 - \beta$ invariant Bootstrap confidence interval for $\Theta_k$ is*

$$\left[ \frac{a-1}{\tilde{T}_{4kB}(1-\beta/2)} + \frac{s_k}{s_0} - \frac{1}{a}\sum_{i=1}^{a}\frac{s_i}{n_i s_0}, \frac{a-1}{\tilde{T}_{4kB}(\beta/2)} + \frac{s_k}{s_0} - \frac{1}{a}\sum_{i=1}^{a}\frac{s_i}{n_i s_0} \right].$$

### 7.4.2 Generalized approach

Similar to $F_1$ in (7.26), the approximate generalized test variable for (7.33) is defined as

$$F_{3k} = U_0 \left[ (\sigma_A^2 + \sigma_k^2) - \frac{(n_k - 1)s_k}{U_k} + \frac{1}{a}\sum_{i=1}^{a}\frac{(n_i - 1)s_i}{n_i U_i} \right]. \tag{7.39}$$

The generalized $p$-value is given by

$$p_{F_{3k}} = 1 - E_{U_1, U_2, \cdots, U_a}\left[ F_{\chi_{a-1}^2}\left( \frac{(a-1)s_0}{c_{2k} - \frac{(n_k-1)s_k}{U_k} + \frac{1}{a}\sum_{i=1}^{a}\frac{(n_i-1)s_i}{n_i U_i}} \right) \right]. \tag{7.40}$$

Apparently, under the scale transformation (7.28), both the hypothesis testing problem (7.33) and approximate generalized test variable $F_{3k}$ are not invariant. Then, we consider the equivalent hypothesis (7.37). The approximate generalized test variable is expressed as

$$F_{3kG} = U_0 \left[ \Theta_k - \frac{(n_k - 1)s_k}{U_k s_0} + \frac{1}{a}\sum_{i=1}^{a}\frac{(n_i - 1)s_i}{n_i U_i s_0} \right].$$

The corresponding generalized $p$-value is

$$p_{F_{3kG}} = 1 - E_{U_1,U_2,\cdots,U_a}\left[F_{\chi^2_{a-1}}\left(\frac{a-1}{\theta_{2k} - \frac{(n_k-1)s_k}{U_k s_0} + \frac{1}{a}\sum_{i=1}^{a}\frac{(n_i-1)s_i}{n_i U_i s_0}}\right)\right]. \tag{7.41}$$

Under the scale transformation

$$\begin{aligned}&\left(\Theta_k, \sigma_i^2\right) \mapsto \left(\Theta_k, l\sigma_i^2\right), \\ &(S_0, S_i) \mapsto (lS_0, lS_i), l > 0, i = 1, 2, \cdots, a,\end{aligned} \tag{7.42}$$

the hypothesis testing problem (7.37) and approximate generalized test variable $F_{3kG}$ are both invariant. Hence, for hypothesis testing problem (7.37), the test based on $p_{F_{3kG}}$ is $p$-invariant under the scale transformation (7.42).

Similar to $F_2$ in (7.31), the approximate generalized pivot quantity for $\sigma_A^2 + \sigma_k^2$ is defined as

$$F_{4k} = \frac{(a-1)s_0}{U_0} - \frac{1}{a}\sum_{i=1}^{a}\frac{(n_i-1)s_i}{n_i U_i} + \frac{(n_k-1)s_k}{U_k}. \tag{7.43}$$

At the confidence level of $1 - \beta$, the approximate generalized lower confidence limit and upper confidence limit for $\sigma_A^2 + \sigma_k^2$ are constructed as $F_{4k}(\beta/2)$ and $F_{4k}(1 - \beta/2)$ respectively.

**Theorem 7.13.** *For $F_{4k}$ in (7.43), we obtain*

$$\begin{aligned}&\lim_{\sigma_1^2,\cdots,\sigma_a^2\to 0} P\left(F_{4k}\left(\frac{\beta}{2}\right) \leq \sigma_A^2 + \sigma_k^2 \leq F_{4k}\left(1 - \frac{\beta}{2}\right)\right) = 1 - \beta, \\ &\lim_{\substack{n_1,\cdots,n_a\to\infty \\ \sigma_1^2,\cdots,\sigma_a^2\to 0}} P\left(F_{4k}\left(\frac{\beta}{2}\right) \leq \sigma_A^2 + \sigma_k^2 \leq F_{4k}\left(1 - \frac{\beta}{2}\right)\right) = 1 - \beta, \\ &\lim_{\substack{n_1,\cdots,n_a\to\infty \\ \sigma_k^2\to 0}} P\left(F_{4k}\left(\frac{\beta}{2}\right) \leq \sigma_A^2 + \sigma_k^2 \leq F_{4k}\left(1 - \frac{\beta}{2}\right)\right) = 1 - \beta, \\ &\lim_{\substack{n_1,\cdots,n_a\to\infty \\ \sigma_A^2\to 0}} P\left(F_{4k}\left(\frac{\beta}{2}\right) \leq \sigma_A^2 + \sigma_k^2 \leq F_{4k}\left(1 - \frac{\beta}{2}\right)\right) = 1 - \beta.\end{aligned} \tag{7.44}$$

The proof is similar to that of Theorem 7.10, so it is omitted.

**Remark 7.4.** *Under the scale transformation (7.42), the approximate generalized pivot quantity for the scale-invariant parameter $\Theta_k$ is expressed as*

$$\tilde{F}_{4k} = \frac{a-1}{U_0} - \frac{1}{a}\sum_{i=1}^{a}\frac{(n_i-1)s_i}{n_i s_0 U_i} + \frac{(n_k-1)s_k}{s_0 U_k}.$$

*Then the $1 - \beta$ invariant generalized confidence interval for $\Theta_k$ is given by $\left[\tilde{F}_{4k}(\beta/2), \tilde{F}_{4k}(1 - \beta/2)\right]$.*

## 7.5 Inference on the ratio of variance components

For $k = 1, 2, \cdots, a$, we consider the one-sided hypothesis for the ratio of variance components in model (7.2) as

$$H_0 : \sigma_A^2 / \sigma_k^2 \leq c_{3k} \quad versus \quad H_1 : \sigma_A^2 / \sigma_k^2 > c_{3k}, \tag{7.45}$$

where $c_{3k}$ is a specified value.

### 7.5.1 Bootstrap approach

For hypothesis testing problem (7.45), we have

$$T_{5k} = \frac{(a-1)S_0}{c_{3k}\sigma_k^2 + \frac{1}{a}\sum_{i=1}^{a}\sigma_i^2/n_i}.$$

Similar to (7.20), the test statistic is given by

$$T_{5k} = \frac{(a-1)S_0}{c_{3k}S_k + \frac{1}{a}\sum_{i=1}^{a}S_i/n_i}. \tag{7.46}$$

Thus, the Bootstrap test statistic based on (7.46) is expressed as

$$T_{5kB} = \frac{(a-1)S_{0B_5}}{c_{3k}S_{kB} + \frac{1}{a}\sum_{i=1}^{a}S_{iB}/n_i}, \tag{7.47}$$

where $S_{0B_5} \overset{asy}{\sim} \frac{1}{a-1}\left(c_{3k}s_k + \frac{1}{a}\sum_{i=1}^{a}\frac{s_i}{n_i}\right)\chi_{a-1}^2$. The Bootstrap $p$-value is computed by $T_{5kB}$ as

$$p_{T_{5k}} = P\left(T_{5kB} > t_{5k}|H_0\right), \tag{7.48}$$

where $t_{5k}$ denotes the observed value of $T_{5k}$ in (7.46). The null hypothesis $H_0$ in (7.45) will be rejected if $p_{T_{5k}}$ is less than the nominal significance level of $\beta$.

**Theorem 7.14.** *Under the transformation (7.18), the distribution of $T_{5kB}$ in (7.47) and $t_{5k}$ in (7.48) are both invariant.*

Similar to Theorem 7.7, it is easy to show the above results, so the proof is omitted.

**Theorem 7.15.** *For hypothesis testing problem (7.45), the Bootstrap test based on $p_{T_{5k}}$ is affine-invariant under the affine transformation (7.24).*

Since the proof is similar to that of Theorem 7.9, we omit it.

To obtain the Bootstrap confidence interval for $\sigma_A^2/\sigma_k^2$, we define

$$T_{6k} = \frac{(a-1)\,S_0}{(\sigma_A^2/\sigma_k^2)S_k + \frac{1}{a}\sum\limits_{i=1}^{a}S_i/n_i}.$$

Similar to (7.25), the Bootstrap pivot quantity based on $T_{6k}$ is constructed as

$$T_{6kB} = \frac{(a-1)\,S_{0B_3}}{\left(\tilde{\sigma}_A^2/\tilde{\sigma}_k^2\right)S_{kB} + \frac{1}{a}\sum\limits_{i=1}^{a}S_{iB}/n_i}, \tag{7.49}$$

Let $T_{6kB}(\beta)$ denote the $100\beta$ empirical percentile of $T_{6kB}$. Then the $1-\beta$ Bootstrap confidence interval for $\sigma_A^2/\sigma_k^2$ is

$$\left[\frac{(a-1)\,s_0}{s_k T_{6kB}(1-\beta/2)} - \frac{\sum\limits_{i=1}^{a}s_i/n_i}{as_k}, \frac{(a-1)\,s_0}{s_k T_{6kB}(\beta/2)} - \frac{\sum\limits_{i=1}^{a}s_i/n_i}{as_k}\right]. \tag{7.50}$$

**Remark 7.5.** *The Bootstrap confidence interval (7.50) for $\sigma_A^2/\sigma_k^2$ is affine-invariant under the affine transformation (7.24).*

### 7.5.2 Generalized approach

For hypothesis testing problem (7.45), the approximate generalized test variable is defined as

$$F_{5k} = U_0\left[\frac{\sigma_A^2}{\sigma_k^2}\frac{(n_k-1)\,s_k}{U_k} + \frac{1}{a}\sum\limits_{i=1}^{a}\frac{(n_i-1)\,s_i}{n_iU_i}\right]. \tag{7.51}$$

Similar to (7.27), the generalized $p$-value is given by

$$p_{F_{5k}} = 1 - E_{U_1,U_2,\cdots,U_a}\left[F_{\chi_{a-1}^2}\left(\frac{(a-1)\,s_0}{c_{3k}\frac{(n_k-1)s_k}{U_k} + \frac{1}{a}\sum\limits_{i=1}^{a}\frac{(n_i-1)s_i}{n_iU_i}}\right)\right]. \tag{7.52}$$

Under the scale transformation (7.28), though the hypothesis testing problem (7.45) remains invariant, the approximate generalized test variable $F_{5k}$ is not. Then we define

$$F_{5kG} = U_0\left[\frac{\sigma_A^2}{\sigma_k^2}\frac{(n_k-1)\,s_k}{U_k s_0} + \frac{1}{a}\sum\limits_{i=1}^{a}\frac{(n_i-1)\,s_i}{n_iU_i s_0}\right].$$

Obviously, $F_{5kG}$ is an approximate generalized test variable, and $F_{5kG}$ is invariant under the scale transformation (7.28). The corresponding generalized $p$-value is

$$p_{F_{5kG}} = 1 - E_{U_1, U_2, \cdots, U_a} \left[ F_{\chi^2_{a-1}} \left( \frac{a-1}{c_{3k} \frac{(n_k-1)s_k}{U_k s_0} + \frac{1}{a} \sum_{i=1}^{a} \frac{(n_i-1)s_i}{n_i U_i s_0}} \right) \right]. \tag{7.53}$$

Therefore, for hypothesis testing problem (7.45), the test based on $p_{F_{5kG}}$ is $p$-invariant under the scale transformation (7.28).

To obtain the generalized confidence interval for $\sigma_A^2 / \sigma_k^2$, the approximate generalized pivot quantity is expressed as

$$F_{6k} = \frac{(a-1)s_0 U_k}{(n_k-1)s_k U_0} - \frac{\frac{1}{a} \sum_{i=1}^{a} (n_i-1)s_i/(n_i U_i)}{(n_k-1)s_k/U_k}. \tag{7.54}$$

At the confidence level of $1-\beta$, the approximate generalized lower confidence limit and upper confidence limit for $\sigma_A^2 / \sigma_k^2$ are constructed as $F_{6k}(\beta/2)$ and $F_{6k}(1-\beta/2)$ respectively.

**Theorem 7.16.** *For $F_{6k}$ in (7.54), we have*

$$\lim_{\sigma_1^2, \cdots, \sigma_a^2 \to 0} P\left( F_{6k}\left(\frac{\beta}{2}\right) \leq \frac{\sigma_A^2}{\sigma_k^2} \leq F_{6k}\left(1-\frac{\beta}{2}\right) \right) = 1-\beta,$$

$$\lim_{n_1, \cdots, n_a \to \infty} P\left( F_{6k}\left(\frac{\beta}{2}\right) \leq \frac{\sigma_A^2}{\sigma_k^2} \leq F_{6k}\left(1-\frac{\beta}{2}\right) \right) = 1-\beta,$$

$$\lim_{\substack{\sigma_1^2, \cdots, \sigma_a^2 \to 0 \\ n_1, \cdots, n_a \to \infty}} P\left( F_{6k}\left(\frac{\beta}{2}\right) \leq \frac{\sigma_A^2}{\sigma_k^2} \leq F_{6k}\left(1-\frac{\beta}{2}\right) \right) = 1-\beta,$$

$$\lim_{\sigma_A^2 \to 0, \sigma_1^2, \cdots, \sigma_{j-1}^2, \sigma_{j+1}^2, \cdots, \sigma_a^2 \to 0} P\left( F_{6k}\left(\frac{\beta}{2}\right) \leq \frac{\sigma_A^2}{\sigma_k^2} \leq F_{6k}\left(1-\frac{\beta}{2}\right) \right) = 1-\beta,$$

$$\lim_{\sigma_A^2 \to 0, n_1, \cdots, n_{j-1}, n_{j+1}, \cdots, n_a \to \infty} P\left( F_{6k}\left(\frac{\beta}{2}\right) \leq \frac{\sigma_A^2}{\sigma_k^2} \leq F_{6k}\left(1-\frac{\beta}{2}\right) \right) = 1-\beta,$$

$$\lim_{\substack{\sigma_A^2 \to 0, \sigma_1^2, \cdots, \sigma_{j-1}^2, \sigma_{j+1}^2, \cdots, \sigma_a^2 \to 0, \\ n_1, \cdots, n_{j-1}, n_{j+1}, \cdots, n_a \to \infty}} P\left( F_{6k}\left(\frac{\beta}{2}\right) \leq \frac{\sigma_A^2}{\sigma_k^2} \leq F_{6k}\left(1-\frac{\beta}{2}\right) \right) = 1-\beta. \tag{7.55}$$

The proof is similar to that given in Theorem 7.10 and thus is omitted.

**Remark 7.6.** *Under the scale transformation (7.28), the $1-\beta$ generalized confidence interval $[F_{6k}(\beta/2), F_{6k}(1-\beta/2)]$ for $\sigma_A^2/\sigma_k^2$ is invariant.*

## 7.6  Monte Carlo simulation

In this section, we study the size and power of the above testing approaches from the numerical perspective by the Monte Carlo simulation. For convenience, we only provide the steps of the Bootstrap approach for hypothesis testing problem (7.10) as follows.

**Step 1:** For given $(n_1, n_2, \cdots, n_a)$, $(\sigma_1^2, \sigma_2^2, \cdots, \sigma_a^2)$ and $(\sigma_A^2, \lambda_1)$, generate $y \sim SN_n(0, \Sigma_Y, \lambda_2)$, where $\Sigma_Y$ and $\lambda_2$ are given in Theorem 7.1. Compute $S_i$, $S_0$ and $Q_0$ in Theorems 7.2, 7.3 and 7.6, and denote them as $s_i$, $s_0$ and $q_0$ respectively, $i = 1, 2, \cdots, a$. Then $\tilde{\Sigma}_Y = \left( s_0 - \frac{1}{a} \sum_{i=1}^{a} s_i / n_i \right) ZZ' + diag\,\{s_i I_{n_i}\}$, where $Z = diag\,\{1_{n_1}, 1_{n_2}, \cdots, 1_{n_a}\}$.

**Step 2:** Compute $T_0$ in (7.13) and denote it as $t_0$.

**Step 3:** Generate $V_B \sim N_n(0, \tilde{\Sigma}_Y)$ and compute $T_{0B}$ in (7.16).

**Step 4:** Repeat Step 3 $k_1$ times and compute $p_{T_0}$ in (7.17). If $p_{T_0} < \beta$, then $l = 1$. Otherwise, $l = 0$.

**Step 5:** Repeat Steps 1–4 $k_2$ times and get $l_1, l_2, \cdots, l_{k_2}$.

Based on the above steps, we can similarly obtain the power of the hypothesis testing problem (7.10) under $H_1$.

In the simulation, let the nominal significance levels $\beta = 0.025, 0.05, 0.075, 0.1$, skewness parameter $\lambda_1 = 1_a$, and the numbers of inner loops $k_1$ and outer loops $k_2$ both be 2500. Let $N_i = (n_1, \cdots, n_a)$ and $\eta_j^2 = (\sigma_1^2, \cdots, \sigma_a^2)$ denote the sample sizes and variance components respectively. Then, $N_i$ and $\eta_j^2$ are set as follows. $N_1 = (3, 3, 4), N_2 = (4, 5, 6), N_3 = (7, 10, 13), N_4 = (12, 20, 28), N_5 = (24, 40, 56),$ $N_6 = (3)_{10}, N_7 = (3, 4, 4, 5, 5)_2, N_8 = (7, 7, 8, 8, 9)_2, N_9 = (9, 9, 10, 10, 12)_2, N_{10} = (11, 11, 12, 13, 13)_2, \eta_1^2 = (1, 1, 1), \eta_2^2 = (1, 1, 0.5), \eta_3^2 = (1, 0.6, 0.3), \eta_4^2 = (1, 0.1, 0.3), \eta_5^2 = (1)_{10}, \eta_6^2 = (1, 0.9, 0.8, 0.7, 0.6, 0.5, 0.4, 0.3, 0.2, 0.1), \eta_7^2 = (1, (0.3, 0.6, 0.9)_3),$ and $\eta_8^2 = (1, (0.1)_2, (0.2)_2, (0.3)_2, (0.4)_2, 0.5),$ where $(u)_m$ denotes "the row vector $u$ is repeated $m$ times by row".

For hypothesis testing problem (7.10), Tables 7.1–7.2 and Tables 7.3–7.4 respectively present the simulated sizes and powers of the Bootstrap approach (BA) under the different nominal significance levels and parameter configurations. As in Tables 7.1–7.2, the BA is satisfactory in controlling the sizes, but its empirical sizes are slightly liberal when the number of variance components is small. From Tables 7.3–7.4, in cases where $\mu$ departs from the null hypothesis, the powers of BA increase significantly. Regardless of the sample sizes and variance components' configurations, the performance of BA is robust in terms of the power.

**Table 7.1:** Sizes for hypothesis testing problem (7.10) ($\mu = \mu_0 = 0, a = 3$).

| | $\beta$ | | | | | | | |
| | 0.05 | 0.1 | 0.05 | 0.1 | 0.05 | 0.1 | 0.05 | 0.1 |
| $\sigma_A^2 = 1$ | $\eta_1^2$ | | $\eta_2^2$ | | $\eta_3^2$ | | $\eta_4^2$ | |
|---|---|---|---|---|---|---|---|---|
| $N_1$ | 0.0632 | 0.1084 | 0.0648 | 0.1160 | 0.0680 | 0.1148 | 0.0704 | 0.1124 |
| $N_2$ | 0.0596 | 0.1044 | 0.0576 | 0.1056 | 0.0596 | 0.1064 | 0.0676 | 0.1124 |
| $N_3$ | 0.0584 | 0.1084 | 0.0596 | 0.1104 | 0.0600 | 0.1068 | 0.0660 | 0.1112 |
| $N_4$ | 0.0560 | 0.1008 | 0.0544 | 0.1028 | 0.0544 | 0.1020 | 0.0584 | 0.1052 |
| $N_5$ | 0.0516 | 0.0980 | 0.0524 | 0.1024 | 0.0540 | 0.1076 | 0.0632 | 0.1128 |
| $\sigma_A^2 = 5$ | $\eta_1^2$ | | $\eta_2^2$ | | $\eta_3^2$ | | $\eta_4^2$ | |
| $N_1$ | 0.0504 | 0.0928 | 0.0512 | 0.0912 | 0.0524 | 0.0956 | 0.0508 | 0.0996 |
| $N_2$ | 0.0468 | 0.0956 | 0.0476 | 0.0972 | 0.0524 | 0.0972 | 0.0556 | 0.1068 |
| $N_3$ | 0.0576 | 0.1096 | 0.0564 | 0.1072 | 0.0532 | 0.1092 | 0.0608 | 0.1060 |
| $N_4$ | 0.0512 | 0.1016 | 0.0496 | 0.1076 | 0.0492 | 0.1052 | 0.0528 | 0.1012 |
| $N_5$ | 0.0504 | 0.1028 | 0.0496 | 0.1012 | 0.0544 | 0.1020 | 0.0508 | 0.1036 |

*Note* : $N_1 = (3,3,4)$, $N_2 = (4,5,6)$, $N_3 = (7,10,13)$, $N_4 = (12,20,28)$, $N_5 = (24,40,56)$, $\eta_1^2 = (1,1,1)$, $\eta_2^2 = (1,1,0.5)$, $\eta_3^2 = (1,0.6,0.3)$, $\eta_4^2 = (1,0.1,0.3)$.

**Table 7.2:** Sizes for hypothesis testing problem (7.10) ($\mu = \mu_0 = 0, a = 10$).

| | $\beta$ | | | | | | | |
| | 0.05 | 0.1 | 0.05 | 0.1 | 0.05 | 0.1 | 0.05 | 0.1 |
| $\sigma_A^2 = 1$ | $\eta_5^2$ | | $\eta_6^2$ | | $\eta_7^2$ | | $\eta_8^2$ | |
|---|---|---|---|---|---|---|---|---|
| $N_6$ | 0.0556 | 0.1012 | 0.0540 | 0.0980 | 0.0532 | 0.0996 | 0.0524 | 0.1032 |
| $N_7$ | 0.0520 | 0.0944 | 0.0536 | 0.0976 | 0.0544 | 0.0952 | 0.0548 | 0.0960 |
| $N_8$ | 0.0480 | 0.0980 | 0.0420 | 0.1024 | 0.0476 | 0.0992 | 0.0488 | 0.1032 |
| $N_9$ | 0.0496 | 0.0936 | 0.0488 | 0.0916 | 0.0476 | 0.0936 | 0.0476 | 0.0936 |
| $N_{10}$ | 0.0492 | 0.1024 | 0.0488 | 0.1000 | 0.0488 | 0.0960 | 0.0484 | 0.0972 |
| $\sigma_A^2 = 5$ | $\eta_5^2$ | | $\eta_6^2$ | | $\eta_7^2$ | | $\eta_8^2$ | |
| $N_6$ | 0.0532 | 0.0980 | 0.0504 | 0.0964 | 0.0528 | 0.0980 | 0.0508 | 0.0984 |
| $N_7$ | 0.0536 | 0.0956 | 0.0520 | 0.0976 | 0.0536 | 0.1008 | 0.0508 | 0.0976 |
| $N_8$ | 0.0500 | 0.1024 | 0.0488 | 0.1028 | 0.0492 | 0.1028 | 0.0472 | 0.1036 |
| $N_9$ | 0.0448 | 0.0920 | 0.0464 | 0.0932 | 0.0460 | 0.0948 | 0.0444 | 0.0924 |
| $N_{10}$ | 0.0496 | 0.0984 | 0.0512 | 0.0988 | 0.0524 | 0.0988 | 0.0532 | 0.1008 |

*Note* : $N_6 = (3)_{10}$, $N_7 = (3,4,4,5,5)_2$, $N_8 = (7,7,8,8,9)_2$, $N_9 = (9,9,10,10,12)_2$, $N_{10} = (11,11,12,13,13)_2$, $\eta_5^2 = (1)_{10}$, $\eta_6^2 = (1,0.9,0.8,0.7,0.6,0.5,0.4,0.3,0.2,0.1)$, $\eta_7^2 = (1,(0.3,0.6,0.9)_3)$, $\eta_8^2 = (1,(0.1)_2,(0.2)_2,(0.3)_2,(0.4)_2,0.5)$.

For hypothesis testing problem (7.19), Tables 7.5–7.6 and Tables 7.7–7.8 respectively present the simulated sizes and powers of the BA and generalized approach (GA) under the different nominal significance levels. It can be seen from Tables 7.5–7.6 that the actual sizes of BA are close to the nominal sizes in most cases, but they are slightly liberal or conservative under certain sample sizes and parameter configurations. The GA appears relatively conservative in the cases of

**Table 7.3:** Powers for hypothesis testing problem (7.10) ($\mu_0 = 0$, $\sigma_A^2 = 5$, $a = 3$).

| | | $\beta$ | | | | | | | |
|---|---|---|---|---|---|---|---|---|---|
| | | 0.05 | 0.1 | 0.05 | 0.1 | 0.05 | 0.1 | 0.05 | 0.1 |
| | $\mu$ | $\eta_1^2$ | | $\eta_2^2$ | | $\eta_3^2$ | | $\eta_4^2$ | |
| $N_1$ | 1 | 0.1196 | 0.2444 | 0.1224 | 0.2428 | 0.1236 | 0.2416 | 0.1320 | 0.2392 |
| | 3 | 0.3832 | 0.6348 | 0.3864 | 0.6436 | 0.3884 | 0.6452 | 0.3800 | 0.6396 |
| | 5 | 0.6676 | 0.8900 | 0.6652 | 0.8912 | 0.6632 | 0.8916 | 0.6584 | 0.8952 |
| | 7 | 0.8480 | 0.9780 | 0.8468 | 0.9800 | 0.8456 | 0.9796 | 0.8540 | 0.9796 |
| $N_2$ | 1 | 0.1252 | 0.2416 | 0.1284 | 0.2416 | 0.1296 | 0.2404 | 0.1292 | 0.2388 |
| | 3 | 0.3800 | 0.6356 | 0.3784 | 0.6412 | 0.3836 | 0.6392 | 0.3844 | 0.6456 |
| | 5 | 0.6684 | 0.8908 | 0.6632 | 0.8908 | 0.6612 | 0.8936 | 0.6724 | 0.8988 |
| | 7 | 0.8468 | 0.9796 | 0.8464 | 0.9796 | 0.8484 | 0.9792 | 0.8520 | 0.9816 |
| $N_3$ | 1 | 0.1320 | 0.2472 | 0.1292 | 0.2520 | 0.1344 | 0.2528 | 0.1324 | 0.2520 |
| | 3 | 0.3948 | 0.6564 | 0.4024 | 0.6544 | 0.4052 | 0.6568 | 0.3996 | 0.6560 |
| | 5 | 0.6772 | 0.8916 | 0.6764 | 0.8936 | 0.6752 | 0.8940 | 0.6816 | 0.8992 |
| | 7 | 0.8480 | 0.9824 | 0.8512 | 0.9824 | 0.8556 | 0.9816 | 0.8556 | 0.9820 |
| $N_4$ | 1 | 0.1380 | 0.2468 | 0.1408 | 0.2508 | 0.1368 | 0.2508 | 0.1368 | 0.2604 |
| | 3 | 0.4028 | 0.6660 | 0.4024 | 0.6620 | 0.4016 | 0.6632 | 0.4044 | 0.6580 |
| | 5 | 0.6844 | 0.9104 | 0.6828 | 0.9092 | 0.6852 | 0.9108 | 0.6772 | 0.9144 |
| | 7 | 0.8700 | 0.9868 | 0.8660 | 0.9848 | 0.8644 | 0.9852 | 0.8664 | 0.9848 |
| $N_5$ | 1 | 0.1416 | 0.2592 | 0.1392 | 0.2588 | 0.1412 | 0.2576 | 0.1440 | 0.2656 |
| | 3 | 0.3996 | 0.6576 | 0.3972 | 0.6588 | 0.3960 | 0.6628 | 0.3960 | 0.6556 |
| | 5 | 0.6736 | 0.8992 | 0.6740 | 0.8968 | 0.6780 | 0.8988 | 0.6788 | 0.9016 |
| | 7 | 0.8576 | 0.9824 | 0.8560 | 0.9816 | 0.8568 | 0.9812 | 0.8608 | 0.9820 |

*Note :* $N_1 = (3,3,4)$, $N_2 = (4,5,6)$, $N_3 = (7,10,13)$, $N_4 = (12,20,28)$, $N_5 = (24,40,56)$, $\eta_1^2 = (1,1,1)$, $\eta_2^2 = (1,1,0.5)$, $\eta_3^2 = (1,0.6,0.3)$, $\eta_4^2 = (1,0.1,0.3)$.

$N_1$, $N_6$ and $N_7$, but its performance improves with the sample sizes increasing. The results of Tables 7.7–7.8 indicate that the BA is uniformly better than the GA in terms of the power for the above parameter configurations, sample sizes and nominal significance levels.

For hypothesis testing problem (7.33), Tables 7.9–7.10 and Tables 7.11–7.12 respectively present the simulated sizes and powers of the BA and GA under the different nominal significance levels. From Tables 7.9–7.10, the BA can maintain the nominal sizes quite well in most cases, but its actual sizes are slightly conservative in the cases of $N_6$, $N_7$ and $N_8$. The performance of GA is liberal in most situations, but it is relatively conservative under the sample size $N_6$. As seen from Tables 7.11–7.12, as $\sigma_A^2 + \sigma_1^2$ departs from the null hypothesis, the powers of two approaches both significantly rise, but the GA outperforms the BA in most cases.

For hypothesis testing problem (7.45), Tables 7.13–7.14 and Tables 7.15–7.16 respectively present the simulated sizes and powers of the BA and GA under the different nominal significance levels. As in Tables 7.13–7.14, the empirical

**Table 7.4:** Powers for hypothesis testing problem (7.10) ($\mu_0 = 0$, $\sigma_A^2 = 5$, $a = 10$).

| | $\mu$ | $\eta_5^2$ | | $\eta_6^2$ | | $\eta_7^2$ | | $\eta_8^2$ | |
|---|---|---|---|---|---|---|---|---|---|
| | | 0.05 | 0.1 | 0.05 | 0.1 | 0.05 | 0.1 | 0.05 | 0.1 |
| $N_6$ | 0.5 | 0.1812 | 0.3164 | 0.1888 | 0.3236 | 0.1828 | 0.3184 | 0.1784 | 0.3152 |
| | 1.0 | 0.4500 | 0.6608 | 0.4612 | 0.6724 | 0.4612 | 0.6728 | 0.4640 | 0.6800 |
| | 1.5 | 0.7696 | 0.9312 | 0.7896 | 0.9372 | 0.7848 | 0.9384 | 0.7952 | 0.9440 |
| | 2.0 | 0.9576 | 0.9944 | 0.9592 | 0.9956 | 0.9632 | 0.9948 | 0.9652 | 0.9956 |
| $N_7$ | 0.5 | 0.1688 | 0.3136 | 0.1700 | 0.3152 | 0.1692 | 0.3116 | 0.1724 | 0.3132 |
| | 1.0 | 0.4588 | 0.6696 | 0.4684 | 0.6780 | 0.4672 | 0.6776 | 0.4660 | 0.6776 |
| | 1.5 | 0.7808 | 0.9300 | 0.7912 | 0.9380 | 0.7884 | 0.9364 | 0.7920 | 0.9416 |
| | 2.0 | 0.9500 | 0.9972 | 0.9532 | 0.9980 | 0.9560 | 0.9972 | 0.9620 | 0.9976 |
| $N_8$ | 0.5 | 0.1832 | 0.3072 | 0.1860 | 0.3080 | 0.1824 | 0.3064 | 0.1876 | 0.3064 |
| | 1.0 | 0.4584 | 0.6728 | 0.4544 | 0.6756 | 0.4580 | 0.6728 | 0.4592 | 0.6736 |
| | 1.5 | 0.7796 | 0.9384 | 0.7856 | 0.9404 | 0.7860 | 0.9408 | 0.7876 | 0.9408 |
| | 2.0 | 0.9620 | 0.9972 | 0.9616 | 0.9972 | 0.9636 | 0.9976 | 0.9644 | 0.9976 |
| $N_9$ | 0.5 | 0.1736 | 0.3068 | 0.1744 | 0.3136 | 0.1720 | 0.3112 | 0.1740 | 0.3128 |
| | 1.0 | 0.4592 | 0.6812 | 0.4628 | 0.6892 | 0.4696 | 0.6820 | 0.4692 | 0.6820 |
| | 1.5 | 0.7948 | 0.9464 | 0.8004 | 0.9492 | 0.8004 | 0.9476 | 0.8036 | 0.9476 |
| | 2.0 | 0.9632 | 0.9948 | 0.9652 | 0.9948 | 0.9624 | 0.9952 | 0.9684 | 0.9960 |
| $N_{10}$ | 0.5 | 0.1860 | 0.3148 | 0.1832 | 0.3152 | 0.1840 | 0.3132 | 0.1824 | 0.3132 |
| | 1.0 | 0.4692 | 0.6836 | 0.4696 | 0.6868 | 0.4664 | 0.6824 | 0.4656 | 0.6844 |
| | 1.5 | 0.8024 | 0.9500 | 0.8072 | 0.9480 | 0.8060 | 0.9492 | 0.8096 | 0.9492 |
| | 2.0 | 0.9656 | 0.9960 | 0.9656 | 0.9968 | 0.9664 | 0.9964 | 0.9672 | 0.9960 |

*Note*: $N_6 = (3)_{10}$, $N_7 = (3,4,4,5,5)_2$, $N_8 = (7,7,8,8,9)_2$, $N_9 = (9,9,10,10,12)_2$, $N_{10} = (11,11,12,13,13)_2$, $\eta_5^2 = (1)_{10}$, $\eta_6^2 = (1,0.9,0.8,0.7,0.6,0.5,0.4,0.3,0.2,0.1)$, $\eta_7^2 = (1,(0.3,0.6,0.9)_3)$, $\eta_8^2 = \left(1,(0.1)_2,(0.2)_2,(0.3)_2,(0.4)_2,0.5\right)$.

sizes of BA are quite liberal when the sample sizes are small, while those of GA are relatively conservative with sample sizes $N_1$ and $N_6$. With the increase of sample sizes, the actual levels of the two proposed approaches are closer to the nominal significance levels. The results of Tables 7.15–7.16 show that in cases where $\frac{\sigma_A^2}{\sigma_1^2}$ departs from the null hypothesis, the powers of two approaches increase apparently, but the BA is uniformly better than the GA in the sense of power.

We also study the sizes and powers of the above approaches under large sample size scenarios and different parameter configurations. Limited by the length of the book, we give the simulation results with sample sizes $N_{11} = (40, 50, 60)$, $N_{12} = (60, 65, 75)$ and $N_{13} = (70, 80, 100)$, see Tables 7.17–7.18. The results show that the proposed approaches are robust in terms of the size and power. We can provide more simulation results at readers' requests.

**Remark 7.7.** *For hypothesis testing problem (7.10), the sizes and powers of the BA are also studied by Monte Carlo simulation when the nominal significance*

**Table 7.5:** Sizes for hypothesis testing problem (7.19) ($\sigma_A^2 = c_1 = 5$, $a = 3$, $\mu = 1$).

|  |  | $\beta$ | | | | | | | |
|---|---|---|---|---|---|---|---|---|---|
|  |  | 0.025 | | 0.05 | | 0.075 | | 0.1 | |
|  |  | BA | GA | BA | GA | BA | GA | BA | GA |
| $N_1$ | $\eta_1^2$ | 0.0260 | 0.0088 | 0.0524 | 0.0252 | 0.0728 | 0.0480 | 0.1044 | 0.0696 |
|  | $\eta_2^2$ | 0.0252 | 0.0088 | 0.0532 | 0.0272 | 0.0756 | 0.0488 | 0.1028 | 0.0708 |
|  | $\eta_3^2$ | 0.0252 | 0.0100 | 0.0556 | 0.0308 | 0.0788 | 0.0556 | 0.1036 | 0.0772 |
|  | $\eta_4^2$ | 0.0236 | 0.0156 | 0.0568 | 0.0380 | 0.0804 | 0.0624 | 0.1072 | 0.0868 |
| $N_2$ | $\eta_1^2$ | 0.0304 | 0.0236 | 0.0532 | 0.0484 | 0.0824 | 0.0696 | 0.1060 | 0.0992 |
|  | $\eta_2^2$ | 0.0292 | 0.0228 | 0.0524 | 0.0488 | 0.0812 | 0.0688 | 0.1076 | 0.0996 |
|  | $\eta_3^2$ | 0.0296 | 0.0228 | 0.0508 | 0.0484 | 0.0828 | 0.0724 | 0.1096 | 0.1008 |
|  | $\eta_4^2$ | 0.0292 | 0.0248 | 0.0572 | 0.0516 | 0.0796 | 0.0736 | 0.1092 | 0.1020 |
| $N_3$ | $\eta_1^2$ | 0.0308 | 0.0304 | 0.0588 | 0.0580 | 0.0812 | 0.0812 | 0.1084 | 0.1052 |
|  | $\eta_2^2$ | 0.0304 | 0.0304 | 0.0588 | 0.0580 | 0.0800 | 0.0788 | 0.1080 | 0.1068 |
|  | $\eta_3^2$ | 0.0312 | 0.0308 | 0.0572 | 0.0568 | 0.0832 | 0.0828 | 0.1068 | 0.1048 |
|  | $\eta_4^2$ | 0.0304 | 0.0304 | 0.0552 | 0.0544 | 0.0816 | 0.0800 | 0.1044 | 0.1036 |
| $N_4$ | $\eta_1^2$ | 0.0208 | 0.0208 | 0.0468 | 0.0468 | 0.0688 | 0.0688 | 0.0936 | 0.0932 |
|  | $\eta_2^2$ | 0.0208 | 0.0208 | 0.0472 | 0.0472 | 0.0704 | 0.0700 | 0.0928 | 0.0924 |
|  | $\eta_3^2$ | 0.0204 | 0.0204 | 0.0444 | 0.0444 | 0.0680 | 0.0680 | 0.0912 | 0.0900 |
|  | $\eta_4^2$ | 0.0196 | 0.0196 | 0.0456 | 0.0456 | 0.0684 | 0.0684 | 0.0912 | 0.0912 |
| $N_5$ | $\eta_1^2$ | 0.0228 | 0.0228 | 0.0472 | 0.0472 | 0.0732 | 0.0732 | 0.0976 | 0.0972 |
|  | $\eta_2^2$ | 0.0232 | 0.0232 | 0.0480 | 0.0480 | 0.0716 | 0.0716 | 0.0968 | 0.0968 |
|  | $\eta_3^2$ | 0.0220 | 0.0220 | 0.0488 | 0.0488 | 0.0724 | 0.0724 | 0.0964 | 0.0964 |
|  | $\eta_4^2$ | 0.0224 | 0.0224 | 0.0488 | 0.0488 | 0.0728 | 0.0728 | 0.1012 | 0.1012 |

*Note :* $N_1 = (3,3,4)$, $N_2 = (4,5,6)$, $N_3 = (7,10,13)$, $N_4 = (12,20,28)$, $N_5 = (24,40,56)$, $\eta_1^2 = (1,1,1)$, $\eta_2^2 = (1,1,0.5)$, $\eta_3^2 = (1,0.6,0.3)$, $\eta_4^2 = (1,0.1,0.3)$.

*levels are 0.025 and 0.075. The results indicate that the BA performs well in terms of the size and power. However, due to space limitations, the simulation results are omitted.*

**Table 7.6:** Sizes for hypothesis testing problem (7.19) ($\sigma_A^2 = c_1 = 5, a = 10, \mu = 1$).

| | | $\beta$ | | | | | | | |
| | | 0.025 | | 0.05 | | 0.075 | | 0.1 | |
| | | BA | GA | BA | GA | BA | GA | BA | GA |
|---|---|---|---|---|---|---|---|---|---|
| $N_6$ | $\eta_5^2$ | 0.0264 | 0.0008 | 0.0464 | 0.0056 | 0.0724 | 0.0128 | 0.1012 | 0.0204 |
| | $\eta_6^2$ | 0.0292 | 0.0032 | 0.0464 | 0.0140 | 0.0744 | 0.0264 | 0.0976 | 0.0400 |
| | $\eta_7^2$ | 0.0276 | 0.0012 | 0.0476 | 0.0116 | 0.0716 | 0.0216 | 0.1000 | 0.0344 |
| | $\eta_8^2$ | 0.0264 | 0.0072 | 0.0472 | 0.0224 | 0.0712 | 0.0344 | 0.1020 | 0.0516 |
| $N_7$ | $\eta_5^2$ | 0.0292 | 0.0104 | 0.0528 | 0.0288 | 0.0796 | 0.0448 | 0.1052 | 0.0640 |
| | $\eta_6^2$ | 0.0296 | 0.0144 | 0.0504 | 0.0356 | 0.0760 | 0.0512 | 0.1048 | 0.0712 |
| | $\eta_7^2$ | 0.0304 | 0.0144 | 0.0532 | 0.0356 | 0.0780 | 0.0516 | 0.1048 | 0.0680 |
| | $\eta_8^2$ | 0.0300 | 0.0188 | 0.0504 | 0.0388 | 0.0796 | 0.0572 | 0.1092 | 0.0796 |
| $N_8$ | $\eta_5^2$ | 0.0312 | 0.0300 | 0.0580 | 0.0544 | 0.0844 | 0.0784 | 0.1080 | 0.1040 |
| | $\eta_6^2$ | 0.0324 | 0.0312 | 0.0588 | 0.0560 | 0.0888 | 0.0872 | 0.1096 | 0.1080 |
| | $\eta_7^2$ | 0.0324 | 0.0312 | 0.0556 | 0.0548 | 0.0820 | 0.0792 | 0.1072 | 0.1032 |
| | $\eta_8^2$ | 0.0324 | 0.0308 | 0.0620 | 0.0612 | 0.0848 | 0.0824 | 0.1076 | 0.1068 |
| $N_9$ | $\eta_5^2$ | 0.0272 | 0.0256 | 0.0576 | 0.0560 | 0.0836 | 0.0820 | 0.1104 | 0.1096 |
| | $\eta_6^2$ | 0.0296 | 0.0288 | 0.0576 | 0.0568 | 0.0808 | 0.0804 | 0.1064 | 0.1048 |
| | $\eta_7^2$ | 0.0296 | 0.0292 | 0.0592 | 0.0584 | 0.0856 | 0.0828 | 0.1104 | 0.1096 |
| | $\eta_8^2$ | 0.0284 | 0.0280 | 0.0560 | 0.0560 | 0.0840 | 0.0836 | 0.1072 | 0.1072 |
| $N_{10}$ | $\eta_5^2$ | 0.0320 | 0.0320 | 0.0524 | 0.0512 | 0.0776 | 0.0756 | 0.1036 | 0.1032 |
| | $\eta_6^2$ | 0.0276 | 0.0276 | 0.0520 | 0.0520 | 0.0768 | 0.0768 | 0.1100 | 0.1088 |
| | $\eta_7^2$ | 0.0292 | 0.0292 | 0.0520 | 0.0516 | 0.0776 | 0.0768 | 0.1068 | 0.1068 |
| | $\eta_8^2$ | 0.0276 | 0.0276 | 0.0504 | 0.0504 | 0.0768 | 0.0764 | 0.1060 | 0.1056 |

*Note* : $N_6 = (3)_{10}$, $N_7 = (3,4,4,5,5)_2$, $N_8 = (7,7,8,8,9)_2$, $N_9 = (9,9,10,10,12)_2$, $N_{10} = (11,11,12,13,13)_2$, $\eta_5^2 = (1)_{10}$, $\eta_6^2 = (1,0.9,0.8,0.7,0.6,0.5,0.4,0.3,0.2,0.1)$, $\eta_7^2 = (1,(0.3,0.6,0.9)_3)$, $\eta_8^2 = (1,(0.1)_2,(0.2)_2,(0.3)_2,(0.4)_2,0.5)$.

## 7.7 Illustrative examples

To verify the reasonableness and effectiveness of the proposed approaches, two examples of the annual average concentrations of fine particulate matter and nitrogen dioxide are presented.

**Example 7.1** There exist annual average concentration data of fine particulate matter (PM 2.5) for major cities in China from 2016 to 2020. The histogram of the data is given in Figure 7.1. It can be seen from Figure 7.1 that the data clearly

**Table 7.7:** Powers for hypothesis testing problem (7.19) ($c_1 = 5$, $a = 3$, $(\sigma_1^2, \sigma_2^2, \sigma_3^2) = \eta_3^2$, $\mu = 1$).

| | $\sigma_A^2$ | $\beta$ | | | | | | | |
|---|---|---|---|---|---|---|---|---|---|
| | | 0.025 | | 0.050 | | 0.075 | | 0.010 | |
| | | BA | GA | BA | GA | BA | GA | BA | GA |
| $N_1$ | 10 | 0.1584 | 0.1060 | 0.2152 | 0.1732 | 0.2688 | 0.2220 | 0.3080 | 0.2632 |
| | 50 | 0.6928 | 0.6280 | 0.7412 | 0.6984 | 0.7696 | 0.7400 | 0.7908 | 0.7636 |
| | 100 | 0.8304 | 0.7912 | 0.8584 | 0.8344 | 0.8784 | 0.8564 | 0.8924 | 0.8724 |
| | 200 | 0.9132 | 0.8888 | 0.9296 | 0.9188 | 0.9400 | 0.9308 | 0.9480 | 0.9368 |
| $N_2$ | 10 | 0.1580 | 0.1488 | 0.2144 | 0.2020 | 0.2716 | 0.2580 | 0.3100 | 0.2976 |
| | 50 | 0.6888 | 0.6780 | 0.7436 | 0.7332 | 0.7776 | 0.7704 | 0.7952 | 0.7876 |
| | 100 | 0.8340 | 0.8256 | 0.8644 | 0.8596 | 0.8824 | 0.8784 | 0.8956 | 0.8932 |
| | 200 | 0.9144 | 0.9120 | 0.9304 | 0.9280 | 0.9416 | 0.9396 | 0.9472 | 0.9468 |
| $N_3$ | 10 | 0.1576 | 0.1564 | 0.2272 | 0.2240 | 0.2736 | 0.2720 | 0.3128 | 0.3104 |
| | 50 | 0.6840 | 0.6820 | 0.7376 | 0.7356 | 0.7724 | 0.7716 | 0.7988 | 0.7988 |
| | 100 | 0.8316 | 0.8308 | 0.8580 | 0.8568 | 0.8768 | 0.8760 | 0.8900 | 0.8896 |
| | 200 | 0.9132 | 0.9120 | 0.9288 | 0.9280 | 0.9428 | 0.9424 | 0.9480 | 0.9480 |
| $N_4$ | 10 | 0.1456 | 0.1452 | 0.2192 | 0.2184 | 0.2664 | 0.2664 | 0.3168 | 0.3160 |
| | 50 | 0.6908 | 0.6904 | 0.7380 | 0.7372 | 0.7688 | 0.7688 | 0.7892 | 0.7884 |
| | 100 | 0.8256 | 0.8252 | 0.8544 | 0.8544 | 0.8720 | 0.8720 | 0.8856 | 0.8856 |
| | 200 | 0.9088 | 0.9084 | 0.9232 | 0.9232 | 0.9344 | 0.9340 | 0.9408 | 0.9404 |
| $N_5$ | 10 | 0.1580 | 0.1580 | 0.2212 | 0.2204 | 0.2740 | 0.2740 | 0.3164 | 0.3164 |
| | 50 | 0.6784 | 0.6780 | 0.7344 | 0.7344 | 0.7676 | 0.7672 | 0.7968 | 0.7968 |
| | 100 | 0.8296 | 0.8296 | 0.8584 | 0.8584 | 0.8760 | 0.8760 | 0.8880 | 0.8880 |
| | 200 | 0.9080 | 0.9080 | 0.9240 | 0.9240 | 0.9352 | 0.9352 | 0.9428 | 0.9428 |

*Note :* $N_1 = (3,3,4)$, $N_2 = (4,5,6)$, $N_3 = (7,10,13)$, $N_4 = (12,20,28)$, $N_5 = (24,40,56)$, $\eta_3^2 = (1,0.6,0.3)$.

show skew distribution characteristics. To verify the conclusion, we first conduct the normality test for the data. It turns out that the $p$-values of the Shapiro-Wilk test, Anderson-Darling test and Cramer-von Mises test are 6.873e-4, 8.978e-4 and 1.981e-3 respectively. Therefore, the annual average concentration data of PM 2.5 are not normally distributed at the nominal significance level of 5%. In addition, we conduct the chi-square goodness-of-fit test to see if the distribution of the data is skew-normal, namely we set $H_0$: the annual average concentration data of PM 2.5 are skew-normally distributed. By calculation, the fitted value of the data is $\chi^2 = 2.1284 < \chi_4^2(0.95) = 9.4877$ with $p$-value 0.7122. Consequently, the null hypothesis $H_0$ is not rejected at the nominal significance level of 5%. That is, the annual average concentration data of PM 2.5 is considered to be a skew-normal distribution. Based on the method of moments estimation, the data is distributed as $SN\left(26.5717, 24.8137^2, 2.6614\right)$, and its density curve is given in Figure 7.1.

Then, the model for annual average concentration data of PM 2.5 is written as (7.2), where $Y$ is the 200-vector of all measurements, $A \sim SN_{46}\left(0, \sigma_A^2 I_{46}, \lambda_1\right)$,

**Table 7.8:** Powers for hypothesis testing problem (7.19) ($c_1 = 5$, $a = 10$, $(\sigma_1^2, \cdots, \sigma_{10}^2) = \eta_6^2, \mu = 1$).

| | $\sigma_A^2$ | $\beta$ | | | | | | | |
|---|---|---|---|---|---|---|---|---|---|
| | | 0.025 | | 0.05 | | 0.075 | | 0.1 | |
| | | BA | GA | BA | GA | BA | GA | BA | GA |
| $N_6$ | 10 | 0.3812 | 0.1356 | 0.4788 | 0.2692 | 0.5408 | 0.3664 | 0.5900 | 0.4296 |
| | 15 | 0.6980 | 0.4032 | 0.7644 | 0.5916 | 0.8092 | 0.6804 | 0.8396 | 0.7328 |
| | 20 | 0.8496 | 0.6324 | 0.8924 | 0.7744 | 0.9164 | 0.8412 | 0.9336 | 0.8708 |
| | 25 | 0.9244 | 0.7644 | 0.9448 | 0.8736 | 0.9616 | 0.9200 | 0.9688 | 0.9400 |
| $N_7$ | 10 | 0.3896 | 0.2920 | 0.4812 | 0.3996 | 0.5476 | 0.4788 | 0.6008 | 0.5344 |
| | 15 | 0.7052 | 0.6132 | 0.7764 | 0.7184 | 0.8148 | 0.7704 | 0.8372 | 0.8020 |
| | 20 | 0.8456 | 0.7896 | 0.8952 | 0.8552 | 0.9168 | 0.8912 | 0.9300 | 0.9128 |
| | 25 | 0.9216 | 0.8820 | 0.9492 | 0.9276 | 0.9608 | 0.9468 | 0.9720 | 0.9588 |
| $N_8$ | 10 | 0.3916 | 0.3876 | 0.4852 | 0.4780 | 0.5464 | 0.5404 | 0.6016 | 0.5944 |
| | 15 | 0.7092 | 0.7060 | 0.7748 | 0.7728 | 0.8200 | 0.8164 | 0.8532 | 0.8512 |
| | 20 | 0.8616 | 0.8600 | 0.9000 | 0.8988 | 0.9192 | 0.9172 | 0.9316 | 0.9296 |
| | 25 | 0.9244 | 0.9228 | 0.9460 | 0.9456 | 0.9576 | 0.9564 | 0.9640 | 0.9628 |
| $N_9$ | 10 | 0.3736 | 0.3716 | 0.4820 | 0.4796 | 0.5456 | 0.5424 | 0.6004 | 0.5980 |
| | 15 | 0.7044 | 0.7012 | 0.7700 | 0.7692 | 0.8120 | 0.8092 | 0.8348 | 0.8340 |
| | 20 | 0.8488 | 0.8476 | 0.8920 | 0.8900 | 0.9148 | 0.9132 | 0.9276 | 0.9264 |
| | 25 | 0.9212 | 0.9208 | 0.9444 | 0.9432 | 0.9580 | 0.9572 | 0.9640 | 0.9628 |
| $N_{10}$ | 10 | 0.3956 | 0.3940 | 0.4932 | 0.4916 | 0.5560 | 0.5548 | 0.6024 | 0.6020 |
| | 15 | 0.7032 | 0.7024 | 0.7772 | 0.7756 | 0.8156 | 0.8152 | 0.8408 | 0.8400 |
| | 20 | 0.8508 | 0.8504 | 0.8904 | 0.8896 | 0.9132 | 0.9120 | 0.9240 | 0.9236 |
| | 25 | 0.9160 | 0.9156 | 0.9388 | 0.9388 | 0.9520 | 0.9512 | 0.9624 | 0.9616 |

*Note :* $N_6 = (3)_{10}$, $N_7 = (3,4,4,5,5)_2$, $N_8 = (7,7,8,8,9)_2$, $N_9 = (9,9,10,10,12)_2$, $N_{10} = (11,11,12,13,13)_2$, $\eta_6^2 = (1,0.9,0.8,0.7,0.6,0.5,0.4,0.3,0.2,0.1)$.

$e \sim N_{200}\left(0, diag\left\{\sigma_i^2 I_{n_i}\right\}\right)$, $i = 1, \cdots, 46$, and $A$ and $e$ are mutually independent. For $i = 1, \cdots, 31$, $n_i = 5$; Otherwise, $n_i = 3$.

Firstly, consider the hypothesis testing problem for fixed effect

$$H_0 : \mu \le 40 \quad versus \quad H_1 : \mu > 40, \tag{7.56}$$

Based on (7.17), the Bootstrap $p$-value is 0.0243 by $10^4$ loops. Thus, the null hypothesis $H_0$ in (7.56) is rejected at the nominal significance level of 5%.

Secondly, consider the hypothesis testing problem for a single variance component

$$H_0 : \sigma_A^2 \le 200 \quad versus \quad H_1 : \sigma_A^2 > 200, \tag{7.57}$$

By (7.22) and (7.27), the Bootstrap $p$-value and generalized $p$-value are 0.1730 and 0.3459 respectively. Hence, these two approaches cannot reject the null hypothesis $H_0$ in (7.57) at the nominal significance level of 5%.

**Table 7.9:** Sizes for hypothesis testing problem (7.33) ($\sigma_A^2 + \sigma_1^2 = c_{21} = 6$, $a = 3$, $\mu = 1$).

| | | $\beta$ | | | | | | | |
| | | 0.025 | | 0.05 | | 0.075 | | 0.1 | |
| | | BA | GA | BA | GA | BA | GA | BA | GA |
|---|---|---|---|---|---|---|---|---|---|
| $N_1$ | $\eta_1^2$ | 0.0228 | 0.0220 | 0.0528 | 0.0540 | 0.0772 | 0.0820 | 0.1032 | 0.1120 |
| | $\eta_2^2$ | 0.0236 | 0.0232 | 0.0524 | 0.0556 | 0.0760 | 0.0856 | 0.1060 | 0.1148 |
| | $\eta_3^2$ | 0.0232 | 0.0288 | 0.0540 | 0.0612 | 0.0788 | 0.0932 | 0.1068 | 0.1244 |
| | $\eta_4^2$ | 0.0232 | 0.0384 | 0.0516 | 0.0676 | 0.0828 | 0.1056 | 0.1092 | 0.1380 |
| $N_2$ | $\eta_1^2$ | 0.0196 | 0.0344 | 0.0484 | 0.0720 | 0.0768 | 0.1040 | 0.1056 | 0.1388 |
| | $\eta_2^2$ | 0.0196 | 0.0360 | 0.0484 | 0.0700 | 0.0776 | 0.1040 | 0.1048 | 0.1352 |
| | $\eta_3^2$ | 0.0180 | 0.0372 | 0.0488 | 0.0732 | 0.0756 | 0.1060 | 0.1060 | 0.1384 |
| | $\eta_4^2$ | 0.0204 | 0.0404 | 0.0536 | 0.0780 | 0.0792 | 0.1096 | 0.1076 | 0.1356 |
| $N_3$ | $\eta_1^2$ | 0.0260 | 0.0408 | 0.0544 | 0.0680 | 0.0796 | 0.0972 | 0.1004 | 0.1248 |
| | $\eta_2^2$ | 0.0288 | 0.0412 | 0.0544 | 0.0692 | 0.0820 | 0.0968 | 0.1020 | 0.1248 |
| | $\eta_3^2$ | 0.0296 | 0.0400 | 0.0528 | 0.0692 | 0.0804 | 0.0972 | 0.1032 | 0.1240 |
| | $\eta_4^2$ | 0.0272 | 0.0360 | 0.0520 | 0.0664 | 0.0800 | 0.1000 | 0.1032 | 0.1236 |
| $N_4$ | $\eta_1^2$ | 0.0192 | 0.0240 | 0.0448 | 0.0528 | 0.0700 | 0.0756 | 0.0892 | 0.1036 |
| | $\eta_2^2$ | 0.0196 | 0.0232 | 0.0448 | 0.0516 | 0.0680 | 0.0764 | 0.0916 | 0.1044 |
| | $\eta_3^2$ | 0.0200 | 0.0236 | 0.0432 | 0.0496 | 0.0652 | 0.0772 | 0.0916 | 0.1032 |
| | $\eta_4^2$ | 0.0188 | 0.0260 | 0.0436 | 0.0516 | 0.0696 | 0.0752 | 0.0876 | 0.0988 |
| $N_5$ | $\eta_1^2$ | 0.0204 | 0.0236 | 0.0488 | 0.0524 | 0.0736 | 0.0760 | 0.0984 | 0.1048 |
| | $\eta_2^2$ | 0.0212 | 0.0240 | 0.0500 | 0.0540 | 0.0716 | 0.0752 | 0.0996 | 0.1032 |
| | $\eta_3^2$ | 0.0228 | 0.0248 | 0.0488 | 0.0544 | 0.0712 | 0.0764 | 0.0988 | 0.1052 |
| | $\eta_4^2$ | 0.0236 | 0.0264 | 0.0484 | 0.0532 | 0.0752 | 0.0792 | 0.1032 | 0.1064 |

*Note* : $N_1 = (3,3,4)$, $N_2 = (4,5,6)$, $N_3 = (7,10,13)$, $N_4 = (12,20,28)$, $N_5 = (24,40,56)$, $\eta_1^2 = (1,1,1)$, $\eta_2^2 = (1,1,0.5)$, $\eta_3^2 = (1,0.6,0.3)$, $\eta_4^2 = (1,0.1,0.3)$.

Next, consider the hypothesis testing problem for the sum of the variance components

$$H_0 : \sigma_A^2 + \sigma_1^2 \leq 250 \quad versus \quad H_1 : \sigma_A^2 + \sigma_1^2 > 250, \qquad (7.58)$$

The Bootstrap $p$-value based on (7.36) is 0.0377, and the generalized $p$-value based on (7.40) is 0.0343. Therefore, at the nominal significance level of 5%, these two approaches can reject the null hypothesis $H_0$ in (7.58).

**Table 7.10:** Sizes for hypothesis testing problem (7.33) ($\sigma_A^2 + \sigma_1^2 = c_{21} = 6$, $a = 10$, $\mu = 1$).

| | | $\beta$ | | | | | | | |
| | | 0.025 | | 0.05 | | 0.075 | | 0.1 | |
| | | BA | GA | BA | GA | BA | GA | BA | GA |
|---|---|---|---|---|---|---|---|---|---|
| $N_6$ | $\eta_5^2$ | 0.0156 | 0.0012 | 0.0364 | 0.0124 | 0.0668 | 0.0296 | 0.0936 | 0.0508 |
| | $\eta_6^2$ | 0.0188 | 0.0096 | 0.0376 | 0.0316 | 0.0680 | 0.0568 | 0.0952 | 0.0800 |
| | $\eta_7^2$ | 0.0176 | 0.0068 | 0.0380 | 0.0268 | 0.0664 | 0.0488 | 0.0944 | 0.0736 |
| | $\eta_8^2$ | 0.0176 | 0.0192 | 0.0376 | 0.0468 | 0.0660 | 0.0704 | 0.0920 | 0.1024 |
| $N_7$ | $\eta_5^2$ | 0.0152 | 0.0212 | 0.0404 | 0.0556 | 0.0708 | 0.0880 | 0.1004 | 0.1168 |
| | $\eta_6^2$ | 0.0176 | 0.0308 | 0.0380 | 0.0660 | 0.0704 | 0.1032 | 0.1048 | 0.1348 |
| | $\eta_7^2$ | 0.0176 | 0.0284 | 0.0404 | 0.0696 | 0.0720 | 0.1012 | 0.1036 | 0.1320 |
| | $\eta_8^2$ | 0.0164 | 0.0332 | 0.0416 | 0.0756 | 0.0704 | 0.1088 | 0.1040 | 0.1448 |
| $N_8$ | $\eta_5^2$ | 0.0164 | 0.0372 | 0.0404 | 0.0696 | 0.0700 | 0.1088 | 0.0968 | 0.1356 |
| | $\eta_6^2$ | 0.0148 | 0.0356 | 0.0408 | 0.0744 | 0.0712 | 0.1052 | 0.0996 | 0.1328 |
| | $\eta_7^2$ | 0.0156 | 0.0376 | 0.0412 | 0.0724 | 0.0668 | 0.1060 | 0.0960 | 0.1328 |
| | $\eta_8^2$ | 0.0168 | 0.0396 | 0.0436 | 0.0776 | 0.0728 | 0.1024 | 0.0924 | 0.1348 |
| $N_9$ | $\eta_5^2$ | 0.0176 | 0.0328 | 0.0448 | 0.0672 | 0.0744 | 0.1012 | 0.1008 | 0.1236 |
| | $\eta_6^2$ | 0.0188 | 0.0332 | 0.0432 | 0.0636 | 0.0716 | 0.1020 | 0.0996 | 0.1264 |
| | $\eta_7^2$ | 0.0196 | 0.0340 | 0.0472 | 0.0696 | 0.0740 | 0.0984 | 0.0988 | 0.1248 |
| | $\eta_8^2$ | 0.0200 | 0.0352 | 0.0456 | 0.0660 | 0.0692 | 0.0960 | 0.0960 | 0.1264 |
| $N_{10}$ | $\eta_5^2$ | 0.0236 | 0.0356 | 0.0492 | 0.0640 | 0.0708 | 0.0932 | 0.0944 | 0.1224 |
| | $\eta_6^2$ | 0.0220 | 0.0336 | 0.0488 | 0.0680 | 0.0728 | 0.0940 | 0.1000 | 0.1256 |
| | $\eta_7^2$ | 0.0236 | 0.0344 | 0.0492 | 0.0660 | 0.0724 | 0.0968 | 0.0968 | 0.1240 |
| | $\eta_8^2$ | 0.0212 | 0.0312 | 0.0452 | 0.0660 | 0.0724 | 0.0940 | 0.0980 | 0.1224 |

*Note :* $N_6 = (3)_{10}$, $N_7 = (3,4,4,5,5)_2$, $N_8 = (7,7,8,8,9)_2$, $N_9 = (9,9,10,10,12)_2$, $N_{10} = (11,11,12,13,13)_2$, $\eta_5^2 = (1)_{10}$, $\eta_6^2 = (1,0.9,0.8,0.7,0.6,0.5,0.4,0.3,0.2,0.1)$, $\eta_7^2 = (1,(0.3,0.6,0.9)_3)$, $\eta_8^2 = \big(1,(0.1)_2,(0.2)_2,(0.3)_2,(0.4)_2,0.5\big)$.

At last, consider the hypothesis testing problem for the ratio of the variance components

$$H_0 : \sigma_A^2/\sigma_1^2 \leq 2 \quad versus \quad H_1 : \sigma_A^2/\sigma_1^2 > 2, \tag{7.59}$$

Based on (7.48) and (7.52), the Bootstrap $p$-value and generalized $p$-value are respectively 0.8045 and 0.8458. Thus, the null hypothesis $H_0$ in (7.59) is not rejected by these two approaches at the nominal significance level of 5%.

**Example 7.2** There exist annual average concentration data of nitrogen dioxide for major cities in China from 2016 to 2020. The histogram of the data is given in Figure 7.2. Similar to Example 7.1, we conduct the normality test for the data. It turns out that the $p$-values of the Shapiro-Wilk test, Anderson-Darling test and Cramer-von Mises test are 0.0239, 0.0335 and 0.0358 respectively. Thus, annual average concentration data of nitrogen dioxide are not normally distributed at

**Table 7.11:** Powers for hypothesis testing problem (7.33) ($c_{21} = 6$, $a = 3$, $(\sigma_1^2, \sigma_2^2, \sigma_3^2) = \eta_3^2, \mu = 1$).

| | $\sigma_A^2$ | $\beta$ | | | | | | | |
|---|---|---|---|---|---|---|---|---|---|
| | | 0.025 | | 0.05 | | 0.075 | | 0.1 | |
| | | BA | GA | BA | GA | BA | GA | BA | GA |
| $N_1$ | 10 | 0.1296 | 0.1560 | 0.2084 | 0.2276 | 0.2624 | 0.2880 | 0.3100 | 0.3420 |
| | 50 | 0.6604 | 0.6836 | 0.7272 | 0.7440 | 0.7632 | 0.7816 | 0.7876 | 0.7988 |
| | 100 | 0.8080 | 0.8244 | 0.8524 | 0.8628 | 0.8736 | 0.8816 | 0.8912 | 0.8948 |
| | 200 | 0.9040 | 0.9096 | 0.8256 | 0.9336 | 0.9392 | 0.9444 | 0.9468 | 0.9524 |
| $N_2$ | 10 | 0.1372 | 0.1816 | 0.1996 | 0.2500 | 0.2532 | 0.3008 | 0.3052 | 0.3528 |
| | 50 | 0.6652 | 0.7044 | 0.7292 | 0.7576 | 0.7632 | 0.7844 | 0.7888 | 0.8104 |
| | 100 | 0.8164 | 0.8428 | 0.8572 | 0.8724 | 0.8792 | 0.8912 | 0.8928 | 0.9068 |
| | 200 | 0.9060 | 0.9196 | 0.9276 | 0.9328 | 0.9368 | 0.9464 | 0.9460 | 0.9492 |
| $N_3$ | 10 | 0.1428 | 0.1696 | 0.2172 | 0.2472 | 0.2700 | 0.3004 | 0.3080 | 0.3376 |
| | 50 | 0.6700 | 0.6944 | 0.7296 | 0.7544 | 0.7696 | 0.7880 | 0.7932 | 0.8080 |
| | 100 | 0.8260 | 0.8356 | 0.8504 | 0.8640 | 0.8740 | 0.8860 | 0.8896 | 0.8968 |
| | 200 | 0.9060 | 0.9148 | 0.9260 | 0.9332 | 0.9384 | 0.9448 | 0.9480 | 0.9532 |
| $N_4$ | 10 | 0.1444 | 0.1608 | 0.2124 | 0.2324 | 0.2704 | 0.2852 | 0.3120 | 0.3328 |
| | 50 | 0.6872 | 0.6972 | 0.7320 | 0.7396 | 0.7672 | 0.7756 | 0.7876 | 0.7956 |
| | 100 | 0.8204 | 0.8264 | 0.8492 | 0.8536 | 0.8692 | 0.8768 | 0.8868 | 0.8932 |
| | 200 | 0.9060 | 0.9104 | 0.9220 | 0.9268 | 0.9336 | 0.9384 | 0.9412 | 0.9436 |
| $N_5$ | 10 | 0.1608 | 0.1664 | 0.2180 | 0.2264 | 0.2760 | 0.2812 | 0.3156 | 0.3196 |
| | 50 | 0.6800 | 0.6872 | 0.7324 | 0.7400 | 0.7676 | 0.7720 | 0.7932 | 0.7984 |
| | 100 | 0.8304 | 0.8320 | 0.8580 | 0.8628 | 0.8760 | 0.8776 | 0.8860 | 0.8896 |
| | 200 | 0.9064 | 0.9068 | 0.9224 | 0.9244 | 0.9324 | 0.9340 | 0.9420 | 0.9440 |

*Note :* $N_1 = (3,3,4)$, $N_2 = (4,5,6)$, $N_3 = (7,10,13)$, $N_4 = (12,20,28)$, $N_5 = (24,40,56)$, $\eta_3^2 = (1,0.6,0.3)$.

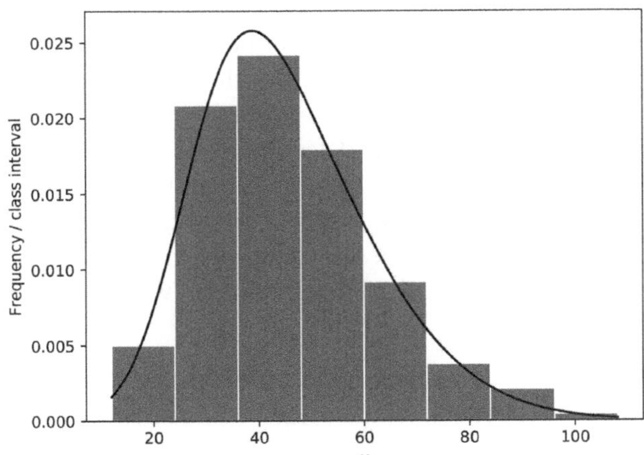

**Figure 7.1:** Histogram of annual average concentration data of PM 2.5 with superimposed skew-normal density curve.

**Table 7.12:** Powers for hypothesis testing problem (7.33) ($c_{21} = 6$, $a = 10$, $(\sigma_1^2, \cdots, \sigma_{10}^2) = \eta_6^2, \mu = 1$).

| | $\sigma_A^2$ | $\beta$ 0.025 BA | GA | 0.05 BA | GA | 0.075 BA | GA | 0.1 BA | GA |
|---|---|---|---|---|---|---|---|---|---|
| $N_6$ | 10 | 0.2172 | 0.2000 | 0.3656 | 0.3444 | 0.4720 | 0.4360 | 0.5348 | 0.5064 |
| | 15 | 0.5112 | 0.4908 | 0.6760 | 0.6468 | 0.7552 | 0.7384 | 0.8024 | 0.7820 |
| | 20 | 0.7144 | 0.7032 | 0.8348 | 0.9208 | 0.8868 | 0.8776 | 0.9100 | 0.9016 |
| | 25 | 0.8200 | 0.8264 | 0.9124 | 0.9068 | 0.9412 | 0.9344 | 0.9568 | 0.9516 |
| $N_7$ | 10 | 0.2216 | 0.3548 | 0.3736 | 0.4696 | 0.4688 | 0.5488 | 0.5420 | 0.6056 |
| | 15 | 0.5236 | 0.6740 | 0.6900 | 0.7612 | 0.7680 | 0.8104 | 0.8104 | 0.8432 |
| | 20 | 0.7160 | 0.8352 | 0.8344 | 0.8796 | 0.8840 | 0.9120 | 0.9116 | 0.9324 |
| | 25 | 0.8228 | 0.9072 | 0.9116 | 0.9424 | 0.9412 | 0.9580 | 0.9564 | 0.9688 |
| $N_8$ | 10 | 0.3232 | 0.4140 | 0.4336 | 0.5068 | 0.5124 | 0.5764 | 0.5684 | 0.6228 |
| | 15 | 0.6332 | 0.7224 | 0.7436 | 0.7876 | 0.7932 | 0.8288 | 0.8276 | 0.8564 |
| | 20 | 0.8056 | 0.8608 | 0.8788 | 0.9000 | 0.9044 | 0.9220 | 0.9224 | 0.9344 |
| | 25 | 0.8972 | 0.9228 | 0.9340 | 0.9484 | 0.9520 | 0.9596 | 0.9584 | 0.9656 |
| $N_9$ | 10 | 0.3364 | 0.4020 | 0.4416 | 0.4940 | 0.5156 | 0.5700 | 0.5784 | 0.6216 |
| | 15 | 0.6576 | 0.7152 | 0.7520 | 0.7792 | 0.7912 | 0.8144 | 0.8188 | 0.8488 |
| | 20 | 0.8188 | 0.8556 | 0.8736 | 0.8936 | 0.9028 | 0.9188 | 0.9212 | 0.9336 |
| | 25 | 0.9036 | 0.9204 | 0.9356 | 0.9464 | 0.9508 | 0.9580 | 0.9608 | 0.9648 |
| $N_{10}$ | 10 | 0.3600 | 0.4084 | 0.4720 | 0.5096 | 0.5388 | 0.5728 | 0.5844 | 0.6120 |
| | 15 | 0.6788 | 0.7148 | 0.7548 | 0.7804 | 0.7996 | 0.8200 | 0.8288 | 0.8484 |
| | 20 | 0.8344 | 0.8576 | 0.8808 | 0.8972 | 0.9064 | 0.9164 | 0.9208 | 0.9304 |
| | 25 | 0.9060 | 0.9212 | 0.9368 | 0.9432 | 0.9492 | 0.9564 | 0.9588 | 0.9656 |

*Note :* $N_6 = (3)_{10}$, $N_7 = (3,4,4,5,5)_2$, $N_8 = (7,7,8,8,9)_2$, $N_9 = (9,9,10,10,12)_2$, $N_{10} = (11,11,12,13,13)_2$, $\eta_6^2 = (1,0.9,0.8,0.7,0.6,0.5,0.4,0.3,0.2,0.1)$.

the nominal significance level of 5%. Furthermore, to verify the skew-normality of the data, we intend to test the null hypothesis $H_0$: annual average concentration data of nitrogen dioxide are skew-normally distributed. This can be done by calculating the fitted value of the data which $\chi^2 = 1.1680 < \chi_3^2(0.95) = 7.8147$ with $p$-value 0.7607. Therefore, the annual average concentration data of nitrogen dioxide is considered to be a skew-normal distribution at the nominal significance level of 5%. Based on the method of moment estimation, the data are distributed as $SN\left(48.2601, 14.0898^2, -1.9895\right)$, whose density curve is given in Figure 7.2.

Then, the model for annual average concentration data of nitrogen dioxide is written as (7.2), where $Y$ is the 167-vector of all measurements,

**Table 7.13:** Sizes for hypothesis testing problem (7.45) ($\sigma_A^2/\sigma_1^2 = c_{31} = 5$, $a = 3$, $\mu = 1$).

| | | $\beta$ | | | | | | | |
| | | 0.025 | | 0.05 | | 0.075 | | 0.1 | |
| | | BA | GA | BA | GA | BA | GA | BA | GA |
|---|---|---|---|---|---|---|---|---|---|
| $N_1$ | $\eta_1^2$ | 0.0720 | 0.0132 | 0.1036 | 0.0324 | 0.1260 | 0.0568 | 0.1480 | 0.0848 |
| | $\eta_2^2$ | 0.0688 | 0.0128 | 0.0996 | 0.0364 | 0.1208 | 0.0636 | 0.1460 | 0.0872 |
| | $\eta_3^2$ | 0.0680 | 0.0152 | 0.0936 | 0.0428 | 0.1176 | 0.0720 | 0.1408 | 0.0940 |
| | $\eta_4^2$ | 0.0628 | 0.0260 | 0.0852 | 0.0552 | 0.1072 | 0.0796 | 0.1320 | 0.1060 |
| $N_2$ | $\eta_1^2$ | 0.0464 | 0.0240 | 0.0724 | 0.0460 | 0.0968 | 0.0740 | 0.1244 | 0.0960 |
| | $\eta_2^2$ | 0.0440 | 0.0240 | 0.0696 | 0.0480 | 0.0944 | 0.0744 | 0.1168 | 0.0968 |
| | $\eta_3^2$ | 0.0400 | 0.0240 | 0.0656 | 0.0488 | 0.0888 | 0.0772 | 0.1144 | 0.0984 |
| | $\eta_4^2$ | 0.0332 | 0.0236 | 0.0588 | 0.0492 | 0.0832 | 0.0764 | 0.1112 | 0.1036 |
| $N_3$ | $\eta_1^2$ | 0.0332 | 0.0284 | 0.0580 | 0.0548 | 0.0776 | 0.0748 | 0.1016 | 0.0996 |
| | $\eta_2^2$ | 0.0320 | 0.0292 | 0.0588 | 0.0548 | 0.0768 | 0.0744 | 0.1028 | 0.0984 |
| | $\eta_3^2$ | 0.0308 | 0.0284 | 0.0580 | 0.0552 | 0.0784 | 0.0764 | 0.0972 | 0.0960 |
| | $\eta_4^2$ | 0.0260 | 0.0256 | 0.0556 | 0.0552 | 0.0740 | 0.0728 | 0.1000 | 0.1000 |
| $N_4$ | $\eta_1^2$ | 0.0228 | 0.0228 | 0.0448 | 0.0432 | 0.0724 | 0.0720 | 0.0924 | 0.0912 |
| | $\eta_2^2$ | 0.0236 | 0.0236 | 0.0444 | 0.0440 | 0.0728 | 0.0716 | 0.0928 | 0.0912 |
| | $\eta_3^2$ | 0.0224 | 0.0220 | 0.0432 | 0.0432 | 0.0696 | 0.0696 | 0.0932 | 0.0932 |
| | $\eta_4^2$ | 0.0196 | 0.0196 | 0.0416 | 0.0416 | 0.0680 | 0.0680 | 0.0908 | 0.0908 |
| $N_5$ | $\eta_1^2$ | 0.0224 | 0.0224 | 0.0480 | 0.0480 | 0.0696 | 0.0692 | 0.0976 | 0.0972 |
| | $\eta_2^2$ | 0.0228 | 0.0224 | 0.0472 | 0.0472 | 0.0720 | 0.0720 | 0.0988 | 0.0988 |
| | $\eta_3^2$ | 0.0224 | 0.0220 | 0.0472 | 0.0468 | 0.0672 | 0.0672 | 0.0992 | 0.0992 |
| | $\eta_4^2$ | 0.0228 | 0.0228 | 0.0492 | 0.0492 | 0.0728 | 0.0728 | 0.0960 | 0.0960 |

*Note* : $N_1 = (3,3,4)$, $N_2 = (4,5,6)$, $N_3 = (7,10,13)$, $N_4 = (12,20,28)$, $N_5 = (24,40,56)$, $\eta_1^2 = (1,1,1)$, $\eta_2^2 = (1,1,0.5)$, $\eta_3^2 = (1,0.6,0.3)$, $\eta_4^2 = (1,0.1,0.3)$.

$A \sim SN_{36}\left(0, \sigma_A^2 I_{36}, \lambda_1\right)$, $e \sim N_{167}\left(0, diag\left\{\sigma_i^2 I_{n_i}\right\}\right)$, $i = 1, \cdots, 36$, and $A$ and $e$ are independent of each other. For $i = 1, \cdots, 30$, $n_i = 5$; For $i = 31, \cdots, 35$, $n_i = 3$; Otherwise, $n_{36} = 2$.

Firstly, consider the hypothesis testing problem for fixed effect

$$H_0 : \mu \leq 34 \quad versus \quad H_1 : \mu > 34, \tag{7.60}$$

Based on (7.17), the Bootstrap $p$-value is 0.0152 by $10^4$ loops. Hence, the null hypothesis $H_0$ in (7.60) can be rejected at the nominal significance level of 5%.

Secondly, consider the hypothesis testing problem for single variance component

$$H_0 : \sigma_A^2 \leq 60 \quad versus \quad H_1 : \sigma_A^2 > 60, \tag{7.61}$$

**Table 7.14:** Sizes for hypothesis testing problem (7.45) ($\sigma_A^2/\sigma_1^2 = c_{31} = 5, a = 10, \mu = 1$).

| | | $\beta$ | | | | | | | |
|---|---|---|---|---|---|---|---|---|---|
| | | 0.025 | | 0.05 | | 0.075 | | 0.1 | |
| | | BA | GA | BA | GA | BA | GA | BA | GA |
| $N_6$ | $\eta_5^2$ | 0.1408 | 0.0008 | 0.1680 | 0.0060 | 0.1856 | 0.0152 | 0.2052 | 0.0364 |
| | $\eta_6^2$ | 0.1208 | 0.0036 | 0.1496 | 0.0176 | 0.1684 | 0.0432 | 0.1840 | 0.0676 |
| | $\eta_7^2$ | 0.1264 | 0.0028 | 0.1564 | 0.0152 | 0.1752 | 0.0384 | 0.1880 | 0.0612 |
| | $\eta_8^2$ | 0.1020 | 0.0084 | 0.1292 | 0.0340 | 0.1548 | 0.0596 | 0.1712 | 0.0852 |
| $N_7$ | $\eta_5^2$ | 0.1424 | 0.0168 | 0.1648 | 0.0396 | 0.1860 | 0.0624 | 0.2000 | 0.0904 |
| | $\eta_6^2$ | 0.1152 | 0.0224 | 0.1432 | 0.0488 | 0.1620 | 0.0704 | 0.1780 | 0.0976 |
| | $\eta_7^2$ | 0.1220 | 0.0224 | 0.1484 | 0.0484 | 0.1668 | 0.0724 | 0.1844 | 0.0968 |
| | $\eta_8^2$ | 0.0984 | 0.0256 | 0.1212 | 0.0516 | 0.1436 | 0.0764 | 0.1604 | 0.1064 |
| $N_8$ | $\eta_5^2$ | 0.0352 | 0.0240 | 0.0596 | 0.0476 | 0.0828 | 0.0732 | 0.1056 | 0.0940 |
| | $\eta_6^2$ | 0.0312 | 0.0256 | 0.0552 | 0.0472 | 0.0784 | 0.0724 | 0.1056 | 0.0956 |
| | $\eta_7^2$ | 0.0320 | 0.0256 | 0.0548 | 0.0472 | 0.0792 | 0.0720 | 0.1016 | 0.0936 |
| | $\eta_8^2$ | 0.0304 | 0.0236 | 0.0504 | 0.0468 | 0.0740 | 0.0716 | 0.0980 | 0.0960 |
| $N_9$ | $\eta_5^2$ | 0.0260 | 0.0224 | 0.0488 | 0.0432 | 0.0728 | 0.0656 | 0.1008 | 0.0916 |
| | $\eta_6^2$ | 0.0252 | 0.0224 | 0.0464 | 0.0428 | 0.0728 | 0.0692 | 0.0984 | 0.0932 |
| | $\eta_7^2$ | 0.0260 | 0.0236 | 0.0480 | 0.0448 | 0.0720 | 0.0684 | 0.0996 | 0.0944 |
| | $\eta_8^2$ | 0.0256 | 0.0244 | 0.0492 | 0.0472 | 0.0732 | 0.0724 | 0.0980 | 0.0960 |
| $N_{10}$ | $\eta_5^2$ | 0.0292 | 0.0264 | 0.0520 | 0.0500 | 0.0772 | 0.0736 | 0.1036 | 0.0992 |
| | $\eta_6^2$ | 0.0292 | 0.0272 | 0.0512 | 0.0472 | 0.0796 | 0.0772 | 0.1036 | 0.1032 |
| | $\eta_7^2$ | 0.0292 | 0.0276 | 0.0528 | 0.0500 | 0.0808 | 0.0772 | 0.1032 | 0.1012 |
| | $\eta_8^2$ | 0.0288 | 0.0280 | 0.0512 | 0.0500 | 0.0800 | 0.0780 | 0.1036 | 0.1028 |

*Note :* $N_6 = (3)_{10}$, $N_7 = (3,4,4,5,5)_2$, $N_8 = (7,7,8,8,9)_2$, $N_9 = (9,9,10,10,12)_2$, $N_{10} = (11,11,12,13,13)_2$, $\eta_5^2 = (1)_{10}$, $\eta_6^2 = (1,0.9,0.8,0.7,0.6,0.5,0.4,0.3,0.2,0.1)$, $\eta_7^2 = (1,(0.3,0.6,0.9)_3)$, $\eta_8^2 = (1,(0.1)_2,(0.2)_2,(0.3)_2,(0.4)_2,0.5)$.

The Bootstrap $p$-value based on (7.22) is 0.1072, and the generalized $p$-value by (7.27) is 0.2271. Thus, the null hypothesis $H_0$ in (7.61) is not rejected by these two approaches at the nominal significance level of 5%.

Next, consider the hypothesis testing problem for the sum of variance components

$$H_0 : \sigma_A^2 + \sigma_1^2 \leq 100 \quad versus \quad H_1 : \sigma_A^2 + \sigma_1^2 > 100, \tag{7.62}$$

By (7.36) and (7.40), the Bootstrap $p$-value and generalized $p$-value are 0.1226 and 0.1264 respectively. Consequently, at the nominal significance level of 5%, these two approaches cannot reject the null hypothesis $H_0$ in (7.62).

**Table 7.15:** Powers for hypothesis testing problem (7.45) ($c_{31} = 5$, $a = 3$, $(\sigma_1^2, \sigma_2^2, \sigma_3^2) = \eta_3^2, \mu = 1$).

| | $\sigma_A^2$ | $\beta$ | | | | | | | |
|---|---|---|---|---|---|---|---|---|---|
| | | 0.025 | | 0.05 | | 0.075 | | 0.1 | |
| | | BA | GA | BA | GA | BA | GA | BA | GA |
| $N_1$ | 10 | 0.1144 | 0.0432 | 0.1596 | 0.0956 | 0.2032 | 0.1396 | 0.2368 | 0.1776 |
| | 50 | 0.3252 | 0.2108 | 0.4240 | 0.3444 | 0.4944 | 0.4372 | 0.5604 | 0.5152 |
| | 100 | 0.4540 | 0.3424 | 0.5716 | 0.5016 | 0.6560 | 0.6168 | 0.7164 | 0.6800 |
| | 200 | 0.5976 | 0.5028 | 0.7188 | 0.6728 | 0.7932 | 0.7592 | 0.8368 | 0.8148 |
| $N_2$ | 10 | 0.0900 | 0.0632 | 0.1372 | 0.1168 | 0.1828 | 0.1648 | 0.2216 | 0.2084 |
| | 50 | 0.3720 | 0.3280 | 0.5020 | 0.4776 | 0.5804 | 0.5684 | 0.6276 | 0.6196 |
| | 100 | 0.5556 | 0.5312 | 0.6688 | 0.6528 | 0.7344 | 0.7284 | 0.7792 | 0.7736 |
| | 200 | 0.7212 | 0.7024 | 0.8024 | 0.7944 | 0.8512 | 0.8440 | 0.8800 | 0.8776 |
| $N_3$ | 10 | 0.0960 | 0.0928 | 0.1544 | 0.1512 | 0.2104 | 0.2088 | 0.2464 | 0.2452 |
| | 50 | 0.5196 | 0.5136 | 0.6148 | 0.6116 | 0.6796 | 0.6772 | 0.7200 | 0.7192 |
| | 100 | 0.7108 | 0.7092 | 0.7792 | 0.7764 | 0.8128 | 0.8116 | 0.8420 | 0.8416 |
| | 200 | 0.8372 | 0.8340 | 0.8828 | 0.8820 | 0.9052 | 0.9052 | 0.9232 | 0.9232 |
| $N_4$ | 10 | 0.1112 | 0.1096 | 0.1736 | 0.1732 | 0.2212 | 0.2212 | 0.2660 | 0.2656 |
| | 50 | 0.6068 | 0.6048 | 0.6820 | 0.6812 | 0.7232 | 0.7228 | 0.7536 | 0.7532 |
| | 100 | 0.7736 | 0.7736 | 0.8224 | 0.8220 | 0.8508 | 0.8504 | 0.8684 | 0.8684 |
| | 200 | 0.8768 | 0.8764 | 0.8988 | 0.8988 | 0.9140 | 0.9140 | 0.9264 | 0.9256 |
| $N_5$ | 10 | 0.1352 | 0.1348 | 0.2012 | 0.2012 | 0.2548 | 0.2548 | 0.2976 | 0.2976 |
| | 50 | 0.6512 | 0.6512 | 0.7024 | 0.7024 | 0.7444 | 0.7444 | 0.7716 | 0.7716 |
| | 100 | 0.8028 | 0.8024 | 0.8416 | 0.8416 | 0.8640 | 0.8640 | 0.8796 | 0.8796 |
| | 200 | 0.8952 | 0.8952 | 0.9140 | 0.9136 | 0.9316 | 0.9316 | 0.9388 | 0.9388 |

*Note :* $N_1 = (3,3,4)$, $N_2 = (4,5,6)$, $N_3 = (7,10,13)$, $N_4 = (12,20,28)$, $N_5 = (24,40,56)$, $\eta_3^2 = (1,0.6,0.3)$.

Finally, consider the hypothesis testing problem for the ratio of the variance components

$$H_0 : \sigma_A^2/\sigma_1^2 \leq 1 \quad versus \quad H_1 : \sigma_A^2/\sigma_1^2 > 1, \tag{7.63}$$

Based on (7.48) and (7.52), the Bootstrap $p$-value and generalized $p$-value are respectively 0.4150 and 0.4723. Therefore, these two approaches cannot reject the null hypothesis $H_0$ in (7.63) at the nominal significance level of 5%.

**Table 7.16:** Powers for hypothesis testing problem (7.45) ($c_{31} = 5$, $a = 10$, $(\sigma_1^2, \cdots, \sigma_{10}^2) = \eta_6^2, \mu = 1$).

| | $\sigma_A^2$ | $\beta$ 0.025 BA | GA | 0.05 BA | GA | 0.075 BA | GA | 0.1 BA | GA |
|---|---|---|---|---|---|---|---|---|---|
| $N_6$ | 15 | 0.2456 | 0.0448 | 0.2936 | 0.1220 | 0.3312 | 0.1868 | 0.3744 | 0.2472 |
| | 20 | 0.2888 | 0.0748 | 0.3388 | 0.1704 | 0.3892 | 0.2480 | 0.4332 | 0.3232 |
| | 30 | 0.3540 | 0.1244 | 0.4208 | 0.2496 | 0.4848 | 0.3484 | 0.5400 | 0.4352 |
| | 40 | 0.4032 | 0.1708 | 0.4884 | 0.3212 | 0.5572 | 0.4328 | 0.6200 | 0.5300 |
| $N_7$ | 15 | 0.2320 | 0.0744 | 0.2740 | 0.1560 | 0.3128 | 0.2232 | 0.3576 | 0.2772 |
| | 20 | 0.2628 | 0.1008 | 0.3216 | 0.2024 | 0.3748 | 0.2796 | 0.4236 | 0.3428 |
| | 30 | 0.3308 | 0.1556 | 0.4008 | 0.2760 | 0.4708 | 0.3724 | 0.5232 | 0.4600 |
| | 40 | 0.3860 | 0.2020 | 0.4696 | 0.3372 | 0.5392 | 0.4556 | 0.6012 | 0.5456 |
| $N_8$ | 15 | 0.2504 | 0.2316 | 0.3664 | 0.3532 | 0.4588 | 0.4460 | 0.5312 | 0.5244 |
| | 20 | 0.3696 | 0.3504 | 0.5144 | 0.5040 | 0.6040 | 0.5960 | 0.6784 | 0.6680 |
| | 30 | 0.5748 | 0.5584 | 0.7212 | 0.7080 | 0.7924 | 0.7864 | 0.8480 | 0.8440 |
| | 40 | 0.7176 | 0.7068 | 0.8372 | 0.8332 | 0.8908 | 0.8864 | 0.9160 | 0.9152 |
| $N_9$ | 15 | 0.3172 | 0.3056 | 0.4488 | 0.4428 | 0.5312 | 0.5272 | 0.5928 | 0.5904 |
| | 20 | 0.4692 | 0.4640 | 0.5972 | 0.5904 | 0.6732 | 0.6720 | 0.7400 | 0.7368 |
| | 30 | 0.6740 | 0.6684 | 0.7916 | 0.7872 | 0.8524 | 0.8500 | 0.8884 | 0.8860 |
| | 40 | 0.8060 | 0.8012 | 0.8888 | 0.8868 | 0.9264 | 0.9244 | 0.9460 | 0.9456 |
| $N_{10}$ | 15 | 0.3648 | 0.3600 | 0.5036 | 0.5016 | 0.5860 | 0.5824 | 0.6448 | 0.6408 |
| | 20 | 0.5460 | 0.5408 | 0.6664 | 0.6612 | 0.7424 | 0.7404 | 0.7956 | 0.7944 |
| | 30 | 0.7648 | 0.7612 | 0.8408 | 0.8392 | 0.8820 | 0.8812 | 0.9076 | 0.9076 |
| | 40 | 0.8628 | 0.8616 | 0.9156 | 0.9152 | 0.9392 | 0.9388 | 0.9528 | 0.9528 |

*Note :* $N_6 = (3)_{10}$, $N_7 = (3,4,4,5,5)_2$, $N_8 = (7,7,8,8,9)_2$, $N_9 = (9,9,10,10,12)_2$, $N_{10} = (11,11,12,13,13)_2$, $\eta_6^2 = (1,0.9,0.8,0.7,0.6,0.5,0.4,0.3,0.2,0.1)$.

**Table 7.17:** Simulation results for hypothesis testing problem (7.10) ($\beta = 0.05$, $a = 3$, $(\sigma_1^2, \sigma_2^2, \sigma_3^2) = (1,0.6,0.3)$).

| | $\mu$ $\lambda_1 = 1_a$ 0 | 2 | 5 | 8 | $\lambda_1 = 3_a$ 0 | 2 | 5 | 8 |
|---|---|---|---|---|---|---|---|---|
| $N_{11}$ | 0.048 | 0.256 | 0.671 | 0.916 | 0.045 | 0.250 | 0.670 | 0.917 |
| $N_{12}$ | 0.041 | 0.251 | 0.678 | 0.916 | 0.037 | 0.248 | 0.670 | 0.920 |
| $N_{13}$ | 0.054 | 0.251 | 0.682 | 0.922 | 0.052 | 0.257 | 0.683 | 0.922 |

*Note :* $N_{11} = (40,50,60)$, $N_{12} = (60,65,75)$, $N_{13} = (70,80,100)$, and the numbers of inner loops $k_1$ and outer loops $k_2$ both be 1000.

**Table 7.18:** Simulation results for hypothesis testing problem on variance component functions $\beta = 0.05$, $a = 3$, $\mu = 1$, $(\sigma_1^2, \sigma_2^2, \sigma_3^2) = (1, 0.6, 0.3)$.

| | | | $\sigma_A^2$ | | | | | | | |
| | | | 5 | | 10 | | 50 | | 200 | |
| Testing problem | | | BA | GA | BA | GA | BA | GA | BA | GA |
|---|---|---|---|---|---|---|---|---|---|---|
| (7.19) | $\lambda_1 = 1_a$ | $N_{11}$ | 0.049 | 0.049 | 0.223 | 0.223 | 0.733 | 0.733 | 0.931 | 0.931 |
| | | $N_{12}$ | 0.044 | 0.044 | 0.242 | 0.242 | 0.741 | 0.741 | 0.917 | 0.917 |
| | | $N_{13}$ | 0.048 | 0.048 | 0.221 | 0.221 | 0.729 | 0.729 | 0.922 | 0.922 |
| | $\lambda_1 = 3_a$ | $N_{11}$ | 0.048 | 0.048 | 0.221 | 0.221 | 0.740 | 0.740 | 0.930 | 0.930 |
| | | $N_{12}$ | 0.042 | 0.042 | 0.238 | 0.238 | 0.742 | 0.742 | 0.924 | 0.924 |
| | | $N_{13}$ | 0.044 | 0.044 | 0.222 | 0.222 | 0.725 | 0.725 | 0.925 | 0.925 |
| (7.33) | $\lambda_1 = 1_a$ | $N_{11}$ | 0.047 | 0.048 | 0.227 | 0.229 | 0.737 | 0.739 | 0.930 | 0.931 |
| | | $N_{12}$ | 0.046 | 0.048 | 0.239 | 0.242 | 0.743 | 0.744 | 0.915 | 0.917 |
| | | $N_{13}$ | 0.045 | 0.046 | 0.219 | 0.222 | 0.731 | 0.732 | 0.925 | 0.926 |
| | $\lambda_1 = 3_a$ | $N_{11}$ | 0.044 | 0.046 | 0.223 | 0.225 | 0.743 | 0.746 | 0.931 | 0.932 |
| | | $N_{12}$ | 0.044 | 0.045 | 0.240 | 0.241 | 0.742 | 0.744 | 0.922 | 0.923 |
| | | $N_{13}$ | 0.046 | 0.046 | 0.223 | 0.227 | 0.724 | 0.727 | 0.924 | 0.925 |
| (7.45) | $\lambda_1 = 1_a$ | $N_{11}$ | 0.047 | 0.047 | 0.190 | 0.190 | 0.723 | 0.723 | 0.925 | 0.925 |
| | | $N_{12}$ | 0.052 | 0.052 | 0.222 | 0.222 | 0.735 | 0.735 | 0.920 | 0.920 |
| | | $N_{13}$ | 0.053 | 0.053 | 0.207 | 0.207 | 0.725 | 0.725 | 0.916 | 0.916 |
| | $\lambda_1 = 3_a$ | $N_{11}$ | 0.050 | 0.050 | 0.193 | 0.193 | 0.731 | 0.730 | 0.924 | 0.924 |
| | | $N_{12}$ | 0.050 | 0.050 | 0.223 | 0.223 | 0.744 | 0.744 | 0.921 | 0.921 |
| | | $N_{13}$ | 0.054 | 0.054 | 0.213 | 0.213 | 0.718 | 0.718 | 0.918 | 0.918 |

*Note* : $N_{11} = (40, 50, 60)$, $N_{12} = (60, 65, 75)$, $N_{13} = (70, 80, 100)$, and the numbers of inner loops $k_1$ and outer loops $k_2$ both be 1000.

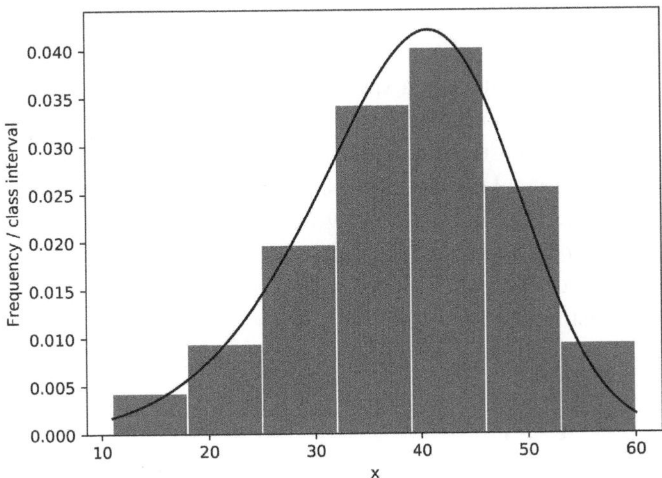

**Figure 7.2:** Histogram of annual average concentration data of nitrogen dioxide with superimposed skew-normal density curve.

# Chapter 8

# Skew-Normal Unbalanced Panel Model with One-Way Error Component

For the skew-normal unbalanced panel model with a one-way error component, the hypothesis testing and interval estimation problems for the regression coefficients and variance component functions are considered. The panel model with a one-way error component is a special type of mixed effects model, which has been widely used in econometrics, market analysis, biomedicine and other fields. The existing studies on such models usually assume that random effects and error terms follow the normal distribution, which easily leads to the lack of robustness of statistical inference. Since the skew-normal distribution is the most common in the fitting distribution of actual skewed data, it is necessary to study the statistical inference of the panel model with a one-way error component under the skew-normal distribution.

## 8.1 Model properties

Let $M_{n \times k}$ be the set of all $n \times k$ matrices over the field of real numbers, and let $M(A)$ denote the subspace that is spanned by the column vectors of matrix $A$. For any matrix $A \in M_{n \times k}$ and positive semidefinite matrix $B \in M_{n \times n}$, $A^-$, $A^{'}$ and $rk(A)$ represent generalized inverse, transpose and rank, respectively. $tr(B)$ and

$B^{\frac{1}{2}}$ represent trace and square root matrix of $B$. $I_n$ and $1_n$ are the n-order identity matrix and n-dimensional column vector with all components = 1, respectively. $diag(\cdot), \rightarrow, \overset{asy}{\sim}, \overset{d}{=}$ and $\overset{\triangle}{=}$ denote diagonal matrice, "approach", "approximately follow", "identically distributed", and "denoted as", respectively.

This chapter considers a skew-normal unbalanced panel model with a one-way error component

$$Y_{it} = \alpha + X'_{it}\beta + \mu_i + v_{it}, i = 1, 2, \cdots, N, t = 1, 2, \cdots, T_i, \tag{8.1}$$

where $Y_{it}$ represents the observed value of the *i*th individual at time $t$, $\mu_i$ represents the random effect of the *i*th individual, $v_{it}$ represents the random error, $X_{it}$ represents the $k \times 1$ observed vector of explanatory variables, $\alpha$ is a scalar, and $\beta$ is a $k \times 1$ vector of regression coefficients. The above model can be written in matrix form as follows.

$$Y = 1_n\alpha + X\beta + Z_\mu\mu + v = Z\Gamma + u, \tag{8.2}$$

where $Y = [Y_{11}, \cdots, Y_{1T_1}, \cdots, Y_{N1}, \cdots, Y_{NT_N}]'$, $X = [X_{11}, \cdots, X_{1T_1}, \cdots, X_{N1}, \cdots, X_{NT_N}]'$, $Z_\mu = diag\{1_{T_1}, 1_{T_2}, \cdots, 1_{T_N}\}$, $\beta = [\beta_1, \beta_2, \cdots, \beta_k]'$, $\mu = [\mu_1, \mu_2, \cdots, \mu_N]'$, $v = \left[v_{11}, \cdots, v_{1T_1}, \cdots, v_{N1}, \cdots, v_{NT_N}\right]'$, $Z = [1_n, X], \Gamma = \left[\alpha, \beta'\right]', u = Z_\mu\mu + v$, $n = \sum_{i=1}^{N} T_i$, $n > N + k$, $N > k + 1$. Assuming that $Z$ is a full column rank matrix, which is easily satisfied in practical applications. Furthermore, assuming that $\mu \sim SN_N(0, \sigma_\mu^2 I_N, \lambda_1)$ and $v \sim N_n(0, \sigma_v^2 I_n)$, where $\mu$ and $v$ are independent of each other.

**Theorem 8.1.** *For the model (8.2), $Y \sim SN_n(\xi_Y, \Sigma_Y, \lambda_2)$, and its moment generating function is denoted by*

$$M_Y(t) = 2\exp(t'\xi_Y + \frac{t'\Sigma_Y t}{2})\Phi(\frac{\sigma_\mu\lambda'_1 Z'_\mu t}{(1 + \lambda'_1\lambda_1)^{\frac{1}{2}}}), \quad t \in R^n, \tag{8.3}$$

*where $\xi_Y = Z\Gamma, \Sigma_Y = \sigma_\mu^2 Z_\mu Z'_\mu + \sigma_v^2 I_n, \lambda_2 = \dfrac{\sigma_\mu \Sigma_Y^{-\frac{1}{2}} Z_\mu \lambda_1}{\left[1 + \lambda'_1(I_N - \sigma_\mu^2 Z'_\mu \Sigma_Y^{-1} Z_\mu)\lambda_1\right]^{\frac{1}{2}}}.$*

The proof of this theorem is analogous to Theorem 8.1 in Ye and Luo (2016), so we omit the proof details.

Let $H_i$ be a $T_i \times (T_i - 1)$ column orthogonal matrix, satisfying $H'_i H_i = I_{T_i-1}$, $H'_i 1_{T_i} = 0$, $i = 1, 2, \cdots, N$. Let $R$ be an $n$-dimensional orthogonal matrix, $C = diag\{\sqrt{T_i}\}$ be a $N \times N$ diagonal matrix, $R_1 = diag\left\{\frac{1_{T_1}}{\sqrt{T_1}}, \frac{1_{T_2}}{\sqrt{T_2}}, \cdots, \frac{1_{T_N}}{\sqrt{T_N}}\right\}$ be a

$N \times N$ diagonal matrix, and $R_2 = diag\{H_1, H_2, \cdots, H_N\}$ be a $N \times N$ diagonal matrix. Consider the QR decomposition of full column rank matrix $Z_\mu$.

$$Z_\mu = R[C,0]' = [R_1, R_2][C,0]'.$$

Multiplying both sides of the model (8.2) by $R_2'$ yields

$$\tilde{Y} = \tilde{X}\beta + \tilde{v}, \tag{8.4}$$

where $\tilde{Y} = R_2'Y$, $\tilde{X} = R_2'X$, $\tilde{v} = R_2'v$, $\tilde{v} \sim N_{n-N}(0, \sigma_v^2 I_{n-N})$. The following Theorem 8.2 can be easily accessed from Wang et al. (2004).

**Theorem 8.2.** *For model* (8.2), *suppose* $c'\beta$ *is any estimable function,* $c \in M(\tilde{X}')$, *and* $\tilde{X}$ *and* $\tilde{Y}$ *are given by Equation* (8.4), *then the following conclusions hold.*

(i) *The ML estimator of* $c'\beta$ *is* $c'\hat{\beta}$, *and* $c'\hat{\beta} \sim N\left(c'\beta, \sigma_v^2 c'(\tilde{X}'\tilde{X})^- c\right)$, *where* $\hat{\beta} = (\tilde{X}'\tilde{X})^- \tilde{X}'\tilde{Y}$.

(ii) *The ML estimator of* $\sigma_v^2$ *is* $\hat{\sigma}_v^2 = \frac{(\tilde{Y}-\tilde{X}\hat{\beta})'(\tilde{Y}-\tilde{X}\hat{\beta})}{n-N}$, *and* $\frac{(n-N-r_0)\hat{\sigma}_v^2}{\sigma_v^2}$ $\sim \chi_{n-N-r_0}^2$, *where* $r_0 = rk(\tilde{X})$, *and* $\chi_{n-N-r_0}^2$ *denotes the chi-square distribution with* $n - N - r_0$ *degrees of freedom.*

(iii) $c'\hat{\beta}$ *is the unique minimum variance unbiased estimator of* $c'\beta$, *and* $c'\hat{\beta}$ *and* $\hat{\sigma}_v^2$ *are independent to each other.*

The proof of Theorem 8.2 is similar to Theorems 4.1.4–4.1.5 in Wang et al. (2004), so the proof is omitted.

**Corollary 8.1.** *When* $c'\beta = s_0$, *we have*

$$\frac{c'\hat{\beta} - s_0}{\hat{\sigma}_v \sqrt{c'(\tilde{X}'\tilde{X})^- c}} \sim t_{n-N-r_0},$$

*where* $t_{n-N-r_0}$ *denotes the t-distribution with* $n - N - r_0$ *degrees of freedom.*

The proof of Corollary 8.1 can be easily obtained by Theorem 8.2, so the proof process is omitted.

Consider the QR decomposition of the full rank matrix $Z$, namely

$$Z = L[M',0]' = [L_1, L_2][M',0]',$$

where $L$ is a $n \times n$ orthogonal matrix, $M$ is a positive upper triangular matrix, and $L_1$ and $L_2$ are column orthogonal matrices of dimensions $n \times (k+1)$ and $n \times (n-k-1)$, respectively. Multiplying both sides of Equation (8.2) by $L_2'$ yields

$$L_2'Y = L_2'Z_\mu\mu + L_2'v.$$

Then, we know that

$$L_2'Y \sim SN_{n-k-1}\left(0, \sigma_\mu^2 L_2' Z_\mu Z_\mu' L_2 + \sigma_v^2 I_{n-k-1}, \lambda_3\right),\qquad(8.5)$$

where $\lambda_3 = \dfrac{\left(L_2'\Sigma_Y L_2\right)^{-1/2} L_2'\Sigma_Y^{1/2}\lambda_2}{\left\{1+\lambda_2'\left[I_n-\Sigma_Y^{1/2}L_2\left(L_2'\Sigma_Y L_2\right)^{-1}L_2'\Sigma_Y^{1/2}\right]\lambda_2\right\}^{1/2}}$. Since $L_2'Z_\mu Z_\mu' L_2$ is a positive semi-definite matrix, there exists a $(n-k-1)$-dimensional orthogonal matrix $P = [P_1, P_2, \cdots, P_d]$, such that

$$P'L_2'Z_\mu Z_\mu' L_2 P = diag\left\{\Delta_1, \cdots, \Delta_1, \cdots, \Delta_d, \cdots, \Delta_d\right\} \triangleq \Lambda,\qquad(8.6)$$

where $0 \le \Delta_1 < \Delta_2 < \cdots < \Delta_d$ are the eigenvalues of $L_2'Z_\mu Z_\mu' L_2$, with multiplicities $r_1, r_2, \cdots, r_d$, and $\sum_{i=1}^{d} r_i = n-k-1$. Since $rk(L_2'Z_\mu Z_\mu' L_2) \le N-1 < n-k-1$, it follows that $\Delta_1 = 0$, and $r_1 = n-k-1-rk(L_2'Z_\mu Z_\mu' L_2)$. Let

$\bar{\Delta} = \dfrac{\sum_{i=2}^{d} r_i \Delta_i}{n-k-1-r_1} = \dfrac{n-tr(L_1'Z_\mu Z_\mu' L_1)}{n-k-1-r_1}$. From Equations (8.5)-(8.6), we have $P_i' L_2' Y \sim$ $SN_{r_i}\left(0, (\Delta_i\sigma_\mu^2 + \sigma_v^2)I_{r_i}, \lambda_4^{(i)}\right)$, where

$$\lambda_4^{(i)} = \dfrac{\left(P_i'\Sigma_L P_i\right)^{-1/2} P_i'\Sigma_L^{1/2}\lambda_3}{\left\{1+\lambda_3'\left[I_{n-k-1} - \Sigma_L^{1/2}P_i\left(P_i'\Sigma_L P_i\right)^{-1}P_i'\Sigma_L^{1/2}\right]\lambda_3\right\}^{1/2}},$$

$$\Sigma_L = \sigma_\mu^2 L_2' Z_\mu Z_\mu' L_2 + \sigma_v^2 I_{n-k-1}.$$

**Theorem 8.3.** *Let* $Q_i = Y' L_2 P_i P_i' L_2' Y$, $i = 1, 2, \cdots, d$. *Then,* $Q_i \sim \left(\Delta_i\sigma_\mu^2 + \sigma_v^2\right)\chi_{r_i}^2$, *and* $Q_1, Q_2, \cdots, Q_d$ *are mutually independent.*

*Proof.* First, let $Q_i^* = \dfrac{Q_i}{\Delta_i\sigma_\mu^2 + \sigma_v^2}$. It is easy to see that $rk\left(P_iP_i'\right) = r_i$, and $\dfrac{P_iP_i'}{\Delta_i\sigma_\mu^2+\sigma_v^2}$ $\left(\sigma_\mu^2 L_2' Z_\mu Z_\mu' L_2 + \sigma_v^2 I_{n-k-1}\right)\dfrac{P_iP_i'}{\Delta_i\sigma_\mu^2+\sigma_v^2} = \dfrac{P_iP_i'}{\Delta_i\sigma_\mu^2+\sigma_v^2}$. By Lemma 7.1 and Equation (8.5), we have $Q_i^* \sim \chi_{r_i}^2$, so $Q_i \sim \left(\Delta_i\sigma_\mu^2 + \sigma_v^2\right)\chi_{r_i}^2$. Second, it is easy to verify that $P_jP_j'\left(\sigma_\mu^2 L_2' Z_\mu Z_\mu' L_2 + \sigma_v^2 I_{n-k-1}\right)P_qP_q' = 0$, where $j, q = 1, 2, \cdots, d, j \ne q$. By Lemma 7.1, we know that $Q_1, Q_2, \cdots, Q_d$ are mutually independent. Therefore, Theorem 8.3 is proved. $\qquad\square$

**Theorem 8.4.** *Let* $V_0 = \dfrac{1}{\bar{\Delta}\sigma_\mu^2+\sigma_v^2}\sum_{j=2}^{d} Q_j$, *then* $V_0 \overset{asy}{\sim} \chi_{n-k-1-r_1}^2$, *where* $Q_j = Y' L_2 P_j P_j' L_2' Y.$

*Proof.* Without loss of generality, assume that in Equation (8.6), $d = n - k - 1$, $P = [p_1, p_2, \cdots, p_{n-k-1}]$, and $\Lambda = diag\{\delta_1, \delta_2, \cdots, \delta_{n-k-1}\}$, where $\delta_1 = \delta_2 = \cdots = \delta_{r_1} = 0$, $0 < \delta_{r_1+1} \leq \delta_{r_1+2} \leq \cdots \leq \delta_{n-k-1}$. Therefore, $Q_j$ and $V_0$ can be respectively rewritten as $Q_j = Y' L_2 p_j p_j' L_2' Y$ and $V_0 = \dfrac{1}{\Delta \sigma_\mu^2 + \sigma_v^2} \sum\limits_{j=r_1+1}^{n-k-1} Q_j$. Let $\varphi_x(\cdot)$ denote the characteristic function of a random variable $x$. According to Theorem 8.3, it can be seen that $\kappa_j = \dfrac{Q_j}{\delta_j \sigma_\mu^2 + \sigma_v^2} \sim \chi_1^2$, $j = 1, 2, \cdots, n - k - 1$, then the characteristic function of $\kappa_j$ is

$$\varphi_{\kappa_j}(t) = E\left[\exp\left(it \frac{Q_j}{\delta_j \sigma_\mu^2 + \sigma_v^2}\right)\right] = \varphi_{Q_j}\left(\frac{t}{\delta_j \sigma_\mu^2 + \sigma_v^2}\right) = (1 - 2it)^{-1/2},$$

then $\varphi_{Q_j}(t) = \left[1 - 2it\left(\delta_j \sigma_\mu^2 + \sigma_v^2\right)\right]^{-1/2}$. Let $\gamma_j = \dfrac{\delta_j \sigma_\mu^2 + \sigma_v^2}{\Delta \sigma_\mu^2 + \sigma_v^2}$, then $V_0 = \sum\limits_{j=r_1+1}^{n-k-1} \gamma_j \kappa_j$. Since

$$\varphi_{\gamma_j \kappa_j}(t) = E\left[\exp\left(it\gamma_j \frac{Q_j}{\delta_j \sigma_\mu^2 + \sigma_v^2}\right)\right] = \varphi_{Q_j}\left(\frac{\gamma_j}{\delta_j \sigma_\mu^2 + \sigma_v^2} t\right) = (1 - 2i\gamma_j t)^{-1/2},$$

it follows that $\varphi_{V_0}(t) = \prod\limits_{j=r_1+1}^{n-k-1} (1 - 2i\gamma_j t)^{-1/2}$. Furthermore, the Taylor expansion of $\varphi_{V_0}(t)$ at $\gamma_{j0} = 1$ is

$$\varphi_{V_0}(t) = (1 - 2it)^{-(n-k-r_1-1)/2} - (1 - 2it)^{-(n-k-r_1+3)/2} t^2 \sum_{j=r_1+1}^{n-k-1} (\gamma_j - 1)^2 + R^*,$$

where $R^*$ denotes the Taylor remainder term.

Since

$$\lim_{\gamma_j \to 1} \left\{ -(1 - 2it)^{-(n-k-r_1+3)/2} t^2 \sum_{j=r_1+1}^{n-k-1} (\gamma_j - 1)^2 + R^* \right\} = 0,$$

the last two terms in the Taylor expansion of $\varphi_{V_0}(t)$ can be ignored. Let $V_0^* \sim \chi_{n-k-1-r_1}^2$, then

$$\varphi_{V_0^*}(t) = (1 - 2it)^{-(n-k-r_1-1)/2}.$$

It is easy to see that the characteristic function of $V_0^*$ is equal to the first term in the Taylor expansion of the characteristic function of $V_0$. Therefore, $V_0 \overset{asy}{\sim} \chi_{n-k-1-r_1}^2$, and Theorem 8.4 is proved. $\qquad\square$

**Corollary 8.2.** *For model (8.2), an unbiased estimator of $\sigma_v^2$ is given by $\tilde{\sigma}_v^2 = \frac{Q_1}{r_1}$,*

*and a feasible estimator of $\sigma_\mu^2$ is given by $\hat{\sigma}_\mu^2 = \dfrac{1}{(n-k-1-r_1)\Delta} \displaystyle\sum_{j=2}^{d} Q_j - \dfrac{Q_1}{r_1 \Delta}.$*

The proof of Corollary 8.2 easily follows from Theorems 8.3-8.4, and is therefore omitted.

## 8.2  Parameter estimation

Consider the hypothesis testing problem for the estimable function $c'\beta$ of regression coefficients

$$H_0 : c'\beta \leq s_0 \quad versus \quad H_1 : c'\beta > s_0, \tag{8.7}$$

where $c \in M(\tilde{X}')$ and $s_0$ is a given value.

According to Wang and Zou (2014), the test statistic and rejection region required to construct a test for hypothesis testing problem (8.7) are consistent with those of the following hypothesis testing problem

$$H_0 : c'\beta = s_0 \quad versus \quad H_1 : c'\beta > s_0.$$

For this purpose, we define the test statistic as

$$T_0 = \frac{c'\hat{\beta} - s_0}{\hat{\sigma}_v \sqrt{c'(\tilde{X}'\tilde{X})^- c}},$$

where $\tilde{X}$, $\tilde{Y}$, $\hat{\beta}$, and $\hat{\sigma}_v$ are given by Theorem 8.2. Under the condition $H_0 : c'\beta = s_0$, based on Theorem 8.2 and Corollary 8.1, we have

$$T_0 \sim t_{n-N-r_0}.$$

Furthermore, based on $T_0$, we can obtain the following $p$-value

$$p_{T_0} = P(T_0 > t_0 | H_0), \tag{8.8}$$

where $t_0$ is the observed value of $T_0$. If $p_{T_0} < \vartheta$, then we reject the null hypothesis $H_0$ in (8.7) at the nominal significance level $\vartheta$.

Let $\eta = \frac{c'\beta}{\hat{\sigma}_{v_0}}$, $\eta_0 = \frac{s_0}{\hat{\sigma}_{v_0}}$, $\tilde{T}_0 = \dfrac{\frac{c'\hat{\beta}}{\hat{\sigma}_{v_0}} - \eta_0}{\frac{\hat{\sigma}_v}{\hat{\sigma}_{v_0}} \sqrt{c'(\tilde{X}'\tilde{X})^- c}}$, $\tilde{p}_{T_0} = P(\tilde{T}_0 > \tilde{t}_0 | H_0)$, where $\hat{\sigma}_{v_0}$ and $\tilde{t}_0$ are the observed values of $\hat{\sigma}_v$ and $\tilde{T}_0$, respectively. We define the affine transformation as

$$Y_{it}^* = dY_{it} + \xi, i = 1, 2, \cdots, N, t = 1, 2, \cdots, T_i, \tag{8.9}$$

where $\xi$ and $d$ are arbitrary given nonzero constants.

**Theorem 8.5.** *For the hypothesis testing problem (8.7), consider the equivalent hypothesis testing problem*

$$H_0 : \eta \leq \eta_0 \quad versus \quad H_1 : \eta > \eta_0, \tag{8.10}$$

*where* $\eta = \frac{c'\beta}{\hat{\sigma}_{v_0}}$, $\eta_0 = \frac{s_0}{\hat{\sigma}_{v_0}}$. *Then, the test based on* $\tilde{p}_{T_0}$ *is invariant under the affine transformation (8.9).*

*Proof.* Using the formula (8.9), we can rewrite $Y_{it}^*$ as

$$Y^* = 1_n\alpha^* + X\beta^* + Z_\mu\mu^* + v^*,$$

where $\alpha^* = d\alpha + \xi$, $\beta^* = d\beta$, $\mu^* = d\mu$, $v^* = dv$, $\sigma_{\mu*}^2 = d^2\sigma_\mu^2$, $\sigma_{v*}^2 = d^2\sigma_v^2$, $\mu^* \sim SN_N(0, \sigma_{\mu*}^2 I_N, \lambda_1)$, $v^* \sim N_n(0, \sigma_{v*}^2 I_n)$. Under the affine transformation (8.9), we have $\tilde{Y}^* = \tilde{X}_*\beta^* + \tilde{v}^*$, where $\tilde{Y}^* = d\tilde{Y}$, $\tilde{X}_* = \tilde{X}$, $\tilde{v}^* = d\tilde{v}$, $\tilde{v}^* \sim N_{n-N}(0, d^2\sigma_v^2 I_{n-N})$. As a result, the ML estimators of $\beta^*$ and $\sigma_{v*}^2$ are $\hat{\beta}^* = d\hat{\beta}$ and $\hat{\sigma}_{v*}^2 = d^2\hat{\sigma}_v^2$, respectively. The observed values of $\hat{\beta}^*$ and $\hat{\sigma}_{v*}^2$ are $\hat{\beta}_0^* = d\hat{\beta}_0$ and $\hat{\sigma}_{v_0*}^2 = d^2\hat{\sigma}_{v_0}^2$, respectively, where $\hat{\beta}_0$ and $\hat{\sigma}_{v_0}^2$ are the observed values of $\hat{\beta}$ and $\hat{\sigma}_v^2$.

It is easy to see that the hypothesis testing problem (8.10) is invariant under the affine transformation (8.9). The test statistic after the affine transformation (8.9) is defined as

$$\tilde{T}_0^* = \frac{\frac{c'\hat{\beta}^*}{\hat{\sigma}_{v_0*}} - \eta_0}{\frac{\hat{\sigma}_{v*}}{\hat{\sigma}_{v_0*}}\sqrt{c'(\tilde{X}_*'\tilde{X}_*)^-c}}.$$

It can be proved that $\tilde{T}_0^* = \tilde{T}_0 \sim t_{n-N-r_0}$ and the observed value of $\tilde{T}_0^*$, $\tilde{t}_0^* = \frac{\frac{c'\hat{\beta}_0^*}{\hat{\sigma}_{v_0*}} - \eta_0}{\sqrt{c'(\tilde{X}_*'\tilde{X}_*)^-c}} = \tilde{t}_0$. Therefore, the distribution and observed value of $\tilde{T}_0$ are invariant under the affine transformation (8.9). As a result, the test based on $\tilde{p}_{T_0}$ is invariant under the affine transformation (8.9). The proof of Theorem 8.5 is complete. $\qquad\square$

**Remark 8.1.** *For the hypothesis testing problem (8.7), the test based on* $p_{T_0}$ *is invariant under the affine transformation (8.9) when* $s_0 = 0$.

**Remark 8.2.** *Consider the left-sided hypothesis testing problem for* $c'\beta$ *as*

$$H_0 : c'\beta \geq s_0 \quad versus \quad H_1 : c'\beta < s_0,$$

*where* $c \in M(\tilde{X}')$ *and* $s_0$ *is a given value. Similar to the right-sided hypothesis testing problem, we can obtain the p-value based on* $T_0$ *as follows.*

$$\bar{p}_{T_0} = P(T_0 < t_0 | H_0).$$

**Remark 8.3.** *For the two-sided hypothesis testing problem for $c'\beta$*

$$H_0 : c'\beta = s_0 \quad versus \quad H_1 : c'\beta \neq s_0,$$

*where $c \in M(\tilde{X}')$ and $s_0$ is a given value, we can obtain the p-value based on $T_0$ as follows.*

$$\hat{p}_{T_0} = 2\min\{P(T_0 > t_0|H_0), P(T_0 < t_0|H_0)\}.$$

**Remark 8.4.** *The confidence interval for the estimable function $c'\beta$ at the confidence level of $1 - \vartheta$ is given by*

$$\left[c'\hat{\beta}_0 - t_{n-N-r_0}(1-\vartheta/2)\hat{\sigma}_{v_0}\sqrt{c'(\tilde{X}'\tilde{X})^-c}, c'\hat{\beta}_0 - t_{n-N-r_0}(\vartheta/2)\hat{\sigma}_{v_0}\sqrt{c'(\tilde{X}'\tilde{X})^-c}\right],$$

*where $\hat{\beta}_0$ and $\hat{\sigma}_{v_0}$ are the observed values of $\hat{\beta}$ and $\hat{\sigma}_v$, respectively. Moreover, the invariant confidence interval for $\eta$ at the confidence level of $1 - \vartheta$ is given by*

$$\left[\frac{c'\hat{\beta}_0}{\hat{\sigma}_{v_0}} - t_{n-N-r_0}(1-\vartheta/2)\sqrt{c'(\tilde{X}'\tilde{X})^-c}, \frac{c'\hat{\beta}_0}{\hat{\sigma}_{v_0}} - t_{n-N-r_0}(\vartheta/2)\sqrt{c'(\tilde{X}'\tilde{X})^-c}\right].$$

## 8.3   Inference on the single variance component

For the one-sided hypothesis testing problem (8.11),we consider

$$H_0 : \sigma_\mu^2 \leq s_1 \quad versus \quad H_1 : \sigma_\mu^2 > s_1, \tag{8.11}$$

where $s_1$ is a given value.

### *8.3.1   Bootstrap approach*

For hypothesis testing problem (8.11), define

$$T_1 = \sum_{j=2}^{d} \frac{Q_j}{s_1\Delta_j + \sigma_v^2}.$$

According to Theorem 8.3, if $\sigma_v^2$ is known, then $T_1$ is the test statistic for the hypothesis testing problem (8.11). However, $\sigma_v^2$ is often unknown in practical problems. Therefore, under the null hypothesis $H_0$ in (8.11), we replace $\sigma_v^2$ with the estimator $\tilde{\sigma}_v^2 = \frac{Q_1}{r_1}$ and get

$$T_1 = \sum_{j=2}^{d} \frac{Q_j}{s_1\Delta_j + \frac{Q_1}{r_1}}. \tag{8.12}$$

However, since it is difficult to obtain the exact distribution of $T_1$, the Bootstrap method can be used to construct the test statistic. Let $q_1, q_2, \cdots, q_d$ be the observed values of $Q_1, Q_2, \cdots, Q_d$, respectively. Based on Equation (8.12), the Bootstrap test statistic for hypothesis test problem (8.11) is defined as follows.

$$T_{1B} = \sum_{j=2}^{d} \frac{Q_{jB_1}}{s_1 \Delta_j + \frac{Q_{1B}}{r_1}}, \tag{8.13}$$

where $Q_{1B} \sim \left(\frac{q_1}{r_1}\right) \chi_{r_1}^2$, $Q_{jB_1} \sim \left(s_1 \Delta_j + \frac{q_1}{r_1}\right) \chi_{r_j}^2$, $j = 2, 3, \cdots, d$. Therefore, based on $T_{1B}$, the following p-value can be obtained

$$p_{T_1} = P\left(T_{1B} > t_1 \big| H_0\right), \tag{8.14}$$

where $t_1$ is the observed value of $T_1$ in Equation (8.12). If $p_{T_1} < \vartheta$, then at the nominal significance level $\vartheta$, we reject the null hypothesis $H_0$ in (8.11).

For the hypothesis test problem (8.11), another Bootstrap test method based on Theorem 8.4 is given in this section. Let $Q_0 = \sum_{j=2}^{d} Q_j$. Define

$$T_2 = \frac{Q_0}{\overline{\Delta} s_1 + \sigma_v^2}.$$

Similar to Equation (8.12), using the estimator $\tilde{\sigma}_v^2 = \frac{Q_1}{r_1}$ to replace $\sigma_v^2$, we have

$$T_2 = \frac{Q_0}{\overline{\Delta} s_1 + \frac{Q_1}{r_1}}.$$

Then, the Bootstrap test statistic can be constructed as follows.

$$T_{2B} = \frac{Q_{0B_1}}{\overline{\Delta} s_1 + \frac{Q_{1B}}{r_1}}, \tag{8.15}$$

where $Q_{0B_1} \overset{asy}{\sim} \left(\overline{\Delta} s_1 + \frac{q_1}{r_1}\right) \chi_{n-k-1-r_1}^2$. Therefore, based on $T_{2B}$, the following p-value can be obtained

$$p_{T_2} = P\left(T_{2B} > t_2 \big| H_0\right), \tag{8.16}$$

where $t_2$ is the observed value of $T_2$. If $p_{T_2} < \vartheta$, then at the nominal significance level $\vartheta$, we reject the null hypothesis $H_0$ in (8.11).

Let $\zeta = \frac{\sigma_\mu^2}{q_1}$, $\zeta_1 = \frac{s_1}{q_1}$, $\tilde{T}_2 = \frac{\frac{Q_0}{q_1}}{\overline{\Delta} \zeta_1 + \frac{Q_1}{r_1 q_1}}$, $\tilde{T}_{2B} = \frac{\frac{Q_{0B_1}}{q_1}}{\overline{\Delta} \zeta_1 + \frac{Q_{1B}}{r_1 q_1}}$, $p_{\tilde{T}_2} = P\left(\tilde{T}_{2B} > \tilde{t}_2 \big| H_0\right)$, $q_0$ and $\tilde{t}_2$ are the observed values of $Q_0$ and $\tilde{T}_2$, respectively.

**Theorem 8.6.** *For hypothesis testing problem* (8.11), *consider the equivalent hypothesis testing problem*

$$H_0 : \zeta \leq \zeta_1 \quad versus \quad H_1 : \zeta > \zeta_1, \tag{8.17}$$

*then the Bootstrap test based on $p_{\tilde{T}_2}$ is invariant under the affine transformation* (8.9).

*Proof.* Similar to the proof of Theorem 8.5, it can be easily shown that under the affine transformation (8.9), $Q_j^* = Y^{*'} L_2 P_j P_j' L_2' Y^* = d^2 Q_j$, $j = 1, 2, \cdots, d$, and $Q_0^* = \sum_{j=2}^{d} Q_j^* = d^2 Q_0$. Let $q_0^* = d^2 q_0$ and $q_j^* = d^2 q_j$ be the observed values of $Q_0^*$ and $Q_j^*$, respectively. Then, $Q_{1B}^* \sim \left(\frac{q_1^*}{r_1}\right) \chi_{r_1}^2$, $Q_{0B_1}^* \overset{asy}{\sim} \left(\overline{\Delta}\zeta_1 q_1^* + \frac{q_1^*}{r_1}\right) \chi_{n-k-1-r_1}^2$.

Furthermore, $Q_{1B}^* \overset{d}{=} d^2 Q_{1B}$ and $Q_{0B_1}^* \overset{d}{=} d^2 Q_{0B_1}$. Similar to the proof of Theorem 8.3, it can be easily shown that $Q_{0B_1}^*$ and $Q_{1B}^*$ are independent of each other. Therefore, we have

$$\tilde{T}_{2B}^* = \frac{\frac{Q_{0B_1}^*}{q_1^*}}{\overline{\Delta}\zeta_1 + \frac{Q_{1B}^*}{r_1 q_1^*}} \overset{d}{=} \frac{\frac{Q_{0B_1}}{q_1}}{\overline{\Delta}\zeta_1 + \frac{Q_{1B}}{r_1 q_1}} = \tilde{T}_{2B}.$$

For the hypothesis testing problem (8.17), it is invariant under the affine transformation (8.9). After the affine transformation, the test statistic becomes $\tilde{T}_2^* = \frac{\frac{Q_0^*}{q_1^*}}{\overline{\Delta}\zeta_1 + \frac{Q_1^*}{r_1 q_1^*}}$, and its observed value is $\tilde{t}_2^* = \tilde{t}_2$. Therefore, the test based on $p_{\tilde{T}_2}$ is invariant under the affine transformation, and Theorem 8.6 is proved. $\qquad\square$

Next, we consider the Bootstrap confidence interval for $\sigma_\mu^2$. According to Theorem 8.4, if $\sigma_v^2$ is known, a natural pivot quantity is given by

$$T_3 = \frac{Q_0}{\overline{\Delta}\sigma_\mu^2 + \sigma_v^2}.$$

However, $\sigma_v^2$ is generally unknown, and we can use $\tilde{\sigma}_v^2 = \frac{Q_1}{r_1}$ as a substitute for $\sigma_v^2$. Then, we have

$$T_3 = \frac{Q_0}{\overline{\Delta}\sigma_\mu^2 + \frac{Q_1}{r_1}}. \tag{8.18}$$

Therefore, based on the construction of $T_3$ in Equation (8.18), we can set up the Bootstrap pivot quantity as

$$T_{3B} = \frac{Q_{0B_2}}{\overline{\Delta}\hat{\sigma}^2_{\mu_0} + \frac{Q_{1B}}{r_1}}, \tag{8.19}$$

where $Q_{0B_2} \overset{asy}{\sim} \left(\frac{q_0}{n-k-1-r_1}\right)\chi^2_{n-k-1-r_1}$, $\hat{\sigma}^2_{\mu_0} = \frac{q_0}{(n-k-1-r_1)\overline{\Delta}} - \frac{q_1}{r_1\overline{\Delta}}$. Note that the distribution of $T_{3B}$ does not depend on any unknown parameters, so we can construct a confidence interval for $\sigma^2_\mu$ based on $T_{3B}$. Let $T_{3B}(\vartheta)$ denote the $100\vartheta$th empirical percentile of $T_{3B}$. Then, the Bootstrap confidence interval for $\sigma^2_\mu$ with confidence level $1 - \vartheta$ is given by

$$\left[\frac{q_0}{\overline{\Delta}T_{3B}(1 - \vartheta/2)} - \frac{q_1}{\overline{\Delta}r_1}, \frac{q_0}{\overline{\Delta}T_{3B}(\vartheta/2)} - \frac{q_1}{\overline{\Delta}r_1}\right].$$

**Remark 8.5.** *To construct a Bootstrap confidence interval for the affine-invariant parameter* $\zeta$, *we define the Bootstrap pivot quantity as*

$$\tilde{T}_{3B} = \frac{Q_{0B_2}/q_1}{\overline{\Delta}\hat{\zeta} + \frac{Q_{1B}}{r_1 q_1}},$$

*where* $\hat{\zeta} = \frac{q_0}{(n-k-1-r_1)\overline{\Delta}q_1} - \frac{1}{r_1\overline{\Delta}}$. *We can then obtain an affine-invariant Bootstrap confidence interval for* $\zeta$ *with confidence level* $1 - \vartheta$ *based on* $\tilde{T}_{3B}$ *as follows.*

$$\left[\frac{q_0}{\overline{\Delta}q_1\tilde{T}_{3B}(1 - \vartheta/2)} - \frac{1}{\overline{\Delta}r_1}, \frac{q_0}{\overline{\Delta}q_1\tilde{T}_{3B}(\vartheta/2)} - \frac{1}{\overline{\Delta}r_1}\right].$$

### *8.3.2  Generalized approach*

Let $V_0 = \frac{Q_0}{\Delta\sigma^2_\mu + \sigma^2_\nu}$, $V_1 = \frac{Q_1}{\sigma^2_\nu}$, $V_j = \frac{Q_j}{\Delta_j\sigma^2_\mu + \sigma^2_\nu}$, $j = 2, 3, \cdots, d$. For hypothesis testing problem (8.11), we define the generalized test variable as

$$F_1 = \sum_{j=2}^{d} V_j \left(\frac{1}{V_1} + \frac{\Delta_j\sigma^2_\mu}{q_1}\right) \sim \sum_{j=2}^{d} \chi^2_{r_j}\left(\frac{1}{\chi^2_{r_1}} + \frac{\Delta_j\sigma^2_\mu}{q_1}\right). \tag{8.20}$$

Clearly, the observed value of $F_1$ is $f_1 = \sum_{j=2}^{d} \frac{q_j}{q_1}$. The distribution of $F_1$ is free of the nuisance parameter and $F_1$ is a stochastically monotonically increasing function of $\sigma^2_\mu$. Therefore, $F_1$ is the generalized test variable for hypothesis testing problem (8.11). Based on $F_1$, we can obtain the generalized $p$-value.

$$
\begin{aligned}
p_{F_1} &= P(F_1 > f_1 | H_0) = P\left( \frac{1}{V_1} > \frac{f_1 - \sum_{j=2}^{d} \frac{\Delta_j s_1 V_j}{q_1}}{\sum_{j=2}^{d} V_j} \right) \\
&= 1 - E_{V_2, V_3, \cdots, V_d} \left[ F_{I\Gamma(r_1/2, 1/2)} \left( \frac{f_1 - \sum_{j=2}^{d} \frac{\Delta_j s_1 V_j}{q_1}}{\sum_{j=2}^{d} V_j} \right) \right].
\end{aligned}
\tag{8.21}
$$

Here, $F_{I\Gamma(r_1/2, 1/2)}$ represents the cumulative distribution function of the inverse gamma distribution with parameters $\frac{r_1}{2}$ and $\frac{1}{2}$, and $E_{V_2, V_3, \cdots, V_d}$ denotes the expectation with respect to $V_2, V_3, \cdots, V_d$. If $p_{F_1} < \vartheta$, then we reject the null hypothesis $H_0$ in (8.11) at the nominal significance level $\vartheta$.

For a testing method, it is natural to require that it remains unchanged in the event of a change of units for the observed data. Therefore, we consider a scaling transformation.

$$
\begin{aligned}
(\beta, \sigma_\mu^2, \sigma_v^2) &\mapsto (a\beta, a^2\sigma_\mu^2, a^2\sigma_v^2), \\
\left(\hat{\beta}, Q_1, Q_2, \cdots, Q_d\right) &\mapsto \left(a\hat{\beta}, a^2 Q_1, a^2 Q_2, \cdots, a^2 Q_d\right), a > 0.
\end{aligned}
\tag{8.22}
$$

Although the generalized test variable $F_1$ remains invariant under the scaling transformation (8.22), the hypothesis testing problem (8.11) itself is not an invariant testing problem under the scaling transformation (8.22). Therefore, we consider an equivalent hypothesis testing problem (8.17). By applying the scaling transformation

$$
\begin{aligned}
(\beta, \zeta, \sigma_v^2) &\mapsto (a\beta, \zeta, a^2\sigma_v^2), \\
\left(\hat{\beta}, Q_1, Q_2, \cdots, Q_d\right) &\mapsto \left(a\hat{\beta}, a^2 Q_1, a^2 Q_2, \cdots, a^2 Q_d\right), a > 0,
\end{aligned}
\tag{8.23}
$$

we can obtain an invariant testing problem (8.17). The generalized $p$-value for this problem can be expressed as

$$
\tilde{p}_{F_1} = 1 - E_{V_2, V_3, \cdots, V_d} \left[ F_{I\Gamma(r_1/2, 1/2)} \left( \frac{f_1 - \sum_{j=2}^{d} \Delta_j \zeta_1 V_j}{\sum_{j=2}^{d} V_j} \right) \right].
$$

Therefore, for hypothesis testing problem (8.17), the test based on $\tilde{p}_{F_1}$ has $p$-invariance under the scaling transformation (8.23).

For the hypothesis testing problem (8.11), the approximate generalized test variable can be defined as

$$
F_2 = V_0 \left( \frac{1}{V_1} + \frac{\overline{\Delta} \sigma_\mu^2}{q_1} \right) \overset{asy}{\sim} \chi^2_{n-k-1-r_1} \left( \frac{1}{\chi^2_{r_1}} + \frac{\overline{\Delta} \sigma_\mu^2}{q_1} \right). \tag{8.24}
$$

It is easy to see that the observed value of $F_2$ is $f_2 = \frac{q_0}{q_1}$. The approximate distribution of $F_2$ is free of the nuisance parameter, and $F_2$ is a stochastically monotonic increasing function of $\sigma_\mu^2$. Therefore, the generalized $p$-value for $F_2$ can be expressed as

$$
p_{F_2} = 1 - E_{V_0} \left[ F_{I\Gamma(r_1/2,1/2)} \left( \frac{f_2 - \frac{\overline{\Delta} s_1 V_0}{q_1}}{V_0} \right) \right]. \tag{8.25}
$$

Similarly, under the scaling transformation (8.23), for the invariant testing problem (8.17), we can obtain the generalized $p$-value based on the approximate generalized test variable $F_2$ as

$$
\tilde{p}_{F_2} = 1 - E_{V_0} \left[ F_{I\Gamma(r_1/2,1/2)} \left( \frac{f_2 - \overline{\Delta} \zeta_1 V_0}{V_0} \right) \right].
$$

Next, we consider the generalized confidence interval for $\sigma_\mu^2$. Define

$$
F_3 = \frac{q_0}{\overline{\Delta} V_0} - \frac{q_1}{\overline{\Delta} V_1} \overset{asy}{\sim} \frac{q_0}{\overline{\Delta} \chi^2_{n-k-1-r_1}} - \frac{q_1}{\overline{\Delta} \chi^2_{r_1}}. \tag{8.26}
$$

It is easy to see that the observed value of $F_3$ is $\sigma_\mu^2$, and the approximate distribution of $F_3$ is free of any unknown parameters. Thus, $F_3$ is an approximate generalized pivot quantity. Based on the empirical percentile of $F_3$, we can obtain the generalized lower and upper confidence limits for $\sigma_\mu^2$ with confidence level $1 - \vartheta$, denoted as $F_3\left(\frac{\vartheta}{2}\right)$ and $F_3\left(1 - \frac{\vartheta}{2}\right)$, respectively.

Because in the frequentist sense, the generalized confidence interval $\left[ F_3\left(\frac{\vartheta}{2}\right), \right.$ $\left. F_3\left(1 - \frac{\vartheta}{2}\right) \right]$ may not be a confidence interval with confidence level $1 - \vartheta$, it is necessary to investigate the coverage probability of this generalized confidence interval.

**Theorem 8.7.** *For the generalized pivot quantity $F_3$ in Equation (8.26), we have*

$$\lim_{\sigma_v^2 \to 0} P\left(F_3\left(\frac{\vartheta}{2}\right) \leq \sigma_\mu^2 \leq F_3\left(1-\frac{\vartheta}{2}\right)\right) = 1-\vartheta,$$

$$\lim_{\sigma_\mu^2 \to 0} P\left(F_3\left(\frac{\vartheta}{2}\right) \leq \sigma_\mu^2 \leq F_3\left(1-\frac{\vartheta}{2}\right)\right) = 1-\vartheta. \tag{8.27}$$

*Proof.* To prove the first equality in Equation (8.27), it suffices to show that

$$\lim_{\sigma_v^2 \to 0} P\left(\sigma_\mu^2 \geq F_3\left(\frac{\vartheta}{2}\right)\right) = 1-\frac{\vartheta}{2},$$

$$\lim_{\sigma_v^2 \to 0} P\left(\sigma_A^2 \leq F_3\left(1-\frac{\vartheta}{2}\right)\right) = 1-\frac{\vartheta}{2}.$$

Let $(V_0^*, V_1^*)$ and $(V_0, V_1)$ be independently and identically distributed random variables. Then, we have

$$P\left(\sigma_\mu^2 \geq F_3\left(\frac{\vartheta}{2}\right)\right) = P\left(P\left(F_3 \leq \sigma_\mu^2\right) \geq \frac{\vartheta}{2}\right)$$

$$= P\left(P\left(\frac{Q_0}{\overline{\Delta V_0}} - \frac{Q_1}{\overline{\Delta V_1}} \leq \sigma_\mu^2 \mid Q_0, Q_1\right) \geq \frac{\vartheta}{2}\right)$$

$$= \tilde{P}\left(P\left(\left(\overline{\Delta}\sigma_\mu^2 + \sigma_v^2\right)\frac{V_0^*}{\overline{\Delta V_0}} - \sigma_v^2\frac{V_1^*}{\overline{\Delta V_1}} \leq \sigma_\mu^2 \mid V_0^*, V_1^*\right) \geq \frac{\vartheta}{2}\right),$$

where $\tilde{P}$ denotes the joint distribution of $(V_0^*, V_1^*)$. Based on this result, we have

$$\lim_{\sigma_v^2 \to 0} P\left(\sigma_\mu^2 \geq F_3\left(\frac{\vartheta}{2}\right)\right) = \tilde{P}\left(P(V_0^* \leq V_0 \mid V_0^*, V_1^*) \geq \frac{\vartheta}{2}\right)$$

$$= \tilde{P}\left(F_{V_0}(V_0^*) \leq 1-\frac{\vartheta}{2}\right) = 1-\frac{\vartheta}{2}.$$

Here, $F_{V_0}$ denotes the cumulative distribution function of $V_0$. Similarly, we can prove that $\lim_{\sigma_v^2 \to 0} P\left(\sigma_\mu^2 \leq F_3\left(1-\frac{\vartheta}{2}\right)\right) = 1-\frac{\vartheta}{2}$. The proof of the other equality in Equation (8.27) follows a similar argument as the first equality, and is therefore omitted. Thus, Theorem 8.7 is proved. $\qquad\square$

**Remark 8.6.** *Consider constructing an invariant generalized confidence interval for the scale-invariant parameter $\zeta$ under the scaling transformation (8.23). We define the approximate generalized pivot quantity*

$$\tilde{F}_3 = \frac{q_0}{\overline{\Delta q_1 V_0}} - \frac{1}{\overline{\Delta V_1}} \overset{asy}{\sim} \frac{q_0}{\overline{\Delta q_1 \chi_{n-k-1-r_1}^2}} - \frac{1}{\overline{\Delta \chi_{r_1}^2}}.$$

*Clearly, based on the empirical percentiles of $\tilde{F}_3$, we can obtain the invariant generalized confidence interval for $\zeta$ with confidence level $1 - \vartheta$. The interval is given by $\left[\tilde{F}_3\left(\frac{\vartheta}{2}\right), \tilde{F}_3\left(1 - \frac{\vartheta}{2}\right)\right]$.*

## 8.4   Inference on the sum of variance components

Consider the problem of one-sided hypothesis testing

$$H_0 : \sigma_\mu^2 + \sigma_v^2 \leq s_2 \quad versus \quad H_1 : \sigma_\mu^2 + \sigma_v^2 > s_2, \tag{8.28}$$

where $s_2$ is a given value.

### 8.4.1   Bootstrap approach

For hypothesis testing problem (8.28), we define

$$T_4 = \sum_{j=2}^{d} \frac{Q_j}{s_2\Delta_j + (1 - \Delta_j)\sigma_v^2}.$$

Similar to Equation (8.12), we can replace $\sigma_v^2$ with the estimator $\tilde{\sigma}_v^2 = \frac{Q_1}{r_1}$ and get

$$T_4 = \sum_{j=2}^{d} \frac{Q_j}{s_2\Delta_j + (1 - \Delta_j)\frac{Q_1}{r_1}}. \tag{8.29}$$

Thus, based on Equation (8.29), we construct the Bootstrap test statistic for hypothesis testing problem (8.28)

$$T_{4B} = \sum_{j=2}^{d} \frac{Q_{jB_2}}{s_2\Delta_j + (1 - \Delta_j)\frac{Q_{1B}}{r_1}}, \tag{8.30}$$

where $Q_{jB_2} \sim \left(s_2\Delta_j + (1 - \Delta_j)\frac{q_1}{r_1}\right)\chi_{r_j}^2$, $j = 2, 3, \ldots, d$. Therefore, based on $T_{4B}$, we can obtain the following $p$-value

$$p_{T_4} = P\left(T_{4B} > t_4 | H_0\right), \tag{8.31}$$

where $t_4$ is the observed value of $T_4$ in Equation (8.29). If $p_{T_4} < \vartheta$, then we reject the null hypothesis $H_0$ in (8.28) at the nominal significance level $\vartheta$.

For hypothesis testing problem (8.28), we give another Bootstrap test method. Define

$$T_5 = \frac{Q_0}{\bar{\Delta}s_2 + (1 - \bar{\Delta})\frac{Q_1}{r_1}}.$$

Similar to Equation (8.15), we can construct the Bootstrap test statistic based on $T_5$. Define

$$T_{5B} = \frac{Q_{0B_3}}{\bar{\Delta}s_2 + (1 - \bar{\Delta})\frac{Q_{1B}}{r_1}}, \tag{8.32}$$

where $Q_{0B_3} \overset{asy}{\sim} \left(\bar{\Delta}s_2 + (1 - \bar{\Delta})\frac{q_1}{r_1}\right) \chi^2_{n-k-1-r_1}$. Therefore, based on $T_{5B}$, we can obtain the following $p$-value

$$p_{T_5} = P\left(T_{5B} > t_5 | H_0\right), \tag{8.33}$$

where $t_5$ is the observed value of $T_5$. If $p_{T_5} < \vartheta$, then we reject the null hypothesis $H_0$ in (8.28) at the nominal significance level $\vartheta$.

Let $\omega = \frac{\sigma_\mu^2 + \sigma_v^2}{q_1}$, $\omega_2 = \frac{s_2}{q_1}$, $\tilde{T}_5 = \frac{\frac{Q_0}{q_1}}{\omega_2\bar{\Delta}+(1-\bar{\Delta})\frac{Q_1}{r_1 q_1}}$, $\tilde{T}_{5B} = \frac{\frac{Q_{0B_3}}{q_1}}{\omega_2\bar{\Delta}+(1-\bar{\Delta})\frac{Q_{1B}}{r_1 q_1}}$,

$p_{\tilde{T}_5} = P\left(\tilde{T}_{5B} > \tilde{t}_5 | H_0\right)$, where $\tilde{t}_5$ is the observed value of $\tilde{T}_5$.

**Theorem 8.8.** *For hypothesis testing problem (8.28), we consider an equivalent hypothesis testing problem as follows.*

$$H_0 : \omega \leq \omega_2 \quad versus \quad H_1 : \omega > \omega_2. \tag{8.34}$$

*The Bootstrap test based on $p_{\tilde{T}_5}$ is invariant under the affine transformation (8.9).*

The proof of Theorem 8.8 is similar to that of Theorem 8.6 and is therefore omitted here.

Consider the Bootstrap confidence interval for $\sigma_\mu^2 + \sigma_v^2$. Let

$$T_6 = \frac{Q_0}{\bar{\Delta}\left(\sigma_\mu^2 + \sigma_v^2\right) + (1 - \bar{\Delta})\frac{Q_1}{r_1}}.$$

Similar to Equation (8.19), we construct a Bootstrap pivot quantity based on $T_6$.

$$T_{6B} = \frac{Q_{0B_2}}{\bar{\Delta}\left(\hat{\sigma}_{\mu_0}^2 + \tilde{\sigma}_{v_0}^2\right) + (1 - \bar{\Delta})\frac{Q_{1B}}{r_1}}, \tag{8.35}$$

where $\tilde{\sigma}_{v_0}^2 = \frac{q_1}{r_1}$. Let $T_{6B}(\vartheta)$ denote the $100\vartheta$ empirical percentile of $T_{6B}$. Then, the Bootstrap confidence interval for $\sigma_\mu^2 + \sigma_v^2$ at the confidence level $1 - \vartheta$ is given by

$$\left[\frac{q_0}{\bar{\Delta}T_{6B}\left(1 - \frac{\vartheta}{2}\right)} - \frac{(1 - \bar{\Delta})q_1}{\bar{\Delta}r_1}, \frac{q_0}{\bar{\Delta}T_{6B}\left(\frac{\vartheta}{2}\right)} - \frac{(1 - \bar{\Delta})q_1}{\bar{\Delta}r_1}\right].$$

**Remark 8.7.** *To construct the Bootstrap confidence interval for the affine-invariant parameter $\omega$, we define the Bootstrap pivot quantity as follows.*

$$\tilde{T}_{6B} = \frac{Q_{0B_2}/q_1}{\bar{\Delta}\hat{\omega} + (1-\bar{\Delta})\frac{Q_{1B}}{r_1 q_1}},$$

*where $\hat{\omega} = \frac{q_0}{(n-k-1-r_1)\bar{\Delta}q_1} - \frac{1}{r_1\bar{\Delta}} + \frac{1}{r_1}$. Furthermore, based on $\tilde{T}_{6B}$, we can obtain the invariant Bootstrap confidence interval for $\omega$ at the confidence level $1 - \vartheta$.*

$$\left[\frac{q_0}{\bar{\Delta}q_1 T_{6B}\left(1-\frac{\vartheta}{2}\right)} - \frac{1-\bar{\Delta}}{\bar{\Delta}r_1}, \frac{q_0}{\bar{\Delta}q_1 T_{6B}\left(\frac{\vartheta}{2}\right)} - \frac{1-\bar{\Delta}}{\bar{\Delta}r_1}\right].$$

### 8.4.2 Generalized approach

For hypothesis testing problem (8.28), we define

$$F_4 = \sum_{j=2}^{d} V_j \left(\frac{1-\Delta_j}{V_1} + \frac{\Delta_j\left(\sigma_\mu^2 + \sigma_v^2\right)}{q_1}\right). \tag{8.36}$$

Similar to $F_1$ in Equation (8.20), it can be shown that $F_4$ is a generalized test variable. Therefore, a generalized $p$-value can be obtained based on $F_4$, namely

$$p_{F_4} = E_{V_2,V_3,\cdots,V_d}\left[F_{I\Gamma(r_1/2,1/2)}\left(\frac{\sum_{j=2}^{d}\frac{q_j - \Delta_j s_2 V_j}{q_1}}{\sum_{j=2}^{d}(1-\Delta_j)V_j}\right)\right]. \tag{8.37}$$

If $p_{F_4} < \vartheta$, then at the nominal significance level $\vartheta$, we reject the null hypothesis $H_0$ in (8.28).

Similar to Equation (8.23), consider a scaling transformation

$$(\beta, \omega, \sigma_v^2) \mapsto (a\beta, \omega, a^2\sigma_v^2),$$

$$\left(\hat{\beta}, Q_1, Q_2, \cdots, Q_d\right) \mapsto \left(a\hat{\beta}, a^2 Q_1, a^2 Q_2, \cdots, a^2 Q_d\right), a > 0. \tag{8.38}$$

The hypothesis testing problem (8.34), which is equivalent to Equation (8.28), is an invariant testing problem, and its generalized $p$-value can be expressed as

$$\tilde{p}_{F_4} = E_{V_2,V_3,\cdots,V_d}\left[F_{I\Gamma(r_1/2,1/2)}\left(\frac{\sum_{j=2}^{d}\left(\frac{q_j}{q_1} - \Delta_j\omega_2 V_j\right)}{\sum_{j=2}^{d}(1-\Delta_j)V_j}\right)\right].$$

Therefore, for hypothesis testing problem (8.34), the test based on $\tilde{p}_{F_4}$ has $p$-invariance under the scaling transformation (8.38).

For hypothesis testing problem (8.28), define the approximate generalized test variable as

$$F_5 = \frac{(\overline{\Delta} - 1)q_1}{\overline{\Delta}V_1} + \frac{q_0}{\overline{\Delta}V_0} - \left(\sigma_\mu^2 + \sigma_\nu^2\right).$$ (8.39)

Therefore, similar to Equation (8.25), its generalized $p$-value can be expressed as

$$p_{F_5} = E_{V_1}\left[F_{I\Gamma((n-k-1-r_1)/2,1/2)}\left(\frac{(1-\overline{\Delta})q_1}{q_0 V_1} + \frac{\overline{\Delta}s_2}{q_0}\right)\right].$$ (8.40)

However, for invariant testing problem (8.34), the approximate generalized test variable $F_5$ is not invariant under the scaling transformation (8.38). Let

$$\tilde{F}_5 = \frac{\overline{\Delta} - 1}{\overline{\Delta}V_1} + \frac{q_0}{\overline{\Delta}q_1 V_0} - \omega.$$

It can be easily proven to be an invariant approximate generalized test variable, and the corresponding $p$-value is

$$p_{\tilde{F}_5} = E_{V_1}\left[F_{I\Gamma((n-k-1-r_1)/2,1/2)}\left(\frac{(1-\overline{\Delta})q_1}{q_0 V_1} + \frac{\overline{\Delta}\omega_2 q_1}{q_0}\right)\right].$$

Therefore, for hypothesis testing problem (8.34), the generalized test based on $p_{\tilde{F}_5}$ is a $p$-invariant test under the scaling transformation (8.38).

Next, we consider the generalized confidence interval for $\sigma_\mu^2 + \sigma_\nu^2$. Similar to Equation (8.26), define the approximate generalized pivot quantity as

$$F_6 = \frac{(\overline{\Delta} - 1)q_1}{\overline{\Delta}V_1} + \frac{q_0}{\overline{\Delta}V_0}.$$ (8.41)

Using the empirical percentile of $F_6$, the generalized lower and upper confidence bounds for $\sigma_\mu^2 + \sigma_\nu^2$ at the confidence level $1 - \vartheta$ can be obtained. They are denoted as $F_6\left(\frac{\vartheta}{2}\right)$ and $F_6\left(1 - \frac{\vartheta}{2}\right)$, respectively.

**Theorem 8.9.** *For the generalized pivot quantity $F_6$ in Equation (8.41), we have*

$$\lim_{\sigma_\nu^2 \to 0} P\left(F_6\left(\frac{\vartheta}{2}\right) \leq \sigma_\mu^2 + \sigma_\nu^2 \leq F_6\left(1 - \frac{\vartheta}{2}\right)\right) = 1 - \vartheta.$$ (8.42)

The proof of Theorem 8.9 is similar to that of Theorem 8.7 and is therefore omitted.

**Remark 8.8.** *Under the scaling transformation (8.38), we construct an invariant generalized confidence interval for the invariant parameter $\omega$. Define the approximate generalized pivot quantity as*

$$\tilde{F}_6 = \frac{\overline{\Delta} - 1}{\overline{\Delta} V_1} + \frac{q_0}{\overline{\Delta} q_1 V_0}.$$

*Using the empirical percentile of $\tilde{F}_6$, the $1 - \vartheta$ invariant generalized confidence interval for $\omega$ can be obtained as $\left[ \tilde{F}_6 \left( \frac{\vartheta}{2} \right), \tilde{F}_6 \left( 1 - \frac{\vartheta}{2} \right) \right]$.*

## 8.5 Inference on the ratio of variance components

Consider the one-sided hypothesis testing problem

$$H_0 : \frac{\sigma_\mu^2}{\sigma_v^2} \leq s_3 \quad versus \quad H_1 : \frac{\sigma_\mu^2}{\sigma_v^2} > s_3, \tag{8.43}$$

where $s_3$ is a given value.

Similar to the testing of the regression coefficient, the required test statistic and rejection region for hypothesis testing problem (8.43) are consistent with the following hypothesis testing problem

$$H_0 : \frac{\sigma_\mu^2}{\sigma_v^2} = s_3 \quad versus \quad H_1 : \frac{\sigma_\mu^2}{\sigma_v^2} > s_3.$$

Based on Theorem 8.3, the test statistic is defined as

$$F_7 = \frac{\sum_{j=2}^{d} \frac{Q_j}{\Delta_j s_3 + 1} / (n - k - 1 - r_1)}{Q_1 / r_1}. \tag{8.44}$$

Under the null hypothesis $H_0 : \frac{\sigma_\mu^2}{\sigma_v^2} = s_3$, it can be known that

$$F_7 \sim F_{n-k-1-r_1, r_1},$$

where $F_{n-k-1-r_1, r_1}$ represents the $F$ distribution with degrees of freedom $n - k - 1 - r_1$ and $r_1$. Based on $F_7$, the $p$-value can be obtained as

$$p_{F_7} = P\left( F_7 > f_7 | H_0 \right), \tag{8.45}$$

where $f_7$ represents the observed value of $F_7$. If $p_{F_7} < \vartheta$, the null hypothesis $H_0$ in (8.43) is rejected at the nominal significance level $\vartheta$.

Based on Theorem 8.4, the approximate test statistic can be given as

$$F_8 = \frac{\frac{Q_0}{\bar{\Delta}s_3+1}/(n-k-1-r_1)}{Q_1/r_1}. \tag{8.46}$$

Under the null hypothesis $H_0 : \frac{\sigma_\mu^2}{\sigma_v^2} = s_3$, it can be obtained that

$$F_8 \overset{asy}{\sim} F_{n-k-1-r_1,r_1}.$$

Based on $F_8$, the following $p$-value can be computed as

$$p_{F_8} = P(F_8 > f_8 | H_0), \tag{8.47}$$

where $f_8$ represents the observed value of $F_8$. If $p_{F_8} < \vartheta$, the null hypothesis $H_0$ in (8.43) is rejected at the nominal significance level $\vartheta$.

**Theorem 8.10.** *For hypothesis testing problem (8.43), the tests based on $p_{F_7}$ and $p_{F_8}$ are both invariant under the affine transformation (8.9).*

Similar to Theorems 8.5 and 8.6, Theorem 8.10 can be easily proven and therefore the proof is omitted.

Next, we consider the confidence interval for $\frac{\sigma_\mu^2}{\sigma_v^2}$. Define the pivot quantity as

$$F_9 = \frac{\frac{Q_0}{\bar{\Delta}\left(\frac{\sigma_\mu^2}{\sigma_v^2}\right)+1}/(n-k-1-r_1)}{Q_1/r_1} \overset{asy}{\sim} F_{n-k-1-r_1,r_1}. \tag{8.48}$$

Based on $F_9$, the $1 - \vartheta$ invariant confidence interval for $\frac{\sigma_\mu^2}{\sigma_v^2}$ can be obtained as

$$\left[ \frac{r_1 q_0}{\bar{\Delta}(n-k-1-r_1)q_1 F_{n-k-1-r_1,r_1}(1-\frac{\vartheta}{2})} - \frac{1}{\bar{\Delta}}, \frac{r_1 q_0}{\bar{\Delta}(n-k-1-r_1)q_1 F_{n-k-1-r_1,r_1}(\frac{\vartheta}{2})} - \frac{1}{\bar{\Delta}} \right].$$

**Remark 8.9.** *For the left-sided and two-sided hypothesis testing problems of a single variance component, sum of variance components, and ratio of variance components, the construction of p-values is similar to that in Remarks 8.2 and 8.3, so the expressions are omitted here.*

## 8.6 Monte Carlo simulation

In this section, the statistical properties of the Type I error probability and power of the test method given in this book are numerically studied through the Monte

Carlo simulation. For convenience, this section only provides an algorithm for simulating the Type I error probability using the Bootstrap method for hypothesis testing problem (8.11).

**Step 1:** Given $N, T_1, T_2, \cdots, T_N, \sigma_\mu^2, \sigma_v^2, \lambda_1, \alpha, \beta, X$, and $Z_\mu$, generate $Y \sim SN_n(\xi_Y, \Sigma_Y, \lambda_2)$. Then, compute $q_j$, $\Delta_j$, and $r_j$ using Theorem 8.3 and Equation (8.6), where $q_j$ is the observed value of $Q_j$, $j = 1, 2, \cdots, d$.

**Step 2:** Compute $T_1$ by Equation (8.12), denoted by $t_1$.

**Step 3:** Generate $Q_{1B} \sim \left(\frac{q_1}{r_1}\right) \chi_{r_1}^2$, $Q_{jB_1} \sim \left(s_1 \Delta_j + \frac{q_1}{r_1}\right) \chi_{r_j}^2$, $j = 2, 3, \cdots, d$, and compute $T_{1B}$ by Equation (8.13).

**Step 4:** Repeat Step 3 $k_1$ times, and obtain $p_{T_1}$ by Equation (8.14). Let $\vartheta$ denote the nominal significance level. If $p_{T_1} < \vartheta$, then $l = 1$. Otherwise, $l = 0$.

**Step 5:** Repeat Steps 1–4 $k_2$ times, and obtain $l_1, l_2, \cdots, l_{k_2}$. Then, the Type I error probability is $\sum_{i=1}^{k_2} \frac{l_i}{k_2}$.

When the alternative hypothesis $H_1$ in (8.12) is true, similar to the above algorithm, the power of the Bootstrap method can be obtained. In the Monte Carlo simulation study, we set the nominal significance level $\vartheta = 0.025, 0.05, 0.075, 0.1$, and both inner loop and outer loop are set to 2500. Without loss of generality, let $N = 8$, $\alpha = 1$, $\lambda_1 = 1_N$, $\beta = (\beta_1, \beta_2, \beta_3) = (-1, -2, 3)'$, and $X_{it}$ is generated from $N_3(0, I_3)$. The sample sizes are set as follows: $N_1 = (T_1, T_2, \cdots, T_8) = (3, 3, 3, 3, 5, 5, 5, 5), N_2 = (5, 5, 6, 6, 6, 6, 7, 7), N_3 = (7, 7, 7, 8, 8, 8, 9, 9), N_4 = (8, 9, 9, 12, 12, 15, 15, 16), N_5 = (11, 12, 13, 14, 16, 17, 18, 19)$. Other parameter settings are shown in Table 8.1.

For hypothesis testing problem (8.7), Tables 8.2–8.3 present the simulation results of the Type I error probability and power of the exact testing method under different nominal significance levels and parameter settings. From Table 8.2, we

**Table 8.1:** Parameter configurations.

| Testing problem | Type I error probability | Power |
|---|---|---|
| (8.7) | $s_0 = 0, \sigma_v^2 = 1, c = (1,1,1)',$ $\sigma_\mu^2 = 0.5, 1, 2, 3$ | $s_0 = 0, \sigma_v^2 = 1, \sigma_\mu^2 = 3, c = (1,1,1)',$ $\beta_1 = -1, \beta_2 = -2, \beta_3 = 3.1, 3.2, 3.3, 3.5$ |
| (8.11) | $s_1 = \sigma_\mu^2 = 1,$ $\sigma_v^2 = 0.5, 1, 2, 3$ | $s_1 = 1, \sigma_v^2 = 1,$ $\sigma_\mu^2 = 2, 4, 5, 6$ |
| (8.28) | $s_2 = \sigma_\mu^2 + \sigma_v^2 = 5,$ $\sigma_v^2 = 0.5, 1, 1.5, 2$ | $s_2 = 5, \sigma_v^2 = 1,$ $\sigma_\mu^2 = 5, 10, 20, 25$ |
| (8.43) | $s_3 = \frac{\sigma_\mu^2}{\sigma_v^2}, \sigma_v^2 = 1,$ $\sigma_\mu^2 = 0.5, 1, 2, 3$ | $s_3 = 1, \sigma_v^2 = 1,$ $\sigma_\mu^2 = 2, 4, 6, 8$ |

**Table 8.2:** Sizes for hypothesis testing problem (8.7) ($c'\beta = s_0 = 0, \beta = (-1,-2,3)'$).

| | | $\vartheta$ | | | |
|---|---|---|---|---|---|
| Sample size | $\sigma_\mu^2$ | 0.025 | 0.05 | 0.075 | 0.1 |
| $N_1$ | 0.5 | 0.0272 | 0.0564 | 0.0856 | 0.1164 |
| | 1 | 0.0280 | 0.0596 | 0.0828 | 0.1192 |
| | 2 | 0.0272 | 0.0552 | 0.0836 | 0.1168 |
| | 3 | 0.0296 | 0.0556 | 0.0872 | 0.1124 |
| $N_2$ | 0.5 | 0.0308 | 0.0572 | 0.0844 | 0.1116 |
| | 1 | 0.0304 | 0.0552 | 0.0836 | 0.1116 |
| | 2 | 0.0312 | 0.0548 | 0.0808 | 0.1128 |
| | 3 | 0.0312 | 0.0544 | 0.0808 | 0.1104 |
| $N_3$ | 0.5 | 0.0252 | 0.0568 | 0.0816 | 0.1008 |
| | 1 | 0.0260 | 0.0540 | 0.0792 | 0.1032 |
| | 2 | 0.0252 | 0.0536 | 0.0788 | 0.1032 |
| | 3 | 0.0244 | 0.0528 | 0.0764 | 0.1048 |
| $N_4$ | 0.5 | 0.0240 | 0.0532 | 0.0764 | 0.0988 |
| | 1 | 0.0248 | 0.0500 | 0.0776 | 0.0960 |
| | 2 | 0.0260 | 0.0476 | 0.0748 | 0.0980 |
| | 3 | 0.0268 | 0.0476 | 0.0732 | 0.0980 |
| $N_5$ | 0.5 | 0.0204 | 0.0504 | 0.0748 | 0.1016 |
| | 1 | 0.0204 | 0.0488 | 0.0752 | 0.1004 |
| | 2 | 0.0212 | 0.0492 | 0.0736 | 0.0996 |
| | 3 | 0.0208 | 0.0492 | 0.0712 | 0.0992 |

Note: $N_1 = (3,3,3,3,5,5,5,5)$, $N_2 = (5,5,6,6,6,6,7,7)$, $N_3 = (7,7,7,8,8,8,9,9)$, $N_4 = (8,9,9,12,12,15,15,16)$, $N_5 = (11,12,13,14,16,17,18,19)$.

can see that the Type I error probability of the proposed method is close to the nominal significance level, but may be slightly liberal in small sample sizes. From Table 8.3, we can see that for the specified parameters, sample sizes, and nominal significance levels, the power of the exact testing method significantly increases as $c'\beta$ deviates from the null hypothesis.

For hypothesis testing problem (8.11), Tables 8.4–8.5 present the simulation results of the Type I error probability and power of the four testing methods $(BA_1, BA_2, GA_1, GA_2)$ based on $p_{T_1}$, $p_{T_2}$, $p_{F_1}$, and $p_{F_2}$. From Table 8.4, we can see that all four methods can control the Type I error probability well, but the $BA_2$ method may be slightly liberal in small sample sizes. $BA_1$ and $GA_2$ methods are better than the $GA_1$ method in most cases, and the $BA_2$ method is better than the $GA_1$ and $GA_2$ methods in most cases. The $BA_1$ method is slightly better than the $BA_2$ and $GA_2$ methods. From Table 8.5, we can see that as $\sigma_\mu^2$ deviates from the null hypothesis, the powers of all four testing methods significantly increase. In most cases, the power of the $BA_1$ method is better than those of the other three methods, the power of the $BA_2$ method is better than those of the $GA_1$ and $GA_2$ methods, and the power of the $GA_1$ method is better than that of the $GA_2$ method.

**Table 8.3:** Powers for hypothesis testing problem (8.7) ($s_0 = 0$, $\beta_1 = -1$, $\beta_2 = -2$).

| Sample size | $\sigma_\mu^2$ | $\vartheta$ | | | |
|---|---|---|---|---|---|
| | | 0.025 | 0.05 | 0.075 | 0.1 |
| $N_1$ | 3.1 | 0.0528 | 0.1012 | 0.1460 | 0.1820 |
| | 3.2 | 0.0980 | 0.1660 | 0.2192 | 0.2688 |
| | 3.3 | 0.1624 | 0.2496 | 0.3128 | 0.3588 |
| | 3.5 | 0.3256 | 0.4416 | 0.5292 | 0.5888 |
| $N_2$ | 3.1 | 0.0608 | 0.1128 | 0.1560 | 0.1964 |
| | 3.2 | 0.1240 | 0.1948 | 0.2540 | 0.3056 |
| | 3.3 | 0.2076 | 0.3052 | 0.3792 | 0.4440 |
| | 3.5 | 0.4552 | 0.5840 | 0.6664 | 0.7276 |
| $N_3$ | 3.1 | 0.0656 | 0.1116 | 0.1524 | 0.1948 |
| | 3.2 | 0.1304 | 0.2128 | 0.2832 | 0.3336 |
| | 3.3 | 0.2456 | 0.3484 | 0.4200 | 0.4800 |
| | 3.5 | 0.5356 | 0.6556 | 0.7272 | 0.7848 |
| $N_4$ | 3.1 | 0.0728 | 0.1228 | 0.1672 | 0.2152 |
| | 3.2 | 0.1652 | 0.2612 | 0.3272 | 0.3860 |
| | 3.3 | 0.3276 | 0.4428 | 0.5212 | 0.5900 |
| | 3.5 | 0.7124 | 0.8052 | 0.8588 | 0.8892 |
| $N_5$ | 3.1 | 0.0816 | 0.1420 | 0.1932 | 0.2364 |
| | 3.2 | 0.2128 | 0.3024 | 0.3712 | 0.4340 |
| | 3.3 | 0.3928 | 0.5284 | 0.6184 | 0.6788 |
| | 3.5 | 0.8232 | 0.8992 | 0.9300 | 0.9452 |

Note: $N_1 = (3,3,3,3,5,5,5,5)$, $N_2 = (5,5,6,6,6,6,7,7)$, $N_3 = (7,7,7,8,8,8,9,9)$, $N_4 = (8,9,9,12,12,15,15,16)$, $N_5 = (11,12,13,14,16,17,18,19)$.

For hypothesis testing problem (8.28), Tables 8.6–8.7 present the simulation results of the Type I error probability and the power of the four testing methods $(BA_1, BA_2, GA_1, GA_2)$ based on $p_{T_4}$, $p_{T_5}$, $p_{F_4}$, and $p_{F_5}$. From Table 8.6, we can see that the Type I error probabilities of the $BA_1$ and $BA_2$ methods are close to the nominal significance levels in most cases, but the $GA_1$ and $GA_2$ methods may be slightly liberal. $BA_1$ and $BA_2$ methods are better than $GA_1$ and $GA_2$ methods in most cases, with the $GA_1$ method better than the $GA_2$ method, and the $BA_1$ method is slightly better than the $BA_2$ method. From Table 8.7, we can see that for the specified parameters, sample sizes, and nominal significance levels, the powers of all four testing methods significantly increase as $\sigma_\mu^2 + \sigma_v^2$ deviates from the null hypothesis. In most cases, the power of the $BA_1$ method is better than those of the $BA_2$ and $GA_1$ methods, and the power of the $GA_2$ method is better than that of the $GA_1$ method. The powers of $GA_1$ and $GA_2$ methods are better than those of the $BA_2$ and $BA_1$ methods in most cases, with the power of the $GA_2$ method consistently better than that of the $BA_2$ method.

For hypothesis testing problem (8.43), Tables 8.8–8.9 present the simulation results of the Type I error probability and the power of exact testing method (EA) and the approximate testing method (AP) under different nominal significance levels and parameter settings. From Table 8.8, we can see that the actual levels of both testing methods are close to the nominal significance levels in most

**Table 8.4:** Sizes for hypothesis testing problem (8.11) ($\sigma_\mu^2 = s_1 = 1$).

| | | $\vartheta$ | | | | | | | |
| | | 0.05 | | | | 0.1 | | | |
| Sample size | $\sigma_\mu^2$ | $BA_1$ | $BA_2$ | $GA_1$ | $GA_2$ | $BA_1$ | $BA_2$ | $GA_1$ | $GA_2$ |
|---|---|---|---|---|---|---|---|---|---|
| $N_1$ | 0.5 | 0.0500 | 0.0564 | 0.0484 | 0.0536 | 0.1104 | 0.1088 | 0.1024 | 0.1052 |
| | 1 | 0.0528 | 0.0552 | 0.0492 | 0.0504 | 0.1044 | 0.1064 | 0.0972 | 0.1004 |
| | 2 | 0.0516 | 0.0564 | 0.0464 | 0.0496 | 0.1012 | 0.1080 | 0.0944 | 0.0964 |
| | 3 | 0.0524 | 0.0556 | 0.0444 | 0.0468 | 0.1044 | 0.1088 | 0.0948 | 0.0956 |
| $N_2$ | 0.5 | 0.0540 | 0.0524 | 0.0504 | 0.0508 | 0.1072 | 0.1052 | 0.1004 | 0.1044 |
| | 1 | 0.0508 | 0.0504 | 0.0472 | 0.0492 | 0.1032 | 0.1028 | 0.0992 | 0.0984 |
| | 2 | 0.0488 | 0.0512 | 0.0484 | 0.0488 | 0.0996 | 0.0984 | 0.0924 | 0.0936 |
| | 3 | 0.0480 | 0.0480 | 0.0440 | 0.0456 | 0.0972 | 0.0960 | 0.0908 | 0.0908 |
| $N_3$ | 0.5 | 0.0492 | 0.0496 | 0.0500 | 0.0484 | 0.1016 | 0.1008 | 0.0992 | 0.1000 |
| | 1 | 0.0484 | 0.0476 | 0.0456 | 0.0472 | 0.1032 | 0.1028 | 0.1020 | 0.0996 |
| | 2 | 0.0492 | 0.0492 | 0.0472 | 0.0484 | 0.0976 | 0.0936 | 0.0900 | 0.0908 |
| | 3 | 0.0472 | 0.0484 | 0.0456 | 0.0460 | 0.0944 | 0.0944 | 0.0908 | 0.0920 |
| $N_4$ | 0.5 | 0.0520 | 0.0584 | 0.0528 | 0.0584 | 0.0988 | 0.1016 | 0.0980 | 0.1012 |
| | 1 | 0.0524 | 0.0504 | 0.0476 | 0.0500 | 0.0988 | 0.1008 | 0.0964 | 0.1000 |
| | 2 | 0.0492 | 0.0464 | 0.0428 | 0.0456 | 0.0984 | 0.0996 | 0.0960 | 0.0984 |
| | 3 | 0.0496 | 0.0468 | 0.0416 | 0.0448 | 0.0968 | 0.0980 | 0.0948 | 0.0972 |
| $N_5$ | 0.5 | 0.0472 | 0.0532 | 0.0512 | 0.0532 | 0.0932 | 0.0944 | 0.0912 | 0.0936 |
| | 1 | 0.0460 | 0.0476 | 0.0480 | 0.0476 | 0.0964 | 0.0956 | 0.0940 | 0.0952 |
| | 2 | 0.0440 | 0.0460 | 0.0428 | 0.0460 | 0.1016 | 0.0996 | 0.0956 | 0.0996 |
| | 3 | 0.0476 | 0.0492 | 0.0428 | 0.0480 | 0.1000 | 0.0984 | 0.0948 | 0.0984 |

Note: $N_1 = (3,3,3,3,5,5,5,5)$, $N_2 = (5,5,6,6,6,6,7,7)$, $N_3 = (7,7,7,8,8,8,9,9)$, $N_4 = (8,9,9,12,12,15,15,16)$, $N_5 = (11,12,13,14,16,17,18,19)$.

cases, but the EA method is better than the AP method in most cases. From Table 8.9, we can see that as $\frac{\sigma_\mu^2}{\sigma_v^2}$ deviates from the null hypothesis, the powers of both testing methods significantly increase, and the power of the EA method is better than that of the AP method in most cases.

**Remark 8.10.** *For hypothesis testing problems (8.11) and (8.28), this book also conducted simulation studies under nominal significance levels of 0.025 and 0.075, and the conclusions were consistent with the nominal significance levels of 0.05 and 0.1. However, due to space limitations, the simulation results are omitted here.*

## 8.7 Illustrative examples

Zhao (2008) provided annual observations of gasoline consumption for OECD countries from 1960 to 1964. For convenience, this section selects partial data from ten countries to verify the rationality and effectiveness of the testing methods given in this book. The histogram of the data is shown in Figure 8.1, which indicates that the data exhibits a skewed distribution characteristics. To verify this conclusion, a normality test is first conducted on the data. The results show

**Table 8.5:** Powers for hypothesis testing problem (8.11) ($s_1 = 1$, $\sigma_v^2 = 1$).

| Sample size | $\sigma_\mu^2$ | $\vartheta$ = 0.05 | | | | $\vartheta$ = 0.1 | | | |
|---|---|---|---|---|---|---|---|---|---|
| | | $BA_1$ | $BA_2$ | $GA_1$ | $GA_2$ | $BA_1$ | $BA_2$ | $GA_1$ | $GA_2$ |
| $N_1$ | 2 | 0.3440 | 0.3456 | 0.3168 | 0.3276 | 0.4556 | 0.4592 | 0.4404 | 0.4456 |
| | 4 | 0.7440 | 0.7324 | 0.7184 | 0.7244 | 0.8136 | 0.8148 | 0.8020 | 0.8048 |
| | 5 | 0.8332 | 0.8332 | 0.8232 | 0.8260 | 0.8816 | 0.8804 | 0.8692 | 0.8736 |
| | 6 | 0.8856 | 0.8840 | 0.8752 | 0.8796 | 0.9280 | 0.9224 | 0.9196 | 0.9180 |
| $N_2$ | 2 | 0.3792 | 0.3824 | 0.3744 | 0.3760 | 0.4876 | 0.4860 | 0.4784 | 0.4792 |
| | 4 | 0.7744 | 0.7732 | 0.7684 | 0.7712 | 0.8428 | 0.8400 | 0.8348 | 0.8368 |
| | 5 | 0.8592 | 0.8592 | 0.8540 | 0.8548 | 0.9076 | 0.9044 | 0.9032 | 0.9028 |
| | 6 | 0.9108 | 0.9092 | 0.9060 | 0.9072 | 0.9356 | 0.9364 | 0.9332 | 0.9356 |
| $N_3$ | 2 | 0.3904 | 0.3856 | 0.3784 | 0.3824 | 0.5044 | 0.5072 | 0.5028 | 0.5044 |
| | 4 | 0.8032 | 0.7992 | 0.7980 | 0.7964 | 0.8648 | 0.8628 | 0.8616 | 0.8624 |
| | 5 | 0.8800 | 0.8748 | 0.8756 | 0.8740 | 0.9140 | 0.9116 | 0.9104 | 0.9108 |
| | 6 | 0.9184 | 0.9156 | 0.9152 | 0.9152 | 0.9428 | 0.9452 | 0.9428 | 0.9444 |
| $N_4$ | 2 | 0.3876 | 0.3800 | 0.3656 | 0.3792 | 0.5004 | 0.4980 | 0.4880 | 0.4972 |
| | 4 | 0.7968 | 0.7924 | 0.7860 | 0.7912 | 0.8628 | 0.8520 | 0.8524 | 0.8520 |
| | 5 | 0.8784 | 0.8748 | 0.8664 | 0.8744 | 0.9260 | 0.9208 | 0.9192 | 0.9208 |
| | 6 | 0.9260 | 0.9240 | 0.9188 | 0.9236 | 0.9560 | 0.9504 | 0.9492 | 0.9504 |
| $N_5$ | 2 | 0.3712 | 0.3708 | 0.3648 | 0.3688 | 0.4936 | 0.4812 | 0.4768 | 0.4800 |
| | 4 | 0.8072 | 0.8044 | 0.7984 | 0.8040 | 0.8660 | 0.8616 | 0.8604 | 0.8616 |
| | 5 | 0.8864 | 0.8832 | 0.8824 | 0.8828 | 0.9284 | 0.9244 | 0.9232 | 0.9244 |
| | 6 | 0.9316 | 0.9312 | 0.9280 | 0.9312 | 0.9548 | 0.9536 | 0.9536 | 0.9536 |

Note: $N_1 = (3,3,3,3,5,5,5,5)$, $N_2 = (5,5,6,6,6,6,7,7)$, $N_3 = (7,7,7,8,8,8,9,9)$, $N_4 = (8,9,9,12,12,15,15,16)$, $N_5 = (11,12,13,14,16,17,18,19)$.

that the *p*-values of the Shapiro-Wilk test, Anderson-Darling test, and Cramer-von Mises test are 0.0014, 0.0009, and 0.0019, respectively. Therefore, at the nominal significance level 5%, the annual observations of gasoline consumption do not follow a normal distribution. Furthermore, to verify the skew-normality of the data, a chi-square goodness-of-fit test is performed, that is, assuming $H_0$: the annual observations of gasoline consumption follow a skew-normal distribution. The calculated test statistic $\chi^2 = 1.7582 < \chi_1^2(0.95) = 3.8415$, and the *p*-value is 0.1848. Therefore, at the nominal significance level of 5%, the null hypothesis $H_0$ cannot be rejected, indicating that the annual observations of gasoline consumption follow a skew-normal distribution. Based on the method of moment estimation, the distribution of the data can be obtained as $SN\left(3.8200, 0.4759^2, 4.3590\right)$, and its density curve is shown in Figure 8.1.

Consider the following gasoline demand equation

$$ln\frac{Gas}{Car} = \alpha + \beta_1 ln\frac{Y}{N} + \beta_2 ln\frac{P_{MG}}{P_{GDP}} + \beta_3 ln\frac{Car}{N} + Z_\mu \mu + v, \qquad (8.49)$$

where $\frac{Gas}{Car}$, $\frac{Y}{N}$, $\frac{P_{MG}}{P_{GDP}}$, and $\frac{Car}{N}$ represent the gasoline consumption per car, real per capita income, real gasoline price, and per capita car ownership, respectively.

**Table 8.6:** Sizes for hypothesis testing problem (8.28) ($s_2 = \sigma_\mu^2 + \sigma_\nu^2 = 5$).

| | | $\vartheta$ | | | | | | | |
| | | 0.05 | | | | 0.1 | | | |
| Sample size | $\sigma_\mu^2$ | $BA_1$ | $BA_2$ | $GA_1$ | $GA_2$ | $BA_1$ | $BA_2$ | $GA_1$ | $GA_2$ |
|---|---|---|---|---|---|---|---|---|---|
| $N_1$ | 0.5 | 0.0484 | 0.0516 | 0.0496 | 0.0540 | 0.1060 | 0.1064 | 0.1072 | 0.1124 |
| | 1 | 0.0456 | 0.0500 | 0.0548 | 0.0556 | 0.1064 | 0.1052 | 0.1128 | 0.1164 |
| | 1.5 | 0.0464 | 0.0496 | 0.0544 | 0.0592 | 0.1028 | 0.1024 | 0.1160 | 0.1196 |
| | 2 | 0.0368 | 0.0424 | 0.0592 | 0.0616 | 0.0956 | 0.0968 | 0.1196 | 0.1236 |
| $N_2$ | 0.5 | 0.0548 | 0.0548 | 0.0580 | 0.0568 | 0.1088 | 0.1112 | 0.1116 | 0.1136 |
| | 1 | 0.0552 | 0.0548 | 0.0576 | 0.0588 | 0.1068 | 0.1040 | 0.1084 | 0.1092 |
| | 1.5 | 0.0508 | 0.0508 | 0.0580 | 0.0588 | 0.1032 | 0.1024 | 0.1148 | 0.1160 |
| | 2 | 0.0480 | 0.0456 | 0.0600 | 0.0612 | 0.0996 | 0.1020 | 0.1220 | 0.1204 |
| $N_3$ | 0.5 | 0.0512 | 0.0500 | 0.0492 | 0.0508 | 0.1000 | 0.1032 | 0.1036 | 0.1068 |
| | 1 | 0.0524 | 0.0540 | 0.0552 | 0.0564 | 0.0996 | 0.0964 | 0.0992 | 0.0988 |
| | 1.5 | 0.0508 | 0.0504 | 0.0548 | 0.0556 | 0.1028 | 0.1008 | 0.1088 | 0.1088 |
| | 2 | 0.0484 | 0.0448 | 0.0552 | 0.0552 | 0.0952 | 0.1016 | 0.1136 | 0.1132 |
| $N_4$ | 0.5 | 0.0516 | 0.0532 | 0.0484 | 0.0540 | 0.0972 | 0.1028 | 0.1012 | 0.1032 |
| | 1 | 0.0536 | 0.0564 | 0.0520 | 0.0580 | 0.0976 | 0.1040 | 0.1040 | 0.1060 |
| | 1.5 | 0.0516 | 0.0544 | 0.0544 | 0.0572 | 0.0980 | 0.1044 | 0.1056 | 0.1080 |
| | 2 | 0.0504 | 0.0544 | 0.0560 | 0.0596 | 0.1012 | 0.1024 | 0.1088 | 0.1088 |
| $N_5$ | 0.5 | 0.0476 | 0.0472 | 0.0460 | 0.0476 | 0.0928 | 0.0968 | 0.0940 | 0.0976 |
| | 1 | 0.0476 | 0.0484 | 0.0460 | 0.0488 | 0.0952 | 0.0972 | 0.0980 | 0.0992 |
| | 1.5 | 0.0480 | 0.0484 | 0.0504 | 0.0528 | 0.0968 | 0.0948 | 0.0972 | 0.1008 |
| | 2 | 0.0480 | 0.0488 | 0.0536 | 0.0540 | 0.0956 | 0.0952 | 0.1000 | 0.1024 |

Note: $N_1 = (3,3,3,3,5,5,5,5)$, $N_2 = (5,5,6,6,6,6,7,7)$, $N_3 = (7,7,7,8,8,8,9,9)$, $N_4 = (8,9,9,12,12,15,15,16)$, $N_5 = (11,12,13,14,16,17,18,19)$.

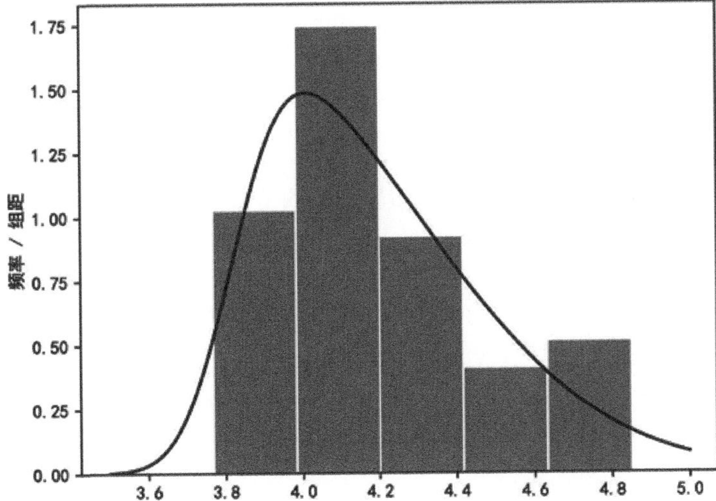


**Figure 8.1:** Histogram of annual observations of gasoline consumption with superimposed skew-normal density curve.

**Table 8.7:** Powers for hypothesis testing problem (8.28) ($s_2 = 5$, $\sigma_v^2 = 1$).

| | | $\vartheta$ | | | | | | | |
| --- | --- | --- | --- | --- | --- | --- | --- | --- | --- |
| | | 0.05 | | | | 0.1 | | | |
| Sample size | $\sigma_\mu^2$ | $BA_1$ | $BA_2$ | $GA_1$ | $GA_2$ | $BA_1$ | $BA_2$ | $GA_1$ | $GA_2$ |
| $N_1$ | 5 | 0.1332 | 0.1252 | 0.1272 | 0.1320 | 0.1996 | 0.2028 | 0.2108 | 0.2148 |
| | 10 | 0.5656 | 0.5592 | 0.5624 | 0.5708 | 0.6584 | 0.6524 | 0.6572 | 0.6608 |
| | 20 | 0.8836 | 0.8792 | 0.8788 | 0.8836 | 0.9248 | 0.9176 | 0.9212 | 0.9228 |
| | 25 | 0.9392 | 0.9324 | 0.9308 | 0.9348 | 0.9596 | 0.9544 | 0.9548 | 0.9572 |
| $N_2$ | 5 | 0.1324 | 0.1264 | 0.1316 | 0.1344 | 0.2140 | 0.2148 | 0.2216 | 0.2200 |
| | 10 | 0.5580 | 0.5580 | 0.5660 | 0.5648 | 0.6564 | 0.6544 | 0.6632 | 0.6620 |
| | 20 | 0.8904 | 0.8880 | 0.8888 | 0.8904 | 0.9244 | 0.9260 | 0.9276 | 0.9280 |
| | 25 | 0.9336 | 0.9340 | 0.9352 | 0.9372 | 0.9592 | 0.9576 | 0.9576 | 0.9588 |
| $N_3$ | 5 | 0.1292 | 0.1232 | 0.1252 | 0.1312 | 0.2124 | 0.2080 | 0.2120 | 0.2140 |
| | 10 | 0.5684 | 0.5704 | 0.5760 | 0.5784 | 0.6724 | 0.6696 | 0.6736 | 0.6760 |
| | 20 | 0.9028 | 0.9000 | 0.9020 | 0.9016 | 0.9300 | 0.9276 | 0.9296 | 0.9296 |
| | 25 | 0.9392 | 0.9376 | 0.9388 | 0.9396 | 0.9568 | 0.9560 | 0.9564 | 0.9576 |
| $N_4$ | 5 | 0.1252 | 0.1272 | 0.1216 | 0.1284 | 0.2132 | 0.2100 | 0.2092 | 0.2160 |
| | 10 | 0.5656 | 0.5616 | 0.5576 | 0.5692 | 0.6708 | 0.6660 | 0.6700 | 0.6716 |
| | 20 | 0.8912 | 0.8852 | 0.8828 | 0.8872 | 0.9284 | 0.9236 | 0.9220 | 0.9244 |
| | 25 | 0.9384 | 0.9356 | 0.9328 | 0.9360 | 0.9620 | 0.9616 | 0.9628 | 0.9624 |
| $N_5$ | 5 | 0.1148 | 0.1224 | 0.1200 | 0.1236 | 0.1996 | 0.1952 | 0.1944 | 0.1980 |
| | 10 | 0.5476 | 0.5468 | 0.5452 | 0.5500 | 0.6584 | 0.6556 | 0.6556 | 0.6612 |
| | 20 | 0.9056 | 0.8988 | 0.8988 | 0.9016 | 0.9324 | 0.9312 | 0.9296 | 0.9320 |
| | 25 | 0.9436 | 0.9416 | 0.9404 | 0.9424 | 0.9600 | 0.9580 | 0.9584 | 0.9580 |

Note: $N_1 = (3,3,3,3,5,5,5,5)$, $N_2 = (5,5,6,6,6,6,7,7)$, $N_3 = (7,7,7,8,8,8,9,9)$, $N_4 = (8,9,9,12,12,15,15,16)$, $N_5 = (11,12,13,14,16,17,18,19)$.

$Z_\mu = diag\{1_{T_1}, 1_{T_2}, \cdots, 1_{T_{10}}\}$, $\mu \sim SN_{10}(0, \sigma_\mu^2 I_{10}, \lambda_1)$, $v \sim N_{45}(0, \sigma_v^2 I_{45})$, $\mu$ and $v$ are mutually independent. When $i = 1, \cdots, 5$, $T_i = 4$. Otherwise, $T_i = 5$.

First, by Theorem 8.2, the maximum likelihood estimate of $\beta = (\beta_1, \beta_2, \beta_3)'$ is given as $\hat{\beta} = (-0.1651, -0.0710, -0.2697)'$. Table 8.10 presents the null hypotheses and p-values for the exact tests of regression coefficients. According to Table 8.10, at the nominal significance level of 5%, the exact test method rejects the null hypotheses of $\beta_3 = 0$ and $\beta_3 \leq -0.5$.

Second, consider the hypothesis testing problem for a single variance component

$$H_0 : \sigma_\mu^2 \leq 0.03 \quad versus \quad H_1 : \sigma_\mu^2 > 0.03. \tag{8.50}$$

From Equations (8.14), (8.16), (8.21) and (8.25), the $p$-values of the $BA_1$, $BA_2$, $GA_1$, and $GA_2$ methods are 0.0004, 0.0196, 0.0300, and 0.0200, respectively. Therefore, at the nominal significance level of 5%, all four methods reject the null hypothesis $H_0$ in (8.50).

**Table 8.8:** Sizes for hypothesis testing problem (8.43) ($s_3 = \frac{\sigma_\mu^2}{\sigma_v^2}$, $\sigma_v^2 = 1$).

| | | $\vartheta$ | | | | | | | |
| | | 0.025 | | 0.05 | | 0.075 | | 0.1 | |
| Sample size | $\sigma_\mu^2$ | EA | AP | EA | AP | EA | AP | EA | AP |
|---|---|---|---|---|---|---|---|---|---|
| $N_1$ | 0.5 | 0.0264 | 0.0272 | 0.0520 | 0.0548 | 0.0832 | 0.0860 | 0.1092 | 0.1108 |
| | 1 | 0.0268 | 0.0288 | 0.0508 | 0.0564 | 0.0844 | 0.0848 | 0.1128 | 0.1116 |
| | 2 | 0.0292 | 0.0292 | 0.0496 | 0.0544 | 0.0784 | 0.0824 | 0.1096 | 0.1116 |
| | 3 | 0.0280 | 0.0296 | 0.0520 | 0.0536 | 0.0780 | 0.0816 | 0.1064 | 0.1060 |
| $N_2$ | 0.5 | 0.0252 | 0.0236 | 0.0476 | 0.0456 | 0.0728 | 0.0740 | 0.1016 | 0.1036 |
| | 1 | 0.0228 | 0.0252 | 0.0492 | 0.0476 | 0.0784 | 0.0780 | 0.1028 | 0.1016 |
| | 2 | 0.0268 | 0.0280 | 0.0508 | 0.0496 | 0.0812 | 0.0792 | 0.1028 | 0.1012 |
| | 3 | 0.0268 | 0.0260 | 0.0512 | 0.0532 | 0.0820 | 0.0780 | 0.1048 | 0.1048 |
| $N_3$ | 0.5 | 0.0256 | 0.0244 | 0.0484 | 0.0496 | 0.0740 | 0.0752 | 0.0988 | 0.1000 |
| | 1 | 0.0248 | 0.0248 | 0.0452 | 0.0480 | 0.0720 | 0.0720 | 0.0984 | 0.0976 |
| | 2 | 0.0248 | 0.0252 | 0.0440 | 0.0456 | 0.0696 | 0.0696 | 0.1036 | 0.1016 |
| | 3 | 0.0244 | 0.0244 | 0.0460 | 0.0444 | 0.0704 | 0.0720 | 0.1016 | 0.0984 |
| $N_4$ | 0.5 | 0.0252 | 0.0264 | 0.0504 | 0.0496 | 0.0764 | 0.0792 | 0.1008 | 0.0980 |
| | 1 | 0.0236 | 0.0280 | 0.0512 | 0.0528 | 0.0780 | 0.0776 | 0.1048 | 0.1024 |
| | 2 | 0.0212 | 0.0280 | 0.0488 | 0.0540 | 0.0768 | 0.0776 | 0.1036 | 0.1020 |
| | 3 | 0.0224 | 0.0280 | 0.0476 | 0.0512 | 0.0736 | 0.0768 | 0.1008 | 0.1012 |
| $N_5$ | 0.5 | 0.0248 | 0.0264 | 0.0496 | 0.0476 | 0.0744 | 0.0740 | 0.0916 | 0.0940 |
| | 1 | 0.0248 | 0.0280 | 0.0476 | 0.0464 | 0.0672 | 0.0692 | 0.0948 | 0.0924 |
| | 2 | 0.0236 | 0.0272 | 0.0472 | 0.0476 | 0.0680 | 0.0696 | 0.0904 | 0.0916 |
| | 3 | 0.0232 | 0.0244 | 0.0456 | 0.0492 | 0.0680 | 0.0704 | 0.0904 | 0.0912 |

Note: $N_1 = (3,3,3,3,5,5,5,5)$, $N_2 = (5,5,6,6,6,6,7,7)$, $N_3 = (7,7,7,8,8,8,9,9)$, $N_4 = (8,9,9,12,12,15,15,16)$, $N_5 = (11,12,13,14,16,17,18,19)$.

Third, consider the hypothesis testing problem for the sum of variance components

$$H_0 : \sigma_\mu^2 + \sigma_v^2 \leq 0.1 \quad versus \quad H_1 : \sigma_\mu^2 + \sigma_v^2 > 0.1. \tag{8.51}$$

From Equations (8.31), (8.33), (8.37), and (8.40), the $p$-values of the $BA_1$, $BA_2$, $GA_1$, and $GA_2$ methods are 0.1828, 0.7016, 0.6340, and 0.6996, respectively. Therefore, at the nominal significance level of 5%, all four methods fail to reject the null hypothesis $H_0$ in (8.51).

Finally, consider the hypothesis testing problem for the ratio of variance components

$$H_0 : \frac{\sigma_\mu^2}{\sigma_v^2} \leq 8 \quad versus \quad H_1 : \frac{\sigma_\mu^2}{\sigma_v^2} > 8. \tag{8.52}$$

**Table 8.9:** Powers for hypothesis testing problem (8.43) ($s_3 = 1$, $\sigma_v^2 = 1$).

| Sample size | $\sigma_\mu^2$ | $\vartheta$ | | | | | | | |
| --- | --- | --- | --- | --- | --- | --- | --- | --- | --- |
| | | 0.025 | | 0.05 | | 0.075 | | 0.1 | |
| | | EA | AP | EA | AP | EA | AP | EA | AP |
| $N_1$ | 2 | 0.1792 | 0.1792 | 0.2576 | 0.2648 | 0.3264 | 0.3312 | 0.3844 | 0.3780 |
| | 4 | 0.5324 | 0.5288 | 0.6312 | 0.6320 | 0.6948 | 0.6888 | 0.7376 | 0.7312 |
| | 6 | 0.7376 | 0.7332 | 0.8136 | 0.8104 | 0.8524 | 0.8496 | 0.8792 | 0.8748 |
| | 8 | 0.8468 | 0.8436 | 0.8976 | 0.8956 | 0.9268 | 0.9212 | 0.9408 | 0.9396 |
| $N_2$ | 2 | 0.2236 | 0.2256 | 0.3184 | 0.3228 | 0.3856 | 0.3856 | 0.4376 | 0.4364 |
| | 4 | 0.6288 | 0.6220 | 0.7060 | 0.7060 | 0.7568 | 0.7580 | 0.7972 | 0.7928 |
| | 6 | 0.8196 | 0.8188 | 0.8696 | 0.8684 | 0.8964 | 0.8964 | 0.9132 | 0.9132 |
| | 8 | 0.9012 | 0.9032 | 0.9348 | 0.9320 | 0.9484 | 0.9496 | 0.9604 | 0.9596 |
| $N_3$ | 2 | 0.2520 | 0.2516 | 0.3400 | 0.3408 | 0.4092 | 0.4068 | 0.4648 | 0.4692 |
| | 4 | 0.6848 | 0.6852 | 0.7676 | 0.7640 | 0.8096 | 0.8076 | 0.8376 | 0.8376 |
| | 6 | 0.8572 | 0.8584 | 0.8980 | 0.8980 | 0.9168 | 0.9144 | 0.9316 | 0.9268 |
| | 8 | 0.9236 | 0.9200 | 0.9480 | 0.9468 | 0.9580 | 0.9564 | 0.9640 | 0.9668 |
| $N_4$ | 2 | 0.2588 | 0.2712 | 0.3624 | 0.3592 | 0.4296 | 0.4224 | 0.4800 | 0.4724 |
| | 4 | 0.7088 | 0.7000 | 0.7720 | 0.7756 | 0.8148 | 0.8100 | 0.8428 | 0.8404 |
| | 6 | 0.8760 | 0.8672 | 0.9100 | 0.9048 | 0.9324 | 0.9276 | 0.9444 | 0.9440 |
| | 8 | 0.9360 | 0.9332 | 0.9616 | 0.9564 | 0.9696 | 0.9668 | 0.9760 | 0.9736 |
| $N_5$ | 2 | 0.2672 | 0.2644 | 0.3580 | 0.3576 | 0.4184 | 0.4120 | 0.4716 | 0.4636 |
| | 4 | 0.7160 | 0.7160 | 0.7852 | 0.7844 | 0.8256 | 0.8224 | 0.8536 | 0.8480 |
| | 6 | 0.8820 | 0.8780 | 0.9188 | 0.9176 | 0.9364 | 0.9352 | 0.9476 | 0.9472 |
| | 8 | 0.9448 | 0.9444 | 0.9640 | 0.9620 | 0.9708 | 0.9712 | 0.9764 | 0.9760 |

Note: $N_1 = (3,3,3,3,5,5,5,5)$, $N_2 = (5,5,6,6,6,6,7,7)$, $N_3 = (7,7,7,8,8,8,9,9)$, $N_4 = (8,9,9,12,12,15,15,16)$, $N_5 = (11,12,13,14,16,17,18,19)$.

**Table 8.10:** $p$-values of exact test for regression coefficients.
8pt

| | The null hypothesis | | | | |
| --- | --- | --- | --- | --- | --- |
| | $\beta_1 = 0$ | $\beta_2 = 0$ | $\beta_3 = 0$ | $\beta_3 \leq -0.2$ | $\beta_3 \leq -0.5$ |
| $p$-value | 0.2690 | 0.8030 | 0.0088 | 0.7619 | 0.0116 |

From Equations (8.45) and (8.47), the $p$-values of the exact test and approximate test are 0.0002 and 0.0093, respectively. Therefore, at the nominal significance level of 5%, both methods reject the null hypothesis $H_0$ in (8.52).

# Chapter 9

# Skew-Normal Two-Way Classification Random Effects Model with Interaction

In this chapter, we consider the statistical inference problems for the fixed effect and variance component functions in the two-way classification random effects model with skew-normal errors. Firstly, the exact test statistic for the fixed effect is constructed. Secondly, using the Bootstrap approach and generalized approach, the one-sided hypothesis testing and interval estimation problems for the single variance component, the sum and ratio of variance components are discussed respectively. Further, the Monte Carlo simulation results indicate that the exact test statistic performs well in the one-sided hypothesis testing problem for the fixed effect. Additionally, the Bootstrap approach is better than the generalized approach in the one-sided hypothesis testing problems for variance component functions in most cases. Finally, the above approaches are applied to the real data examples of the consumer price index and value-added index of three industries to verify their rationality and effectiveness.

## 9.1 Model properties

Let $M_{n \times n}$ be the set of all $n \times n$ matrices over the real field $\Re$, and use $A'$, $tr(A)$ and $rk(A)$ to denote the transpose, trace and rank of matrix $A$ respectively. Besides, $P_A = A(A'A)^- A'$ and $\bar{J}_n = 1_n 1_n'/n$.

Firstly, we consider the two-way classification random effects model with skew-normal errors

$$y = 1_n \mu + Z_\alpha \alpha + Z_\beta \beta + Z_\gamma \gamma + \varepsilon, \tag{9.1}$$

where $y$ is a $n \times 1$ random vector, $\mu$ is the fixed effect, $\alpha$, $\beta$ and $\gamma$ are the random effects, $\varepsilon$ is a $n \times 1$ vector of random errors, $n = abc$, $Z_\alpha = I_a \otimes 1_b \otimes 1_c$, $Z_\beta = 1_a \otimes I_b \otimes 1_c$, and $Z_\gamma = I_a \otimes I_b \otimes 1_c$. Besides, $1_m$ is a $m \times 1$ vector with every element unity, $I_m$ is an identity matrix of order $m$, and $\otimes$ denotes the Kronecker product. Assume that $\alpha \sim N_a(0, \sigma_\alpha^2 I_a)$, $\beta \sim N_b(0, \sigma_\beta^2 I_b)$, $\gamma \sim N_{ab}(0, \sigma_\gamma^2 I_{ab})$, $\varepsilon \sim SN_n(0, \sigma_{\varepsilon^2} I_n, \alpha_\varepsilon)$, and all random vectors are mutually independent, where $SN_m(\mu_0, \Sigma_0, \alpha_0)$ denotes the $m$-dimensional skew-normal distribution with location parameter $\mu_0$, positive definite scale parameter $\Sigma_0$, and skewness parameter $\alpha_0$. In particular, when $\alpha_\varepsilon = 0$, model (9.1) is reduced to the normal two-way classification random effects model (Karlsson and Skoglund, 2004; Fan and Wang, 2007; Gilder et al., 2007).

Based on Ye et al. (2015), Theorem 9.1 is given as follows.

**Theorem 9.1.** *For model (9.1), let* $Q = y'Ay/\sigma_*^2$ *with non-negative definite* $A \in M_{n \times n}$, $k = rk(A)$, *and* $\sigma_*^2 = \frac{1}{k}[\sigma_\varepsilon^2 tr(A) + \sigma_\alpha^2 tr(AZ_\alpha Z_\alpha') + \sigma_\beta^2 tr(AZ_\beta Z_\beta') + \sigma_\gamma^2 tr(AZ_\gamma Z_\gamma')]$. *Then the necessary and sufficient conditions under which* $Q \sim S\chi_k^2(\lambda, \delta_1, \delta_2)$, *for some* $\delta_1 \in \Re$ *including* $\delta_1 = 0$, *are*

*(i)* $\Omega A$ *is idempotent of rank $k$,*

*(ii)* $\lambda = \mu_y' A \mu_y / \sigma_*^2$,

*(iii)* $\delta_1 = \alpha_1' \Omega^{1/2} A \mu_y / (d\sigma_*)$, *and*

*(iv)* $\delta_2 = \alpha_1' P_1 P_1' \alpha_1 / d^2$,
*where* $\mu_y = 1_n \mu$, $\Sigma_y = \sigma_\alpha^2 Z_\alpha Z_\alpha' + \sigma_\beta^2 Z_\beta Z_\beta' + \sigma_\gamma^2 Z_\gamma Z_\gamma' + \sigma_\varepsilon^2 I_n = \sigma_*^2 \Omega$,
$d = (1 + \alpha_1' P_2 P_2' \alpha_1)^{1/2}$, $\alpha_1 = \dfrac{\sigma_\varepsilon \Sigma_y^{-1/2} \alpha_\varepsilon}{[1 + \alpha_\varepsilon'(I_n - \sigma_\varepsilon^2 \Sigma_y^{-1})\alpha_\varepsilon]^{1/2}}$, *and* $P = (P_1, P_2)$ *is an orthogonal matrix in* $M_{n \times n}$ *such that*

$$\Omega^{1/2} A \Omega^{1/2} = P \begin{pmatrix} I_k & 0 \\ 0 & 0 \end{pmatrix} P' = P_1 P_1'.$$

**Theorem 9.2.** *For model (9.1), let* $A_1 = (I_a - \bar{J}_a) \otimes \bar{J}_b \otimes \bar{J}_c$, $A_2 = \bar{J}_a \otimes (I_b - \bar{J}_b) \otimes \bar{J}_c$, $A_3 = (I_a - \bar{J}_a) \otimes (I_b - \bar{J}_b) \otimes \bar{J}_c$, $A_4 = I_a \otimes I_b \otimes (I_c - \bar{J}_c)$. *Then we have*

$$V_i = \frac{T_i}{\sigma_i^2} \sim \chi_{n_i}^2, i = 1, \cdots, 4, \tag{9.2}$$

*and* $V_i(i = 1, \cdots, 4)$ *are mutually independent, where* $T_i = y'A_i y$, $\sigma_1^2 = bc\sigma_\alpha^2 + c\sigma_\gamma^2 + \sigma_\varepsilon^2$, $\sigma_2^2 = ac\sigma_\beta^2 + c\sigma_\gamma^2 + \sigma_\varepsilon^2$, $\sigma_3^2 = c\sigma_\gamma^2 + \sigma_\varepsilon^2$, $\sigma_4^2 = \sigma_\varepsilon^2$, $n_1 = a - 1$, $n_2 = b - 1$, $n_3 = (a-1)(b-1)$, *and* $n_4 = ab(c-1)$.

*Proof.* For model (9.1), the scale parameter matrix of $y$ is

$$\Sigma_y = \sigma_\alpha^2 Z_\alpha Z'_\alpha + \sigma_\beta^2 Z_\beta Z'_\beta + \sigma_\gamma^2 Z_\gamma Z'_\gamma + \sigma_\varepsilon^2 I_n$$
$$= \sigma_\alpha^2 (I_a \otimes J_b \otimes J_c) + \sigma_\beta^2 (J_a \otimes I_b \otimes J_c) + \sigma_\gamma^2 (I_a \otimes I_b \otimes J_c) + \sigma_\varepsilon^2 I_n.$$

It can be concluded that $\Sigma_y$ is as follows after spectral decomposition

$$\Sigma_y = \sum_{i=1}^{4} \sigma_i^2 A_i + \sigma_0^2 \bar{J}_n,$$

where $\sigma_0^2 = bc\sigma_\alpha^2 + ac\sigma_\beta^2 + c\sigma_\gamma^2 + \sigma_\varepsilon^2$, $\sigma_1^2 = bc\sigma_\alpha^2 + c\sigma_\gamma^2 + \sigma_\varepsilon^2$, $\sigma_2^2 = ac\sigma_\beta^2 + c\sigma_\gamma^2 + \sigma_\varepsilon^2$, $\sigma_3^2 = c\sigma_\gamma^2 + \sigma_\varepsilon^2$, and $\sigma_4^2 = \sigma_\varepsilon^2$. Accordingly, $A_1 = (I_a - \bar{J}_a) \otimes \bar{J}_b \otimes \bar{J}_c$, $A_2 = \bar{J}_a \otimes (I_b - \bar{J}_b) \otimes \bar{J}_c$, $A_3 = (I_a - \bar{J}_a) \otimes (I_b - \bar{J}_b) \otimes \bar{J}_c$, and $A_4 = I_a \otimes I_b \otimes (I_c - \bar{J}_c)$.

For Theorem 9.2, it suffices to show that $\lambda_i = 0$, $A_i \Omega_i A_i = A_i$, and $T_i(i = 1, \cdots, 4)$ are mutually independent based on Theorem 9.1, where $\Omega_i = \sigma_i^{-2} \Sigma_y$, $i = 1, \cdots, 4$. By Theorem 9.1, we have

$$\lambda_1 = \mu'_y A_1 \mu_y / \sigma_1^2 = \mu' 1'_n A_1 1_n \mu / \sigma_1^2 = 0.$$

Further, we obtain

$$A_1 \Omega_1 A_1 = A_1 \left[ \sigma_\alpha^2 bc(I_a \otimes \bar{J}_b \otimes \bar{J}_c) + \sigma_\beta^2 ac(\bar{J}_a \otimes I_b \otimes \bar{J}_c) + \sigma_\gamma^2 c(I_a \otimes I_b \otimes \bar{J}_c) + \sigma_\varepsilon^2 I_n \right] A_1 / \sigma_1^2$$
$$= \frac{bc\sigma_\alpha^2 + c\sigma_\gamma^2 + \sigma_\varepsilon^2}{\sigma_1^2} A_1 = A_1.$$

In the same way, $\lambda_i = 0$ and $A_i \Omega_i A_i = A_i$ are also available for $i = 2, 3, 4$.

Since

$$A_1 \Sigma_y A_2 = A_1 (\sigma_\alpha^2 Z_\alpha Z'_\alpha + \sigma_\beta^2 Z_\beta Z'_\beta + \sigma_\gamma^2 Z_\gamma Z'_\gamma + \sigma_\varepsilon^2 I_n) A_2 = 0,$$

$T_1$ and $T_2$ are mutually independent by Proposition 2.2 in Ye et al. (2015), namely $V_1$ and $V_2$ are mutually independent. Similarly, $V_i$ $(i = 1, \cdots, 4)$ are mutually independent, so the results in Theorem 9.2 are obtained. $\qquad\square$

## 9.2 Inference on the fixed effect

In this section, the one-sided hypothesis testing problem for the fixed effect in model (9.1) is considered. The hypothesis of interest is

$$H_0 : \mu \leq \mu_0 \quad versus \quad H_1{:}\mu > \mu_0, \tag{9.3}$$

where $\mu_0$ is a specified value. Without loss of generality, we assume $\mu_0 = 0$, then the hypothesis testing problem (9.3) is transformed to

$$H_0 : \mu \leq 0 \quad versus \quad H_1{:}\mu > 0. \tag{9.4}$$

By Theorem 9.1, we have

$$V_0 = y' P_{Z_\gamma} y / \sigma_*^2 \sim S\chi_{n_0}^2(\lambda, \delta_1, \delta_2),$$

where $P_{Z_\gamma} = I_a \otimes I_b \otimes \bar{J}_c$, $\sigma_*^2 = c\sigma_\alpha^2 + c\sigma_\beta^2 + c\sigma_\gamma^2 + \sigma_\varepsilon^2$, $n_0 = ab$, $\lambda = \mu_y' P_{Z_\gamma} \mu_y / \sigma_*^2$, $\mu_y = 1_n \mu$, $\delta_1 = \alpha_1' \Omega^{1/2} P_{Z_\gamma} \mu_y / (d\sigma_*)$, $\delta_2 = \alpha_1' P_1 P_1' \alpha_1 / d^2$, and $\Omega$, $d$, $\alpha_1$ and $P_1$ are given in Theorem 9.1. By Theorem 9.2, we have

$$V_4 = y' A_4 y / \sigma_4^2 \sim \chi_{n_4}^2.$$

Furthermore, by Proposition 2.2 in Ye et al. (2015), it is easy to infer that $V_0$ and $V_4$ are mutually independent. Based on Definition 10.2, the exact test statistic is constructed as

$$F = \frac{(c-1)y' P_{Z_\gamma} y / \sigma_*^2}{y' A_4 y / \sigma_4^2} \sim SF_{n_0,n_4}(\lambda, \delta_1, \delta_2). \tag{9.5}$$

Under the null hypothesis $H_0$ in (9.4), we obtain

$$F \sim F_{n_0,n_4}, \tag{9.6}$$

where $F_{n_0,n_4}$ represents the $F$ distribution with degrees of freedom $n_0$ and $n_4$. By $F$ in (9.6), the p-value is computed as

$$p = P(F > F_{n_0,n_4}(\delta)|H_0), \tag{9.7}$$

where $\delta$ is the nominal significance level and $F_{n_0,n_4}(\delta)$ is the $100\delta$ empirical percentile of $F_{n_0,n_4}$. The null hypothesis is rejected whenever the above p-value is less than the nominal significance level of $\delta$.

## 9.3 Inference on the single variance component

Using the Bootstrap approach and generalized approach, the hypothesis testing problems for the single variance component in model (9.1) are discussed. The hypotheses of interest are

$$H_0 : \sigma_\alpha^2 \leq c_0 \quad versus \quad H_1{:}\sigma_\alpha^2 > c_0, \tag{9.8}$$

$$H_0 : \sigma_\beta^2 \leq c_0 \ \text{versus} \ H_1{:}\sigma_\beta^2 > c_0, \tag{9.9}$$

$$H_0 : \sigma_\gamma^2 \leq c_0 \ \text{versus} \ H_1{:}\sigma_\gamma^2 > c_0, \tag{9.10}$$

where $c_0$ is a specified value.

### 9.3.1 Bootstrap approach

Firstly, the unbiased estimator of $\sigma_i^2$ is given by (9.2) as follows.

$$\hat{\sigma}_i^2 = \frac{T_i}{n_i}, i = 1, \cdots, 4. \tag{9.11}$$

If $\sigma_3^2$ is known, then $V_1$ in (9.2) will be the test statistic for hypothesis testing problem (9.8). However, $\sigma_3^2$ is often unknown in practical applications. Under the null hypothesis $H_0$ in (9.8), by replacing the parameter $\sigma_3^2$ with its estimator $\hat{\sigma}_3^2$ in $V_1$, the corresponding test statistic is given by

$$F_1 = \frac{T_1}{bcc_0 + T_3/n_3}. \tag{9.12}$$

Obviously, it is difficult to obtain the exact distribution of $F_1$, so the Bootstrap approach is used to construct the test statistic. Thus, the Bootstrap test statistic based on (9.12) is expressed as

$$F_{1B} = \frac{T_{1B}}{bcc_0 + T_{3B}/n_3}, \tag{9.13}$$

where $T_{1B} \sim (bcc_0 + t_3/n_3)\chi_{n_1}^2$, $T_{3B} \sim (t_3/n_3)\chi_{n_3}^2$, and $t_3$ is the observed value of $T_3$. By $F_{1B}$ in (9.13), the Bootstrap p-value is computed as

$$p_1 = P(F_{1B} > f_1|H_0), \tag{9.14}$$

where $f_1$ denotes the observed value of $F_1$ in (9.12). The null hypothesis $H_0$ in (9.8) is rejected whenever the above p-value is less than the nominal significance level of $\delta$.

**Remark 9.1.** *When $\sigma_\beta^2 = \sigma_\gamma^2 = 0$ and $\alpha_\varepsilon = 0$, model (9.1) is reduced to the normal one-way classification random effects model, then $F_{1B}$ in (9.13) degenerates into the result of Yang et al. (2012).*

Similarly, the Bootstrap test statistics for hypothesis testing problems (9.9) and (9.10) are respectively represented as

$$F_{2B} = \frac{T_{2B}}{acc_0 + T_{3B}/n_3}, F_{3B} = \frac{T_{3B}}{cc_0 + T_{4B}/n_4},$$

where $T_{2B} \sim (acc_0 + t_3/n_3)\chi_{n_2}^2$ and $T_{3B} \sim (t_3/n_3)\chi_{n_3}^2$ in $F_{2B}$, and $T_{3B} \sim (cc_0 + t_4/n_4)\chi_{n_3}^2$ and $T_{4B} \sim (t_4/n_4)\chi_{n_4}^2$ in $F_{3B}$. Here $t_4$ is the observed value of $T_4$. Based on $F_{2B}$ and $F_{3B}$, the Bootstrap p-values are respectively computed as

$$p_2 = P(F_{2B} > f_2|H_0), p_3 = P(F_{3B} > f_3|H_0).$$

Similar to $f_1$ in (9.14), $f_2$ and $f_3$ are observed values of test statistics.

**Remark 9.2.** *The Bootstrap pivot quantity of $\sigma_\alpha^2$ can be constructed as $\tilde{F}_{1B}$ based on $F_{1B}$. Suppose that $\tilde{F}_{1B}(\omega)$ is the $100\omega$ empirical percentile of $\tilde{F}_{1B}$, then the $100(1-\delta)\%$ Bootstrap confidence interval for $\sigma_\alpha^2$ is given by*

$$\left[ \frac{t_1}{bc\tilde{F}_{1B}(1-\delta/2)} - \frac{t_3}{n_3bc}, \frac{t_1}{bc\tilde{F}_{1B}(\delta/2)} - \frac{t_3}{n_3bc} \right],$$

*where $t_1$ is the observed value of $T_1$. Likewise, the Bootstrap confidence intervals for $\sigma_\beta^2$ and $\sigma_\gamma^2$ are also obtained.*

### 9.3.2 Generalized approach

For hypothesis testing problem (9.8), the generalized test variable has the form

$$F_4 = V_1(1/V_3 + bc\sigma_\alpha^2/t_3). \tag{9.15}$$

It is apparent that $f_4 = t_1/t_3$, the observed value of $F_4$, is free of any unknown parameters. The distribution of $F_4$ is free of the nuisance parameters. From the expression in (9.15), $F_4$ is stochastically increasing in $\sigma_\alpha^2$. Hence, $F_4$ is a generalized test variable for hypothesis testing problem (9.8). Then, based on $F_4$, the generalized p-value can be computed as

$$\begin{aligned}
p_4 &= P(F_4 \geq t_1/t_3|H_0) = P\left( V_1 \geq \frac{V_3 t_1}{bcV_3 c_0 + t_3} \right) \\
&= 1 - E_{V_3}\left[ F_{\chi_{n_1}^2}\left( \frac{V_3 t_1}{bcV_3 c_0 + t_3} \right) \right],
\end{aligned} \tag{9.16}$$

where $F_{\chi_{n_1}^2}$ is the cumulative distribution function of a chi-square distribution with $n_1$ degrees of freedom, and the expectation of (9.16) is taken with respect to $V_3$. The null hypothesis $H_0$ in (9.8) will be rejected if $p_4$ is less than the nominal significance level of $\delta$.

**Remark 9.3.** *When $\alpha_\varepsilon = 0$, model (9.1) is reduced to the normal two-way classification random effects model, then $p_4$ in (9.16) degenerates into the result of Weerahandi (1991).*

Next, to obtain the generalized confidence interval for $\sigma_\alpha^2$, we define

$$F_4^* = \frac{1}{bc}\left( \frac{t_1\sigma_1^2}{T_1} - \frac{t_3\sigma_3^2}{T_3} \right).$$

Obviously, the distribution of $F_4^*$ is free of any unknown parameters, and the observed value of $F_4^*$ is free of nuisance parameters. Thus, $F_4^*$ is a generalized pivot quantity. According to the quantile of $F_4^*$, the generalized upper confidence limit and lower confidence limit of $\sigma_\alpha^2$ are obtained at the confidence level of $1 - \delta$, which are written as $F_4^*(1 - \delta/2)$ and $F_4^*(\delta/2)$ respectively.

**Remark 9.4.** *When $\sigma_\beta^2 = \sigma_\gamma^2 = 0$ and $\alpha_\varepsilon = 0$, the generalized confidence interval* $[F_4^*(\delta/2), F_4^*(1 - \delta/2)]$ *degenerates into the result of Weerahandi (1993).*

Similarly, the generalized test variables of hypothesis testing problems (9.9) and (9.10) are respectively expressed as

$$F_5 = V_2(1/V_3 + ac\sigma_\beta^2/t_3), F_6 = V_3(1/V_4 + c\sigma_\gamma^2/t_4).$$

Based on $F_5$ and $F_6$, the generalized p-values for hypothesis testing problems (9.9) and (9.10) are respectively computed as follows.

$$p_5 = 1 - E_{V_3}\left[F_{\chi_{n_2}^2}\left(\frac{V_3 t_2}{acV_3 c_0 + t_3}\right)\right], p_6 = 1 - E_{V_4}\left[F_{\chi_{n_3}^2}\left(\frac{V_4 t_3}{cV_4 c_0 + t_4}\right)\right].$$

Further, the generalized pivot quantities for $\sigma_\beta^2$ and $\sigma_\gamma^2$ are repectively given by

$$F_5^* = \frac{1}{ac}\left(\frac{t_2\sigma_2^2}{T_2} - \frac{t_3\sigma_3^2}{T_3}\right), F_6^* = \frac{1}{c}\left(\frac{t_3\sigma_3^2}{T_3} - \frac{t_4\sigma_4^2}{T_4}\right).$$

Similar to $\sigma_\alpha^2$, the generalized confidence intervals for $\sigma_\beta^2$ and $\sigma_\gamma^2$ can be obtained easily.

## 9.4    Inference on the sum of variance components

In this section, the Bootstrap approach and generalized approach are applied into the hypothesis testing problem for the sum of three variance components in model (9.1). The hypothesis of interest is

$$H_0 : \sigma_\alpha^2 + \sigma_\beta^2 + \sigma_\gamma^2 \leq c_1 \ \ versus \ \ H_1 : \sigma_\alpha^2 + \sigma_\beta^2 + \sigma_\gamma^2 > c_1, \tag{9.17}$$

where $c_1$ is a specified value.

### *9.4.1    Bootstrap approach*

Under the null hypothesis $H_0$ in (9.17), by replacing the parameters $\sigma_2^2$, $\sigma_3^2$ and $\sigma_4^2$ with their estimators $\hat{\sigma}_2^2$, $\hat{\sigma}_3^2$ and $\hat{\sigma}_4^2$ in $V_1$ respectively, the corresponding test statistic is given by

$$F_7 = \frac{T_1}{bcc_1 - \frac{b}{a}\left(\frac{T_2}{n_2} - \frac{T_3}{n_3}\right) - \frac{(b-1)T_3}{n_3} + \frac{bT_4}{n_4}}. \tag{9.18}$$

By (9.18), the Bootstrap test statistic for hypothesis testing problem (9.17) is defined as

$$F_{7B} = \frac{T_{1B}}{bcc_1 - \frac{b}{a}\left(\frac{T_{2B}}{n_2} - \frac{T_{3B}}{n_3}\right) - \frac{(b-1)T_{3B}}{n_3} + \frac{bT_{4B}}{n_4}}, \tag{9.19}$$

where $T_{1B} \sim \left(bcc_1 - \frac{b}{a}\left(\frac{t_2}{n_2} - \frac{t_3}{n_3}\right) - \frac{(b-1)t_3}{n_3} + \frac{bt_4}{n_4}\right)\chi^2_{n_1}$, $T_{2B} \sim (t_2/n_2)\chi^2_{n_2}$, $T_{3B} \sim (t_3/n_3)\chi^2_{n_3}$, $T_{4B} \sim (t_4/n_4)\chi^2_{n_4}$, and $t_2$ is the observed value of $T_2$. By $F_{7B}$ in (9.19), the Bootstrap p-value is computed as

$$p_7 = P(F_{7B} > f_7 | H_0), \tag{9.20}$$

where $f_7$ denotes the observed value of $F_7$ in (9.18). The null hypothesis $H_0$ in (9.17) is rejected whenever the above p-value is less than the nominal significance level of $\delta$.

**Remark 9.5.** *Similar to Remark 9.2, the Bootstrap pivot quantity of $\sigma_\alpha^2 + \sigma_\beta^2 + \sigma_\gamma^2$ can be constructed as $\tilde{F}_{7B}$ based on $F_{7B}$. Let $\tilde{F}_{7B}(\omega)$ be the $100\omega$ empirical percentile of $\tilde{F}_{7B}$. The $100(1-\delta)\%$ Bootstrap confidence interval for $\sigma_\alpha^2 + \sigma_\beta^2 + \sigma_\gamma^2$ is given by*

$$\left[\frac{t_1}{bc\tilde{F}_{7B}(1-\delta/2)} + \frac{1}{ac}\left(\frac{t_2}{n_2} - \frac{t_3}{n_3}\right) + \frac{(b-1)t_3}{bcn_3} - \frac{t_4}{cn_4},\right.$$
$$\left.\frac{t_1}{bc\tilde{F}_{7B}(\delta/2)} + \frac{1}{ac}\left(\frac{t_2}{n_2} - \frac{t_3}{n_3}\right) + \frac{(b-1)t_3}{bcn_3} - \frac{t_4}{cn_4}\right].$$

### 9.4.2 Generalized approach

For hypothesis testing problem (9.17), the generalized test variable is defined as

$$F_8 = \frac{1}{bc}\left(\frac{t_1}{V_1} - \frac{t_3}{V_3}\right) + \frac{1}{ac}\left(\frac{t_2}{V_2} - \frac{t_3}{V_3}\right) + \frac{1}{c}\left(\frac{t_3}{V_3} - \frac{t_4}{V_4}\right) - (\sigma_\alpha^2 + \sigma_\beta^2 + \sigma_\gamma^2),$$

It is obvious that $f_8 = 0$, the observed value of $F_8$, is free of any unknown parameters. The distributions of $V_i (i = 1, \cdots, 4)$ have no unknown parameters, thus the distribution of $F_8$ is free of nuisance parameters. In addition, $F_8$ is stochastically decreasing in $\sigma_\alpha^2 + \sigma_\beta^2 + \sigma_\gamma^2$. Therefore, $F_8$ is a generalized test variable for hypothesis testing problem (9.17) and the generalized p-value is computed as

$$p_8 = P(F_8 \leq 0 | H_0)$$

$$= 1 - E_{V_2, V_3, V_4}\left[F_{\chi^2_{n_1}}\left(t_1\left(bcc_1 - \frac{b}{a}\left(\frac{t_2}{V_2} - \frac{t_3}{V_3}\right) - b\left(\frac{t_3}{V_3} - \frac{t_4}{V_4}\right) + \frac{t_3}{V_3}\right)^{-1}\right)\right]. \tag{9.21}$$

The null hypothesis $H_0$ in (9.17) will be rejected if $p_8$ is less than the nominal significance level of $\delta$.

To obtain the confidence interval for $\sigma_\alpha^2 + \sigma_\beta^2 + \sigma_\gamma^2$, the generalized pivot quantity is defined as

$$F_8^* = \frac{1}{bc}\left(\frac{t_1}{V_1} - \frac{t_3}{V_3}\right) + \frac{1}{ac}\left(\frac{t_2}{V_2} - \frac{t_3}{V_3}\right) + \frac{1}{c}\left(\frac{t_3}{V_3} - \frac{t_4}{V_4}\right).$$

Let $F_8^*(\omega)$ be the $100\omega$ empirical percentile of $F_8^*$, then the $100(1-\delta)\%$ generalized confidence interval for $\sigma_\alpha^2 + \sigma_\beta^2 + \sigma_\gamma^2$ is given by $[F_8^*(\delta/2), F_8^*(1-\delta/2)]$.

## 9.5   Inference on the ratio of variance components

Consider the hypothesis testing problems

$$H_0 : \sigma_\alpha^2/\sigma_\beta^2 \leq c_2 \; \textit{versus} \; H_1 : \sigma_\alpha^2/\sigma_\beta^2 > c_2, \tag{9.22}$$

$$H_0 : \sigma_\alpha^2/\sigma_\gamma^2 \leq c_2 \; \textit{versus} \; H_1 : \sigma_\alpha^2/\sigma_\gamma^2 > c_2, \tag{9.23}$$

$$H_0 : \sigma_\beta^2/\sigma_\gamma^2 \leq c_2 \; \textit{versus} \; H_1 : \sigma_\beta^2/\sigma_\gamma^2 > c_2, \tag{9.24}$$

where $c_2$ is a specified value.

### 9.5.1   Bootstrap approach

Similar to Ye et al. (2021), by replacing $\sigma_2^2$ and $\sigma_3^2$ with their estimators $\hat{\sigma}_2^2$ and $\hat{\sigma}_3^2$ in $V_1$ under $H_0$ from (9.22), then we get

$$F_9 = \frac{T_1}{bc_2(T_2/n_2 - T_3/n_3)/a + T_3/n_3}. \tag{9.25}$$

Based on (9.25), the Bootstrap test statistic for hypothesis testing problem (9.22) is defined as

$$F_{9B} = \frac{T_{1B}}{bc_2(T_{2B}/n_2 - T_{3B}/n_3)/a + T_{3B}/n_3},$$

where $T_{1B} \sim \left(\frac{bc_2(t_2/n_2 - t_3/n_3)}{a} + \frac{t_3}{n_3}\right)\chi_{n_1}^2$, $T_{2B} \sim (t_2/n_2)\chi_{n_2}^2$, and $T_{3B} \sim (t_3/n_3)\chi_{n_3}^2$. By $F_{9B}$, the Bootstrap $p$-value is computed as

$$p_9 = P(F_{9B} > f_9 | H_0), \tag{9.26}$$

where $f_9$ is the observed value of $F_9$ in (9.25). The null hypothesis $H_0$ is rejected whenever $p_9$ is less than the nominal significance level of $\delta$.

Likewise, the Bootstrap test statistics for hypothesis testing problems (9.23) and (9.24) can be respectively defined as

$$F_{10B} = \frac{T_{1B}}{bc_2(T_{3B}/n_3 - T_{4B}/n_4) + T_{3B}/n_3}, F_{11B} = \frac{T_{2B}}{ac_2(T_{3B}/n_3 - T_{4B}/n_4) + T_{3B}/n_3}.$$

Then the Bootstrap p-values based on $F_{10B}$ and $F_{11B}$ are respectively computed as

$$p_{10} = P(F_{10B} > f_{10}|H_0), p_{11} = P(F_{11B} > f_{11}|H_0),$$

where $f_{10}$ and $f_{11}$ are observed values of the test statistics.

**Remark 9.6.** *The Bootstrap pivot quantity of $\sigma_\alpha^2/\sigma_\beta^2$ can be constructed as $\tilde{F}_{9B}$ based on $F_{9B}$. Let $\tilde{F}_{9B}(\omega)$ be the $100\omega$ empirical percentile of $\tilde{F}_{9B}$, Then the $100(1-\delta)\%$ Bootstrap confidence interval for $\sigma_\alpha^2/\sigma_\beta^2$ is*

$$\left[ \left( b\left( \frac{t_2}{n_2} - \frac{t_3}{n_3} \right) \right)^{-1} \left( \frac{at_1}{\tilde{F}_{9B}(1-\delta/2)} - \frac{at_3}{n_3} \right), \left( b\left( \frac{t_2}{n_2} - \frac{t_3}{n_3} \right) \right)^{-1} \left( \frac{at_1}{\tilde{F}_{9B}(\delta/2)} - \frac{at_3}{n_3} \right) \right].$$

*In the same way, the $100(1-\delta)\%$ Bootstrap confidence intervals for $\sigma_\alpha^2/\sigma_\gamma^2$ and $\sigma_\beta^2/\sigma_\gamma^2$ are also available.*

## 9.5.2 Generalized approach

For hypothesis testing problem (9.22), the generalized test variable is

$$F_{12} = \frac{aV_2(t_1V_3 - t_3V_1)}{bV_1(t_2V_3 - t_3V_2)} - \frac{\sigma_\alpha^2}{\sigma_\beta^2}. \tag{9.27}$$

By (9.27), the generalized p-value is computed as

$$p_{12} = P(F_{12} \le 0|H_0) = 1 - E_{V_2,V_3}\left[ F_{\chi_{n_1}^2}\left( \frac{at_1V_2V_3}{(a-bc_2)t_3V_2 + bc_2t_2V_3} \right) \right]. \tag{9.28}$$

The null hypothesis $H_0$ in (9.22) is rejected if $p_{12}$ is less than the nominal significance level of $\delta$.

To obtain the confidence interval for $\sigma_\alpha^2/\sigma_\beta^2$, we define

$$F_{12}^* = \frac{aV_2(t_1V_3 - t_3V_1)}{bV_1(t_2V_3 - t_3V_2)},$$

where $\sigma_\alpha^2/\sigma_\beta^2$ is the observed value of $F_{12}^*$. Therefore, the generalized confidence interval can be constructed by the quantile of $F_{12}^*$.

Similar to (9.27), the generalized test variables for hypothesis testing problems (9.23) and (9.24) are respectively

$$F_{13} = \frac{V_4(t_1 V_3 - t_3 V_1)}{b V_1(t_3 V_4 - t_4 V_3)} - \frac{\sigma_\alpha^2}{\sigma_\gamma^2}, F_{14} = \frac{V_4(t_2 V_3 - t_3 V_2)}{a V_1(t_3 V_4 - t_4 V_3)} - \frac{\sigma_\beta^2}{\sigma_\gamma^2}.$$

Thus, based on $F_{13}$ and $F_{14}$, the generalized p-values for hypothesis testing problems (9.23) and (9.24) are respectively computed as

$$p_{13} = 1 - E_{V_3, V_4}\left[ F_{\chi_{n_1}^2}\left( \frac{t_1 V_3 V_4}{(bc_2 + 1)t_3 V_4 - bc_2 t_4 V_3} \right) \right],$$

$$p_{14} = 1 - E_{V_3, V_4}\left[ F_{\chi_{n_2}^2}\left( \frac{t_2 V_3 V_4}{(ac_2 + 1)t_3 V_4 - ac_2 t_4 V_3} \right) \right].$$

Further, the generalized confidence intervals for $\sigma_\alpha^2/\sigma_\gamma^2$ and $\sigma_\beta^2/\sigma_\gamma^2$ can be obtained easily.

## 9.6  Monte Carlo simulation

The Type I error probability and power of the above testing approaches are investigated from the numerical perspective by using the Monte Carlo simulation. For convenience, here we only provide the algorithm of the Bootstrap approach for hypothesis testing problem (9.8) as follows.

**Step 1:** For a given $(a, b, c, \sigma_\alpha^2, \sigma_\gamma^2, \sigma_\varepsilon^2, c_0)$, generate $t_1 \sim (bc\sigma_\alpha^2 + c\sigma_\gamma^2 + \sigma_\varepsilon^2)\chi_{n_1}^2$ and $t_3 \sim (c\sigma_\gamma^2 + \sigma_\varepsilon^2)\chi_{n_3}^2$.

**Step 2:** Compute $F_1$ in (9.12), denoted by $f_1$.

**Step 3:** Generate $T_{1B} \sim (bcc_0 + t_3/n_3)\chi_{n_1}^2$ and $T_{3B} \sim (t_3/n_3)\chi_{n_3}^2$, then compute $F_{1B}$ in (9.13).

**Step 4:** Repeat Step 3 $l_1$ times and compute $p_1$ by (9.14). If $p_1 < \delta$, then $Q = 1$. Otherwise, $Q = 0$.

**Step 5:** Repeat Steps 1–4 $l_2$ times and get $Q_1, \cdots, Q_{l_2}$. Then the Type I error probability is $\sum_{i=1}^{l_2} Q_i/l_2$.

Based on the above algorithm, the power of hypothesis testing problem (9.8) under $H_1$ can be obtained similarly.

In this simulation, the parameters and sample sizes are set as follows. Firstly, let the nominal significance level $\delta$ be 0.025, 0.05, 0.075, 0.1, and the number of inner loops $l_1$ and outer loops $l_2$ both be 2500. Secondly, considering the hypothesis testing problem of fixed effect in (9.4), the sample sizes $(a, b, c)$ are

**Table 9.1:** Type I error probabilities for (9.4) ($\sigma_\beta^2 = \sigma_\varepsilon^2 = 1, \mu = \mu_0 = 0$).

| $a$ | $b$ | $c$ | $\alpha^*$ | $\sigma_\alpha^2$ | $\sigma_\gamma^2$ | $\delta$ | | | |
|---|---|---|---|---|---|---|---|---|---|
| | | | | | | 0.025 | 0.05 | 0.075 | 0.1 |
| 2 | 2 | 2 | 0 | 0.1 | 6 | 0.0208 | 0.0448 | 0.0720 | 0.0972 |
| | | | | 0.5 | 6.5 | 0.0216 | 0.0452 | 0.0712 | 0.0960 |
| | | | | 1 | 7 | 0.0212 | 0.0452 | 0.0708 | 0.0956 |
| | | | | 1.5 | 8 | 0.0224 | 0.0432 | 0.0700 | 0.0960 |
| 2 | 3 | 4 | 0.5 | 0.1 | 6 | 0.0240 | 0.0452 | 0.0604 | 0.0808 |
| | | | | 0.5 | 6.5 | 0.0240 | 0.0444 | 0.0608 | 0.0828 |
| | | | | 1 | 7 | 0.0232 | 0.0464 | 0.0608 | 0.0820 |
| | | | | 1.5 | 8 | 0.0236 | 0.0480 | 0.0620 | 0.0844 |
| 3 | 4 | 5 | 1 | 0.1 | 6 | 0.0256 | 0.0548 | 0.0820 | 0.1088 |
| | | | | 0.5 | 6.5 | 0.0276 | 0.0564 | 0.0800 | 0.1060 |
| | | | | 1 | 7 | 0.0292 | 0.0564 | 0.0820 | 0.1076 |
| | | | | 1.5 | 8 | 0.0308 | 0.0568 | 0.0828 | 0.1104 |
| 5 | 6 | 6 | 2 | 0.1 | 6 | 0.0268 | 0.0576 | 0.0796 | 0.1064 |
| | | | | 0.5 | 6.5 | 0.0284 | 0.0532 | 0.0836 | 0.1048 |
| | | | | 1 | 7 | 0.0272 | 0.0592 | 0.0836 | 0.1084 |
| | | | | 1.5 | 8 | 0.0268 | 0.0596 | 0.0864 | 0.1108 |

(2,2,2), (2,3,4), (3,4,5) and (5,6,6). Let $\alpha_\varepsilon = \alpha^* 1_n$ and $\alpha^* = 0, 0.5, 1, 1.5, 2$, then we set $\sigma_\beta^2 = \sigma_\varepsilon^2 = 1$, $\sigma_\alpha^2 = 0.1, 0.5, 1, 1.5$, and $\sigma_\gamma^2 = 6, 6.5, 7, 8$. Finally, considering the hypothesis testing problems of variance component functions, the sample sizes $(a, b, c)$ are (3,4,5), (5,6,7), (6,8,10) and (8,10,12). For hypothesis testing problem (9.8), we suppose $c_0 = 0.1$, $\sigma_\alpha^2 = \sigma_\beta^2 = 0.1$, $\sigma_\gamma^2 = 0.1, 1, 2.5, 4, 6$, and $\sigma_\varepsilon^2 = 0.5, 2.5, 4, 6, 8$. For hypothesis testing problem (9.17), let $c_1 = 8$, $\sigma_\beta^2 = 0.5$, $\sigma_\alpha^2 = 4, 4.5, 5, 5.5, 6$, and $\sigma_\varepsilon^2 = 0.5, 1, 1.5, 2, 2.5$.

For hypothesis testing problem (9.4), Tables 9.1 and 9.2 respectively give the simulated Type I error probabilities and powers. As in Table 9.1, the exact test statistic is slightly conservative when the sample size is small. Additionally, the actual levels of the exact test statistic are near the nominal significance levels as the sample size increases. As in Table 9.2, the powers of this approach increase significantly.

For hypothesis testing problem (9.8), Table 9.3 presents the simulated Type I error probabilities of the Bootstrap approach (BA) and generalized approach (GA) at different nominal significance levels. When the sample size is small, the Type I error probabilities of BA is slightly liberal, while those of GA is slightly conservative. With the increase of sample size, the actual levels of the two proposed approaches are closer to the nominal significance levels. Additionally, the Type I error probabilities of BA are better than those of GA in most cases. Table 9.4 presents the simulated powers of BA and GA at different nominal significance levels. The powers of BA are consistently better than those of GA.

**Table 9.2:** Powers of the test for (9.4) ($\sigma_\alpha^2 = \sigma_\beta^2 = \sigma_\gamma^2 = 1, \mu_0 = 0$).

| $a$ | $b$ | $c$ | $\alpha^*$ | $\sigma_\varepsilon^2$ | $\mu$ | $\delta$ | | | |
|---|---|---|---|---|---|---|---|---|---|
| | | | | | | 0.025 | 0.05 | 0.075 | 0.1 |
| 2 | 2 | 2 | 0 | 1 | 1 | 0.0393 | 0.0784 | 0.1148 | 0.1444 |
| | | | | 1.5 | 2 | 0.0864 | 0.1532 | 0.2028 | 0.2504 |
| | | | | 2 | 3 | 0.1600 | 0.2592 | 0.3496 | 0.4196 |
| | | | | 2.5 | 4 | 0.2564 | 0.4012 | 0.5140 | 0.6088 |
| 2 | 3 | 4 | 0.5 | 1 | 1 | 0.0760 | 0.1248 | 0.1588 | 0.1884 |
| | | | | 1.5 | 2 | 0.2424 | 0.3356 | 0.4028 | 0.4604 |
| | | | | 2 | 3 | 0.5376 | 0.6432 | 0.7040 | 0.7456 |
| | | | | 2.5 | 4 | 0.7904 | 0.8592 | 0.8928 | 0.9208 |
| 3 | 4 | 5 | 1 | 1 | 1 | 0.1416 | 0.1976 | 0.2428 | 0.2784 |
| | | | | 1.5 | 2 | 0.4360 | 0.5268 | 0.5844 | 0.6284 |
| | | | | 2 | 3 | 0.8104 | 0.8608 | 0.8868 | 0.9056 |
| | | | | 2.5 | 4 | 0.9660 | 0.9796 | 0.9852 | 0.9896 |
| 5 | 6 | 6 | 2 | 1 | 1 | 0.2280 | 0.2944 | 0.3352 | 0.3712 |
| | | | | 1.5 | 2 | 0.7092 | 0.7736 | 0.8084 | 0.8384 |
| | | | | 2 | 3 | 0.9752 | 0.9844 | 0.9868 | 0.9896 |
| | | | | 2.5 | 4 | 0.9996 | 1.0000 | 1.0000 | 1.0000 |

**Table 9.3:** Type I error probabilities for (9.8) ($\sigma_\beta^2 = \sigma_\alpha^2 = c_0 = 0.1$).

| $a$ | $b$ | $c$ | $\sigma_\gamma^2$ | $\sigma_\varepsilon^2$ | \multicolumn{8}{c}{$\delta$} | | | | | | | |
|---|---|---|---|---|---|---|---|---|---|---|---|---|
| | | | | | \multicolumn{2}{c}{0.025} | \multicolumn{2}{c}{0.05} | \multicolumn{2}{c}{0.075} | \multicolumn{2}{c}{0.1} |
| | | | | | BA | GA | BA | GA | BA | GA | BA | GA |
| 3 | 4 | 5 | 0.1 | 0.5 | 0.0268 | 0.0184 | 0.0516 | 0.0384 | 0.0756 | 0.0596 | 0.1004 | 0.0816 |
| | | | 1 | 2.5 | 0.0352 | 0.0212 | 0.0604 | 0.0432 | 0.0856 | 0.0660 | 0.1084 | 0.0892 |
| | | | 2.5 | 4 | 0.0344 | 0.0224 | 0.0596 | 0.0452 | 0.0848 | 0.0700 | 0.1060 | 0.0940 |
| | | | 4 | 6 | 0.0328 | 0.0232 | 0.0584 | 0.0480 | 0.0848 | 0.0716 | 0.1044 | 0.0964 |
| | | | 6 | 8 | 0.0316 | 0.0244 | 0.0580 | 0.0476 | 0.0848 | 0.0736 | 0.1032 | 0.0964 |
| 5 | 6 | 7 | 0.1 | 0.5 | 0.0252 | 0.0228 | 0.0512 | 0.0452 | 0.0756 | 0.0712 | 0.0996 | 0.0952 |
| | | | 1 | 2.5 | 0.0260 | 0.0240 | 0.0516 | 0.0452 | 0.0756 | 0.0708 | 0.1012 | 0.0956 |
| | | | 2.5 | 4 | 0.0268 | 0.0236 | 0.0512 | 0.0476 | 0.0788 | 0.0724 | 0.1012 | 0.0944 |
| | | | 4 | 6 | 0.0264 | 0.0244 | 0.0512 | 0.0476 | 0.0768 | 0.0740 | 0.1012 | 0.0972 |
| | | | 6 | 8 | 0.0264 | 0.0244 | 0.0496 | 0.0488 | 0.0752 | 0.0744 | 0.1004 | 0.0980 |
| 6 | 8 | 10 | 0.1 | 0.5 | 0.0252 | 0.0244 | 0.0496 | 0.0472 | 0.0752 | 0.0736 | 0.1004 | 0.0972 |
| | | | 1 | 2.5 | 0.0252 | 0.0244 | 0.0500 | 0.0464 | 0.0760 | 0.0712 | 0.1008 | 0.0956 |
| | | | 2.5 | 4 | 0.0264 | 0.0248 | 0.0504 | 0.0480 | 0.0764 | 0.0728 | 0.1012 | 0.0976 |
| | | | 4 | 6 | 0.0260 | 0.0240 | 0.0496 | 0.0488 | 0.0756 | 0.0736 | 0.1012 | 0.0976 |
| | | | 6 | 8 | 0.0260 | 0.0244 | 0.0504 | 0.0484 | 0.0752 | 0.0740 | 0.1004 | 0.0984 |
| 8 | 10 | 12 | 0.1 | 0.5 | 0.0252 | 0.0244 | 0.0504 | 0.0476 | 0.0752 | 0.0724 | 0.1000 | 0.0984 |
| | | | 1 | 2.5 | 0.0260 | 0.0232 | 0.0504 | 0.0488 | 0.0748 | 0.0728 | 0.1000 | 0.0972 |
| | | | 2.5 | 4 | 0.0252 | 0.0244 | 0.0508 | 0.0492 | 0.0764 | 0.0728 | 0.1004 | 0.0980 |
| | | | 4 | 6 | 0.0248 | 0.0236 | 0.0512 | 0.0488 | 0.0748 | 0.0744 | 0.1000 | 0.0984 |
| | | | 6 | 8 | 0.0256 | 0.0248 | 0.0500 | 0.0496 | 0.0748 | 0.0748 | 0.1004 | 0.0988 |

For hypothesis testing problem (9.17), Tables 9.5 and 9.6 respectively give the simulated Type I error probabilities and powers of BA and GA at different nominal significance levels. From Table 9.5, the BA and GA are relatively conser-

**Table 9.4:** Powers of the test for (9.8) ($\sigma_\beta^2 = \sigma_\varepsilon^2 = c_0 = 0.1$).

| | | | | | $\delta$ | | | | | | | |
| $a$ | $b$ | $c$ | $\sigma_\alpha^2$ | $\sigma_\gamma^2$ | 0.025 | | 0.05 | | 0.075 | | 0.1 | |
| | | | | | BA | GA | BA | GA | BA | GA | BA | GA |
|---|---|---|---|---|---|---|---|---|---|---|---|---|
| 3 | 4 | 5 | 0.5 | 1 | 0.1444 | 0.1056 | 0.2120 | 0.1748 | 0.2628 | 0.2232 | 0.3048 | 0.2680 |
| | | | 1 | 1.5 | 0.2160 | 0.1596 | 0.2960 | 0.2544 | 0.3496 | 0.3108 | 0.3980 | 0.3612 |
| | | | 1.5 | 2 | 0.2428 | 0.1988 | 0.3320 | 0.2956 | 0.3916 | 0.3564 | 0.4380 | 0.4048 |
| | | | 2 | 2.5 | 0.2644 | 0.2176 | 0.3548 | 0.3168 | 0.4140 | 0.3848 | 0.4616 | 0.4348 |
| | | | 2.5 | 3 | 0.2752 | 0.2284 | 0.3692 | 0.3340 | 0.4288 | 0.4032 | 0.4760 | 0.4552 |
| 5 | 6 | 7 | 0.5 | 1 | 0.3032 | 0.2828 | 0.3924 | 0.3724 | 0.4612 | 0.4444 | 0.5164 | 0.5064 |
| | | | 1 | 1.5 | 0.4872 | 0.4656 | 0.5752 | 0.5620 | 0.6360 | 0.6228 | 0.6744 | 0.6644 |
| | | | 1.5 | 2 | 0.5632 | 0.5456 | 0.6468 | 0.6404 | 0.6964 | 0.6884 | 0.7340 | 0.7268 |
| | | | 2 | 2.5 | 0.6028 | 0.5920 | 0.6860 | 0.6776 | 0.7284 | 0.7248 | 0.7688 | 0.7604 |
| | | | 2.5 | 3 | 0.6284 | 0.6216 | 0.7116 | 0.7008 | 0.7492 | 0.7432 | 0.7848 | 0.7804 |
| 6 | 8 | 10 | 0.5 | 1 | 0.4392 | 0.4284 | 0.5316 | 0.5200 | 0.5956 | 0.5864 | 0.6288 | 0.6224 |
| | | | 1 | 1.5 | 0.6568 | 0.6492 | 0.7228 | 0.7164 | 0.7672 | 0.7608 | 0.7964 | 0.7936 |
| | | | 1.5 | 2 | 0.7368 | 0.7296 | 0.7920 | 0.7888 | 0.8256 | 0.8220 | 0.8528 | 0.8512 |
| | | | 2 | 2.5 | 0.7808 | 0.7728 | 0.8256 | 0.8232 | 0.8576 | 0.8556 | 0.8768 | 0.8744 |
| | | | 2.5 | 3 | 0.8004 | 0.7932 | 0.8488 | 0.8464 | 0.8744 | 0.8716 | 0.8964 | 0.8940 |
| 8 | 10 | 12 | 0.5 | 1 | 0.5988 | 0.5940 | 0.6760 | 0.6724 | 0.7256 | 0.7204 | 0.7612 | 0.7588 |
| | | | 1 | 1.5 | 0.8184 | 0.8092 | 0.8604 | 0.8584 | 0.8952 | 0.8916 | 0.9100 | 0.9096 |
| | | | 1.5 | 2 | 0.8852 | 0.8824 | 0.9164 | 0.9156 | 0.9388 | 0.9372 | 0.9464 | 0.9464 |
| | | | 2 | 2.5 | 0.9144 | 0.9128 | 0.9428 | 0.9416 | 0.9556 | 0.9548 | 0.9636 | 0.9636 |
| | | | 2.5 | 3 | 0.9344 | 0.9336 | 0.9528 | 0.9524 | 0.9652 | 0.9640 | 0.9720 | 0.9720 |

vative and liberal respectively with a small sample size. However, most of the results are significantly improved as the sample size increases. Also, the Type I error probabilities of BA are better than those of GA in most cases. From Table 9.6, as $\sigma_\alpha^2 + \sigma_\beta^2 + \sigma_\gamma^2$ departs from the null hypothesis and the sample size increases, the powers of BA and GA both increase, but the latter is consistently better than the former.

**Remark 9.7.** *In the above simulations, we only provide the results under zero and positive skewness parameter. When the skewness parameter is negative, the simulation results are similar to those of the positive skewness parameter, so it is omitted.*

**Remark 9.8.** *For hypothesis testing problem (9.22), we also give the simulations under the parameter setting of $c_2 = 5$, $\sigma_\gamma^2 = 0.1$, $\sigma_\beta^2 = 4, 4.5, 5, 5.5, 6$, and $\sigma_\varepsilon^2 = 0.1, 0.5, 1, 1.5, 2$. The results show that the Type I error probabilities and powers of BA are both better than those of GA with a small sample size. As the sample size increases, the above two approaches can efficiently control the Type I error probability. However, due to space limitations, the simulation results are not shown.*

**Table 9.5:** Type I error probabilities for (9.17) ($\sigma_\alpha^2 + \sigma_\beta^2 + \sigma_\gamma^2 = c_1 = 8, \sigma_\beta^2 = 0.5$).

| | | | | | $\delta$ | | | | | | | |
| | | | | | 0.025 | | 0.05 | | 0.075 | | 0.1 | |
| $a$ | $b$ | $c$ | $\sigma_\alpha^2$ | $\sigma_\varepsilon^2$ | BA | GA | BA | GA | BA | GA | BA | GA |
|---|---|---|---|---|---|---|---|---|---|---|---|---|
| 3 | 4 | 5 | 4 | 0.5 | 0.0236 | 0.0504 | 0.0544 | 0.1004 | 0.0880 | 0.1460 | 0.1172 | 0.1820 |
| | | | 4.5 | 1 | 0.0204 | 0.0480 | 0.0512 | 0.0920 | 0.0832 | 0.1352 | 0.1100 | 0.1748 |
| | | | 5 | 1.5 | 0.0172 | 0.0444 | 0.0496 | 0.0864 | 0.0752 | 0.1276 | 0.1052 | 0.1688 |
| | | | 5.5 | 2 | 0.0168 | 0.0416 | 0.0464 | 0.0820 | 0.0740 | 0.1208 | 0.0992 | 0.1592 |
| | | | 6 | 2.5 | 0.0196 | 0.0396 | 0.0428 | 0.0764 | 0.0712 | 0.1128 | 0.0976 | 0.1460 |
| 5 | 6 | 7 | 4 | 0.5 | 0.0100 | 0.0396 | 0.0336 | 0.0816 | 0.0600 | 0.1208 | 0.0896 | 0.1484 |
| | | | 4.5 | 1 | 0.0112 | 0.0372 | 0.0356 | 0.0756 | 0.0608 | 0.1140 | 0.0876 | 0.1436 |
| | | | 5 | 1.5 | 0.0144 | 0.0364 | 0.0400 | 0.0720 | 0.0624 | 0.1064 | 0.0908 | 0.1412 |
| | | | 5.5 | 2 | 0.0176 | 0.0332 | 0.0416 | 0.0688 | 0.0656 | 0.1012 | 0.0924 | 0.1360 |
| 5 | 6 | 7 | 6 | 2.5 | 0.0204 | 0.0320 | 0.0456 | 0.0640 | 0.0692 | 0.0944 | 0.0956 | 0.1280 |
| 6 | 8 | 10 | 4 | 0.5 | 0.0112 | 0.0392 | 0.0312 | 0.0764 | 0.0576 | 0.1120 | 0.0872 | 0.1408 |
| | | | 4.5 | 1 | 0.0140 | 0.0352 | 0.0380 | 0.0720 | 0.0616 | 0.1044 | 0.0896 | 0.1340 |
| | | | 5 | 1.5 | 0.0192 | 0.0316 | 0.0420 | 0.0716 | 0.0680 | 0.0984 | 0.0924 | 0.1288 |
| | | | 5.5 | 2 | 0.0224 | 0.0312 | 0.0452 | 0.0660 | 0.0700 | 0.0952 | 0.0952 | 0.1240 |
| | | | 6 | 2.5 | 0.0232 | 0.0304 | 0.0464 | 0.0632 | 0.0724 | 0.0924 | 0.0964 | 0.1192 |
| 8 | 10 | 12 | 4 | 0.5 | 0.0152 | 0.0328 | 0.0388 | 0.0704 | 0.0612 | 0.1040 | 0.0884 | 0.1316 |
| | | | 4.5 | 1 | 0.0196 | 0.0332 | 0.0420 | 0.0688 | 0.0672 | 0.0976 | 0.0908 | 0.1252 |
| | | | 5 | 1.5 | 0.0220 | 0.0336 | 0.0448 | 0.0640 | 0.0720 | 0.0924 | 0.0952 | 0.1248 |
| | | | 5.5 | 2 | 0.0232 | 0.0320 | 0.0460 | 0.0620 | 0.0724 | 0.0892 | 0.0960 | 0.1204 |
| | | | 6 | 2.5 | 0.0232 | 0.0312 | 0.0476 | 0.0612 | 0.0732 | 0.0892 | 0.0964 | 0.1164 |

**Table 9.6:** Powers of the test for (9.17) ($c_1 = 8, \sigma_\gamma^2 = \sigma_\varepsilon^2 = 0.5$).

| | | | | | $\delta$ | | | | | | | |
| | | | | | 0.025 | | 0.05 | | 0.075 | | 0.1 | |
| $a$ | $b$ | $c$ | $\sigma_\alpha^2$ | $\sigma_\beta^2$ | BA | GA | BA | GA | BA | GA | BA | GA |
|---|---|---|---|---|---|---|---|---|---|---|---|---|
| 3 | 4 | 5 | 6 | 4.5 | 0.0936 | 0.1464 | 0.1508 | 0.2204 | 0.1948 | 0.2832 | 0.2284 | 0.3340 |
| | | | 6.5 | 5 | 0.1068 | 0.1844 | 0.1616 | 0.2656 | 0.1976 | 0.3332 | 0.2364 | 0.3896 |
| | | | 7 | 5.5 | 0.1100 | 0.2212 | 0.1680 | 0.3096 | 0.2144 | 0.3840 | 0.2512 | 0.4408 |
| | | | 8 | 6 | 0.1152 | 0.2780 | 0.1848 | 0.3788 | 0.2344 | 0.4496 | 0.2764 | 0.5024 |
| | | | 10 | 8 | 0.1492 | 0.4280 | 0.2204 | 0.5260 | 0.2628 | 0.5868 | 0.2912 | 0.6272 |
| 5 | 6 | 7 | 6 | 4.5 | 0.1040 | 0.1656 | 0.1708 | 0.2512 | 0.2212 | 0.3272 | 0.2696 | 0.3876 |
| | | | 6.5 | 5 | 0.1156 | 0.2220 | 0.1856 | 0.3232 | 0.2468 | 0.4020 | 0.3064 | 0.4620 |
| | | | 7 | 5.5 | 0.1196 | 0.2836 | 0.1988 | 0.3904 | 0.2700 | 0.4720 | 0.3192 | 0.5256 |
| | | | 8 | 6 | 0.1380 | 0.3744 | 0.2352 | 0.4856 | 0.3004 | 0.5484 | 0.3428 | 0.6032 |
| | | | 10 | 8 | 0.1800 | 0.5660 | 0.2612 | 0.6604 | 0.3104 | 0.7284 | 0.3408 | 0.7740 |
| 6 | 8 | 10 | 6 | 4.5 | 0.1056 | 0.1900 | 0.1780 | 0.2856 | 0.2408 | 0.3588 | 0.3008 | 0.4192 |
| | | | 6.5 | 5 | 0.1320 | 0.2624 | 0.2092 | 0.3712 | 0.2832 | 0.4436 | 0.3424 | 0.5008 |
| | | | 7 | 5.5 | 0.1324 | 0.3404 | 0.2264 | 0.4484 | 0.3060 | 0.5180 | 0.3584 | 0.5712 |
| | | | 8 | 6 | 0.1552 | 0.4420 | 0.2652 | 0.5420 | 0.3452 | 0.6116 | 0.3916 | 0.6652 |
| | | | 10 | 8 | 0.1972 | 0.6640 | 0.2880 | 0.7548 | 0.3392 | 0.8032 | 0.3700 | 0.8328 |
| 8 | 10 | 12 | 6 | 4.5 | 0.0996 | 0.2340 | 0.1820 | 0.3312 | 0.2528 | 0.4108 | 0.3260 | 0.4684 |
| | | | 6.5 | 5 | 0.1340 | 0.3292 | 0.2244 | 0.4356 | 0.3116 | 0.5048 | 0.3832 | 0.5548 |
| | | | 7 | 5.5 | 0.1400 | 0.4256 | 0.2472 | 0.5204 | 0.3368 | 0.5884 | 0.4044 | 0.6376 |
| | | | 8 | 6 | 0.1676 | 0.5328 | 0.2940 | 0.6256 | 0.3776 | 0.6912 | 0.4364 | 0.7432 |
| | | | 10 | 8 | 0.2052 | 0.7744 | 0.3012 | 0.8324 | 0.3608 | 0.8704 | 0.3992 | 0.8892 |

## 9.7  Illustrative examples

In this section, to illustrate the rationality and effectiveness of the proposed approaches, we apply them to the examples of consumer price index (CPI) and value-added index of three industries.

**Example 9.1** The above approaches are applied to the study of CPI for Jiangsu, Zhejiang and Shanghai from January to June in 2020. The frequency histogram of CPI is given in Figure 9.1. For testing the normality of the data, the p-values from the R output of the Shapiro-Wilk test, Anderson-Darling test and Cramer-von Mises test are 1.186e-07, 2.536e-11 and 6.91e-09 respectively. We can conclude that the CPI is not normally distributed at the nominal significance level of 5%. Further, the chi-square goodness-of-fit test is used to test the null hypothesis that the CPI is skew-normally distributed. The value of the test statistic $\chi^2 = 4.3412 < \chi_2^2(0.95) = 5.9915$, so the null hypothesis is not rejected at the nominal significance level of 5%. Hence, the distribution of CPI can be considered approximately skew-normal. Based on the method of moment estimation, the CPI is approximately distributed as $SN(96.9298, 6.6284^2, 22.3439)$ and its density curve is given in Figure 9.1.

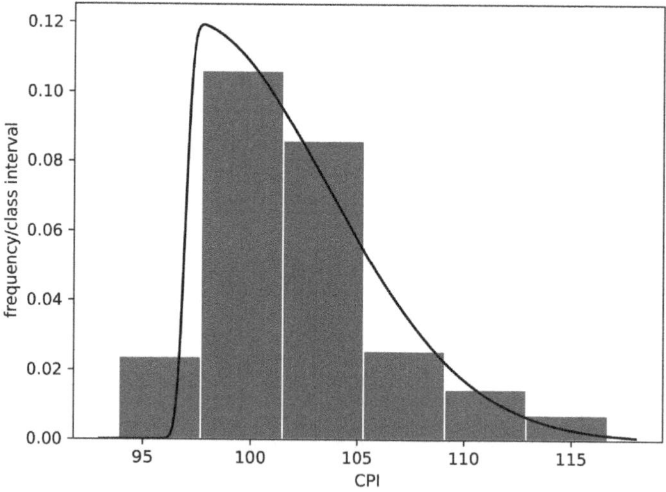


**Figure 9.1:** CPI histogram and probability density curve.

In model (9.1), $y$ is a $144 \times 1$ observed values. Assume that $\alpha \sim N_8(0, \sigma_\alpha^2 I_8)$, $\beta \sim N_6(0, \sigma_\beta^2 I_6)$, $\gamma \sim N_{48}(0, \sigma_\gamma^2 I_{48})$, $\varepsilon \sim SN_{144}(0, \sigma_\varepsilon^2 I_{144}, \alpha_\varepsilon)$, and all random vectors are mutually independent.

Firstly, consider the hypothesis testing problem for the fixed effect

$$H_0 : \mu \leq 0 \ \ versus \ \ H_1{:}\mu > 0. \tag{9.29}$$

By (9.5), $F = 1.6608 > F_{0.05}(48, 96) = 1.4889$. Hence, the null hypothesis $H_0$ in (9.29) is rejected at the nominal significance level of 5%.

Secondly, consider the hypothesis testing problem for the single variance component

$$H_0 : \sigma_\alpha^2 \leq 2 \ \ versus \ \ H_1{:}\sigma_\alpha^2 > 2. \tag{9.30}$$

From (9.14) and (9.16), the Bootstrap p-value and generalized p-value are respectively 0.3681 and 0.3778 by $10^4$ loops. Hence, the null hypothesis $H_0$ in (9.30) is not rejected by the above two approaches at the nominal significance level of 5%.

Thirdly, consider the hypothesis testing problem for the sum of variance components

$$H_0 : \sigma_\alpha^2 + \sigma_\beta^2 + \sigma_\gamma^2 \leq 10 \ \ versus \ \ H_1{:}\sigma_\alpha^2 + \sigma_\beta^2 + \sigma_\gamma^2 > 10. \tag{9.31}$$

The Bootstrap p-value by (9.20) is 0.0426, and the generalized p-value by (9.21) is 0.0307. Therefore, the above two p-values indicate that these two approaches both reject the null hypothesis $H_0$ in (9.31).

Finally, consider the hypothesis testing problem for the ratio of variance components

$$H_0 : \sigma_\alpha^2/\sigma_\beta^2 \leq 5 \ \ versus \ \ H_1{:}\sigma_\alpha^2/\sigma_\beta^2 > 5. \tag{9.32}$$

The Bootstrap p-value and generalized p-value are respectively 0.9425 and 0.9486 based on (9.26) and (9.28). Thus, the null hypothesis $H_0$ in (9.32) is not rejected by the two approaches at the nominal significance level of 5%.

**Example 9.2** The proposed approaches are applied to the value-added index of three industries in northwest China from 2010 to 2018. Similar to Example 9.1, Shapiro-Wilk, Anderson-Darling and Cramer-von Mises tests are used to conduct the normality test for the data. It shows that the p-values of the value-added indexes of three industries are 0.0003, 8.43e-05 and 0.0004 respectively. Therefore, the data is not normally distributed at the nominal significance level of 5%. Furthermore, to verify the skew-normality of the data, we intend to test the null hypothesis $H_0$: the value-added index of three industries are skew-normally distributed. The fitted value of the data is $\chi^2 = 5.2167 < \chi_2^2(0.95) = 5.9915$. Thus, the value-added index of three industries in northwest China is considered to follow the skew-normal distribution $SN(104.2468, 5.9352^2, 2.7602)$ at the nominal significance level of 5% and its density curve is given in Figure 9.2.

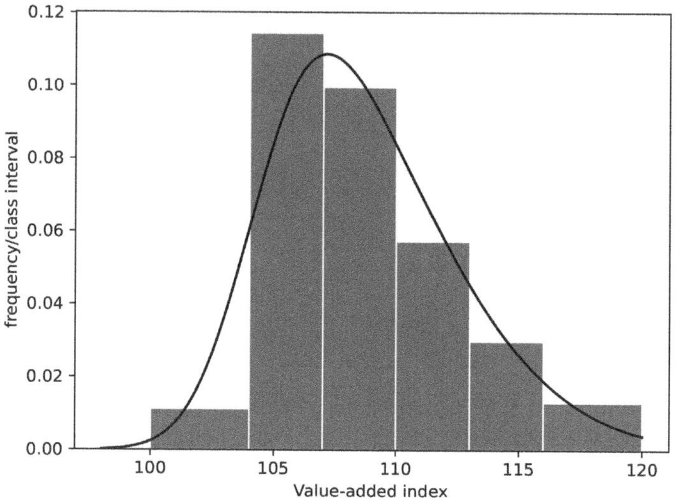

**Figure 9.2:** Value-added index histogram and probability density curve.

In model (9.1), $y$ is a $135 \times 1$ observed values. Assume that $\alpha \sim N_3(0, \sigma_\alpha^2 I_3)$, $\beta \sim N_9(0, \sigma_\beta^2 I_9)$, $\gamma \sim N_{27}(0, \sigma_\gamma^2 I_{27})$, $\varepsilon \sim SN_{135}(0, \sigma_\varepsilon^2 I_{135}, \alpha_\varepsilon)$, and all random vectors are mutually independent.

First of all, consider the hypothesis testing problem for the fixed effect

$$H_0 : \mu \leq 0 \ \ versus \ \ H_1{:}\mu > 0. \tag{9.33}$$

By (9.5), $F = 2.4090 > F_{0.05}(27, 108) = 1.5893$. Therefore, the null hypothesis $H_0$ in (9.33) is rejected at the nominal significance level of 5%.

Next, consider the hypothesis testing problem for the single variance component

$$H_0 : \sigma_\alpha^2 \leq 2 \ \ versus \ \ H_1{:}\sigma_\alpha^2 > 2. \tag{9.34}$$

For $10^4$ loops, the Bootstrap p-value by (9.14) is 0.0099, and the generalized p-value by (9.16) is 0.0113. Hence, the above two p-values indicate that these two approaches both reject the null hypothesis $H_0$ in (9.34).

Then, consider the hypothesis testing problem for the sum of variance components

$$H_0 : \sigma_\alpha^2 + \sigma_\beta^2 + \sigma_\gamma^2 \leq 12 \ \ versus \ \ H_1{:}\sigma_\alpha^2 + \sigma_\beta^2 + \sigma_\gamma^2 > 12. \tag{9.35}$$

By (9.20) and (9.21), the Bootstrap p-value and generalized p-value are respectively 0.0292 and 0.0223. As a result, the null hypothesis $H_0$ in (9.35) is rejected by the two approaches at the nominal significance level of 5%.

Finally, consider the hypothesis testing problem for the ratio of variance components

$$H_0 : \sigma_\alpha^2/\sigma_\beta^2 \leq 5 \ \ versus \ \ H_1:\sigma_\alpha^2/\sigma_\beta^2 > 5. \tag{9.36}$$

Based on (9.26) and (9.28), the Bootstrap p-value and generalized p-value are respectively 0.9869 and 0.6793. Thus, the null hypothesis $H_0$ in (9.36) is not rejected by the two approaches at the nominal significance level of 5%.

# Chapter 10

# Skew-Normal Mixed Effects Model

In many practical problems, longitudinal data are more common and more frequently show various characteristics of a skewed distribution, such as skew-normal distribution, skew-t distribution and skew-elliptical distribution. Among many skewed distributions, the skew-normal distribution can be said to be the most common in the actual longitudinal data fitting distribution. Obviously, if we simply follow the traditional normal distribution assumption to conduct statistical inference research on mixed effect models at this time, it is easy to lead to the lack of robustness of statistical inference methods and misleading conclusions (Zhang and Davidian, 2001). From this point of view, the existing classical theories and methods on the normal mixed effect model are still not enough to make more accurate statistical inferences on the actual longitudinal data. It is necessary to study the statistical modeling of longitudinal data deeply under the assumption of skew-normal distribution.

In view of this, this chapter will build on the common distribution characteristics of actual longitudinal data, under the assumption of a skew-normal distribution, study the statistical inference theory of mixed effect models, establish several new and effective statistical inference methods, and apply them to the analysis of skew-normal longitudinal data of economic and social reality problems. This can provide effective statistical methods and tools for actual longitudinal data analysis, which helps to improve the accuracy of data analysis and solve practical problems, and has important practical significance.

# 10.1 Skew-normal mixed effect model with two random effects

Let $M_{n \times k}$ be the set of all $n \times k$ matrices over the real field $\Re$ and $\Re^n = M_{n \times 1}$. For any $B \in M_{n \times k}$, use $B'$, $B^+$, $B^-$, $rk(B)$, and $\mathcal{M}(B)$ to denote the transpose, the Moore-Penrose inverse, the generalized inverse, the rank, and the column space of $B$, respectively. Let $P_B = B(B'B)^- B'$ and $N_B = I_n - P_B$. For any non-negative definite matirx $T \in M_{n \times n}$ and $m > 0$, use $tr(T)$ and $\rho(T)$ to denote the trace and the inverse of the largest eigenvalue of $T$, respectively, and use $T^m$ and $T^{-m}$ to denote the $m$th non-negative definite roots of $T$ and $T^+$, respectively. Also for $B \in M_{m \times n}$ and $C \in M_{p \times q}$, use $B \otimes C$ to denote the Kronecker product of $B$ and $C$.

We consider the linear mixed model with skew-normal random effects given by

$$y = X\beta + Z\varepsilon + \varepsilon_0, \tag{10.1}$$

where $y$ is a $n \times 1$ random vector, $X$ and $Z$ are $n \times p$ and $n \times k$ design matrices, respectively, $\beta$ is a $p \times 1$ vector of fixed effects, $\varepsilon$ is a $k \times 1$ vector of random effects, and $\varepsilon_0$ is a $n \times 1$ vector of random errors. In this chapter, we assume that $\varepsilon \sim SN_k(0, \sigma_1^2 I_k, \alpha)$, $\varepsilon_0 \sim N_n(0, \sigma_0^2 I_n)$, and $\varepsilon$ and $\varepsilon_0$ are mutually independent, where $SN_m(\mu, \Sigma, \alpha)$ denotes a $m$-dimensional multivariate skew-normal distribution, with location parameter $\mu$, positive definite scale parameter $\Sigma$, and skewness parameter $\alpha$, $N_m(\mu, \Sigma)$ denotes a $m$-dimensional multivariate normal distribution, with mean vector $\mu$ and covariance matrix $\Sigma$. When $\sigma_0^2 = 0$ and $\alpha = 0$, this model is respectively reduced to the skew-normal regression model and usual normal linear mixed model.

This section will systematically explore statistical properties such as density function, moment generation function (MGF), mean vector, covariance matrix, and independence condition for the skew-normal mixed effects model (10.1). On this basis, the necessary and sufficient conditions for the observation vector quadratic form of the skew-normal mixed effect model to follow the noncentral skew chi-square distribution are proved, and the Cochran theorem under the model is given. Finally, based on the noncentral skew-F distribution, construct test statistics for regression coefficients and variance components, and prove that these test methods are exact tests.

## 10.1.1 *Quadratic form and its Cochran's theorem*

**Theorem 10.1.** *Suppose that the model $y$ is given in (10.1). Then*
*(i) The MGF of $y$ is*

$$M_y(t) = 2\exp\left(t'\mu_y + \frac{t'\Sigma_y t}{2}\right) \Phi\left\{\frac{\sigma_1 \alpha' Z' t}{(1 + \alpha'\alpha)^{1/2}}\right\}, \qquad t \in \Re^n, \tag{10.2}$$

*where $\mu_y = X\beta$ and $\Sigma_y = \sigma_0^2 I_n + \sigma_1^2 ZZ'$. $\Phi(\cdot)$ denotes the standard normal cumulative distribution function.*

*(ii) The density function of y is*

$$f_y(x;\mu_y,\Sigma_y,\alpha_1) = 2\phi_n(x;\mu_y,\Sigma_y)\Phi(\alpha_1'\Sigma_y^{-1/2}(x-\mu_y)), \qquad x \in \Re^n, \qquad (10.3)$$

*where $\phi_n(x;\mu,\Sigma_y)$ is the n-dimensional normal density function and*
$\alpha_1 = \dfrac{\sigma_1\Sigma_y^{-1/2}Z\alpha}{[1+\alpha'(I_k-\sigma_1^2 Z'\Sigma_y^{-1}Z)\alpha]^{1/2}}$. *We denote $Y \sim SN_n(\mu_y,\Sigma_y,\alpha_1)$.*
*(iii) The mean vector and covariance matrix of y are*

$$E(y) = \mu_y + \sqrt{\frac{2}{\pi}}\frac{\Sigma_y^{1/2}\alpha_1}{(1+\alpha_1'\alpha_1)^{1/2}}, \qquad Cov(y) = \Sigma_y^{1/2}\left(I_n - \frac{2\alpha_1\alpha_1'}{\pi(1+\alpha_1'\alpha_1)}\right)\Sigma_y^{1/2}.$$

$$(10.4)$$

The proof of this theorem is similar to those of Theorems 2.1–2.2 and Corollary 2.1, so the proof process is omitted.

**Corollary 10.1.** *Let $V_1 \sim SN_n(\mu_1,\Sigma_1,\alpha)$ and $V_2 \sim N_n(\mu_2,\Sigma_2)$. If $V_1$ and $V_2$ are independent, then for any a, $b \in \Re$,*

$$aV_1 + bV_2 \sim SN_n(a\mu_1 + b\mu_2, a^2\Sigma_1 + b^2\Sigma_2, \alpha_*), \qquad (10.5)$$

*where $\alpha_* = \dfrac{a(a^2\Sigma_1+b^2\Sigma_2)^{-1/2}\Sigma_1^{1/2}\alpha}{\left\{1+\alpha'\left[I_n-a^2\Sigma_1^{1/2}(a^2\Sigma_1+b^2\Sigma_2)^{-1}\Sigma_1^{1/2}\right]\alpha\right\}^{1/2}}$.*

The proof techniques applied in Theorem 2.2 can similarly prove Corollary 10.1.

**Remark 10.1.** *Corollary 10.1 is an extension of the result of Azzalini (2005) to the multivariate version, where $V_1 \sim SN(0,1,\alpha)$, $V_2 \sim N(0,1)$, $aV_1 + bV_2 \sim SN(0, a^2 + b^2, \alpha_*)$, and $\alpha_* = \dfrac{a\alpha}{[a^2+b^2(1+\alpha'\alpha)]^{1/2}}$.*

**Theorem 10.2.** *Suppose that the model y is given in (10.1). For any $B_i \in M_{k_i \times n}$, $i = 1,2$, then $B_1 y$ and $B_2 y$ are independent if and only if*
*(i) $B_1\Sigma_y B_2' = 0$ and*
*(ii) either $B_1\Sigma_y^{1/2}\alpha_1 = 0$ or $B_2\Sigma_y^{1/2}\alpha_1 = 0$,*

*where $\Sigma_y = \sigma_0^2 I_n + \sigma_1^2 ZZ'$ and $\alpha_1 = \dfrac{\sigma_1\Sigma_y^{-1/2}Z\alpha}{[1+\alpha'(I_k-\sigma_1^2 Z'\Sigma_y^{-1}Z)\alpha]^{1/2}}$.*

The proof of this theorem is similar to Theorem 2.3, so the proof process is omitted.

**Theorem 10.3.** *For the model y given in* (10.1), *let* $Q = y'Ay/\sigma^2$ *with symmetric* $A \in M_{n \times n}$, $m = rk(A)$, *and* $\sigma^2 = \frac{1}{m}[\sigma_0^2 tr(A) + \sigma_1^2 tr(AZZ')]$. *Then the MGF of Q is*

$$
M_Q(t) = \frac{2\exp\left\{-\frac{1}{2\sigma^2}\mu_y'\Omega^{-1}\mu_y + \frac{1}{2\sigma^2}\mu_y'\Omega^{-1}(I_n - 2t\Omega A)^{-1}\mu_y\right\}}{|I_n - 2t\Omega A|^{1/2}}
$$

$$
\times \Phi\left\{\frac{\alpha_1'\Omega^{-1/2}[(I_n - 2t\Omega A)^{-1} - I_n]\mu_y/\sigma}{[1 + \alpha_1'\Omega^{-1/2}(I_n - 2t\Omega A)^{-1}\Omega^{1/2}\alpha_1]^{1/2}}\right\}, \tag{10.6}
$$

$$
E(Q) = m + \mu_y'A\mu_y/\sigma^2 + \frac{4\mu_y'A\Omega^{1/2}\alpha_1}{[2\pi\sigma^2(1 + \alpha_1'\alpha_1)]^{1/2}}, \tag{10.7}
$$

$$
Var(Q) = 4\mu_y'A\Omega A\mu_y/\sigma^2 + 2tr(\Omega A)^2 - \frac{8(\alpha_1'\Omega^{1/2}A\mu_y)^2}{\pi\sigma^2(1 + \alpha_1'\alpha_1)}
$$

$$
+ \frac{16\alpha_1'\Omega^{1/2}A\Omega A\mu_y(1 + \alpha_1'\alpha_1) - 8\alpha_1'\Omega^{1/2}A\mu_y(\alpha_1'\Omega^{1/2}A\Omega^{1/2}\alpha_1)}{[2\pi\sigma^2(1 + \alpha_1'\alpha_1)^3]^{1/2}}, \tag{10.8}
$$

*for* $t \in \Re$ *such that* $2|t| < \rho(\Omega A)$, *where* $\mu_y = X\beta$, $\Sigma_y = \sigma_0^2 I_n + \sigma_1^2 ZZ' = \sigma^2\Omega$,

*and* $\alpha_1 = \dfrac{\sigma_1 \Sigma_y^{-1/2} Z\alpha}{[1 + \alpha'(I_k - \sigma_1^2 Z'\Sigma_y^{-1}Z)\alpha]^{1/2}}$.

The proof of this theorem is similar to those of Theorem 2.5 and Corollary 2.3, so the proof process is omitted.

**Lemma 10.1.** *Assume* $\mu_y \in R^n$, $\lambda > 0$, $\sigma^2 > 0$, *m is a positive integer*, $m \leq n$, $\Omega$ *is a $n \times n$ positive definite matrix*, $rk(A) = m$. *If*

$$
\frac{2\exp\left\{-\frac{1}{2\sigma^2}\mu_y'\Omega^{-1}\mu_y + \frac{1}{2\sigma^2}\mu_y'\Omega^{-1}(I_n - 2t\Omega A)^{-1}\mu_y\right\}}{|I_n - 2t\Omega A|^{1/2}}
$$

$$
= \frac{\exp\left\{t(1 - 2t)^{-1}\lambda\right\}}{(1 - 2t)^{m/2}}
$$

*where* $t \in R$, $|t| < min\{1, \rho(\Omega A)\}$. *The following conclusions are given by*
*(i)* $\Omega A$ *is idempotent of rank m,*
*(ii)* $\lambda = \mu_y'A\mu_y/\sigma^2$.

The proof of this Lemma is similar to that of Lemma 2.3, so the proof process is omitted.

**Theorem 10.4.** *For the model y given in* (10.1), *let* $Q = y'Ay/\sigma^2$ *with symmetric* $A \in M_{n \times n}$, $m = rk(A)$, *and* $\sigma^2 = \frac{1}{m}[\sigma_0^2 tr(A) + \sigma_1^2 tr(AZZ')]$. *Then the necessary and sufficient conditions under which* $Q \sim S\chi_m^2(\lambda, \delta_1, \delta_2)$, *for some* $\delta_1 \in \Re$ *including* $\delta_1 = 0$, *are*

*(i) $\Omega A$ is idempotent of rank m,*

*(ii) $\lambda = \mu_y' A \mu_y / \sigma^2$,*

*(iii) $\delta_1 = \alpha_1' \Omega^{1/2} A \mu_y / (d\sigma)$, and*

*(iv) $\delta_2 = \alpha_1' P_1 P_1' \alpha_1 / d^2$,*

*where $\mu_y = X\beta$, $\Sigma_y = \sigma_0^2 I_n + \sigma_1^2 ZZ' = \sigma^2 \Omega$, $\alpha_1 = \dfrac{\sigma_1 \Sigma_y^{-1/2} Z\alpha}{[1+\alpha'(I_k - \sigma_1^2 Z'\Sigma_y^{-1}Z)\alpha]^{1/2}}$, $d = (1+\alpha_1' P_2 P_2' \alpha_1)^{1/2}$, and $P = (P_1, P_2)$ is an orthogonal matrix in $M_{n\times n}$ such that*

$$\Omega^{1/2} A \Omega^{1/2} = P \begin{pmatrix} I_m & 0 \\ 0 & 0 \end{pmatrix} P' = P_1 P_1'. \tag{10.9}$$

Similar to the proof process of Theorem 2.6, the above theorem can be proven based on Lemma 10.1.

**Example 10.1** Consider the one-way classification model with skew-normal random effects given by

$$y = 1_{ab}\mu + (I_a \otimes 1_b)\varepsilon + \varepsilon_0,$$

where $\mu \in \Re$ is a fixed effect, $\varepsilon \sim SN_a(0, \sigma_1^2 I_a, \alpha)$, $\varepsilon_0 \sim N_{ab}(0, \sigma_0^2 I_{ab})$, $\varepsilon$ and $\varepsilon_0$ are mutually independent. Denote $X = 1_{ab}$ and $Z = I_a \otimes 1_b$. Let $Q = y'Ay/\sigma^2$, where $A = P_Z = I_a \otimes \bar{J}_b$, $\sigma^2 = \sigma_0^2 + b\sigma_1^2$ and $\bar{J}_m = 1_m 1_m'/m$.

Specifically, let $a = b = 2$, $\sigma_1^2 = 1$, $\sigma_0^2 = 2$, and $\alpha = 1_2$. We aim to find the distribution of $Q$. It is easy to calculate that

$$A = \frac{1}{2}\begin{pmatrix} 1 & 1 & 0 & 0 \\ 1 & 1 & 0 & 0 \\ 0 & 0 & 1 & 1 \\ 0 & 0 & 1 & 1 \end{pmatrix}, \Omega = \frac{1}{4}\begin{pmatrix} 3 & 1 & 0 & 0 \\ 1 & 3 & 0 & 0 \\ 0 & 0 & 3 & 1 \\ 0 & 0 & 1 & 3 \end{pmatrix}, \Omega A = \frac{1}{2}\begin{pmatrix} 1 & 1 & 0 & 0 \\ 1 & 1 & 0 & 0 \\ 0 & 0 & 1 & 1 \\ 0 & 0 & 1 & 1 \end{pmatrix}.$$

Note that $\Omega A$ is idempotent of rank 2, (i) of Theorem 10.4 is satisfied. Also

$$\lambda = \mu_y' A \mu_y / \sigma^2 = \mu^2 1_4'(I_2 \otimes \bar{J}_2)1_4/4 = \mu^2,$$

so (ii) of Theorem 10.4 holds. Since $\Omega^{1/2} A \Omega^{1/2}$ is idempotent of rank 2, we obtain the orthogonal matrix $P$ such that $\Omega^{1/2} A \Omega^{1/2} = P\,\mathrm{diag}(1,1,0,0)P'$, where

$$P = (P_1, P_2) = \begin{pmatrix} \frac{\sqrt{2}}{2} & 0 & \frac{\sqrt{2}}{2} & 0 \\ \frac{\sqrt{2}}{2} & 0 & -\frac{\sqrt{2}}{2} & 0 \\ 0 & \frac{\sqrt{2}}{2} & 0 & \frac{\sqrt{2}}{2} \\ 0 & \frac{\sqrt{2}}{2} & 0 & -\frac{\sqrt{2}}{2} \end{pmatrix} \quad \text{with} \quad P_1 = \begin{pmatrix} \frac{\sqrt{2}}{2} & 0 \\ \frac{\sqrt{2}}{2} & 0 \\ 0 & \frac{\sqrt{2}}{2} \\ 0 & \frac{\sqrt{2}}{2} \end{pmatrix}.$$

Note that

$$\alpha_1 = \frac{\sigma_1 \Omega^{-1/2} Z\alpha/\sigma}{[1+\alpha'(I_a - \sigma_1^2 Z'\Omega^{-1}Z/\sigma^2)\alpha]^{1/2}} = \frac{\sqrt{2}}{4}1_4,$$

$$d = (1+\alpha_1'P_2P_2'\alpha_1)^{1/2} = 1,$$

$$\alpha_2 = P_1'\alpha_1/d = \frac{1}{2}1_2,$$

$$v = P_1'\Omega^{1/2}A\mu_y/\sigma = \frac{\sqrt{2}}{2}\mu 1_2,$$

so that $\delta_1 = \alpha_2'v = \frac{\sqrt{2}}{2}\mu$ and $\delta_2 = \alpha_2'\alpha_2 = \frac{1}{2}$. Thus it is easy to check that (iii) and (iv) of Theorem 10.4 are satisfied. Therefore by Theorem 10.4, $Q \sim S\chi_2^2(\lambda,\delta_1,\delta_2)$.

**Definition 10.1.** *Let $U$ be a random vector in $\Re^n$ such that $U \sim SN_n(v,I_n,\zeta)$. Partition $U$, $v$, $\zeta$ into $\ell+1$ parts, respectively, i.e.,*

$$U = \begin{pmatrix} U_1 \\ \vdots \\ U_\ell \\ U_{\ell+1} \end{pmatrix}, \qquad v = \begin{pmatrix} v_1 \\ \vdots \\ v_\ell \\ v_{\ell+1} \end{pmatrix}, \qquad \zeta = \begin{pmatrix} \zeta_1 \\ \vdots \\ \zeta_\ell \\ \zeta_{\ell+1} \end{pmatrix}, \qquad (10.10)$$

*where $U_i$, $v_i$, $\zeta_i \in \Re^{m_i}$ for $i = 1,2,\cdots,\ell+1$, and $U_{\ell+1}$, $v_{\ell+1}$, $\zeta_{\ell+1} \in \Re^{m_{\ell+1}}$ with $m_{\ell+1} = n - \sum_{i=1}^{\ell} m_i \geq 0$. Then the joint distribution of $(U_1'U_1,\cdots,U_\ell'U_\ell)'$, denoted by*

$$(U_1'U_1,\cdots,U_\ell'U_\ell)' \sim GS\chi_{m_1,\cdots,m_\ell}^2(\lambda_1,\cdots,\lambda_\ell;\eta_{11},\cdots,\eta_{1\ell};\eta_{21},\cdots,\eta_{2\ell};\eta_2),$$
$$(10.11)$$

*is defined as the generalized noncentral skew chi-square distribution with parameters $m_1,\cdots,m_\ell$, $\lambda_1,\cdots,\lambda_\ell$, $\eta_{11},\cdots,\eta_{1\ell}$, $\eta_{21},\cdots,\eta_{2\ell}$, and $\eta_2$, where $\lambda_i = v_i'v_i$, $\eta_{1i} = \zeta_i'v_i$, $\eta_{2i} = \zeta_i'\zeta_i$, $i = 1,\cdots,\ell$, and $\eta_2 = \zeta'\zeta$. In particular, when $\ell = 1$, $m = m_1$, and $\lambda = \lambda_1$, the distribution of $U_1'U_1$ is*

$$U_1'U_1 \sim GS\chi_m^2(\lambda;\eta_{11};\eta_{21};\eta_2).$$

**Remark 10.2.** *The relationship between $S\chi_m^2(\lambda,\delta_1,\delta_2)$ in Definition 2.2 and $GS\chi_m^2(\lambda;\eta_{11};\eta_{21};\eta_2)$ in Definition 10.1 is given below*

$$\delta_1 = \eta_{11}/(1+\eta_2-\eta_{21})^{1/2}, \quad \delta_2 = \eta_{21}/(1+\eta_2-\eta_{21}),$$

*and $\eta_2 = \eta_{21} + \eta_{22}$.*

**Lemma 10.2.** *For the model* $y$ *given in* (10.1), *let* $Q_i = y'A_i y/\sigma_{*i}^2$ *with non-negative definite* $A_i \in M_{n\times n}$, $m_i = rk(A_i)$, *and* $\sigma_{*i}^2 = \frac{1}{m_i}[\sigma_0^2 tr(A_i) + \sigma_1^2 tr(A_i ZZ')]$, $i = 1, \cdots, \ell$. *Then the MGF of* $Q = (Q_1, Q_2, \cdots, Q_\ell)'$ *is*

$$
M_Q(t) = \frac{2\exp\left\{ -\frac{1}{2}\mu_y'\Sigma_y^{-1}\mu_y + \frac{1}{2}\mu_y'\Sigma_y^{-1}(I_n - 2\Sigma_y\tilde{A})^{-1}\mu_y \right\}}{|I_n - 2\Sigma_y\tilde{A}|^{1/2}}
$$

$$
\times \Phi\left\{ \frac{\alpha_1'\Sigma_y^{-1/2}[(I_n - 2\Sigma_y\tilde{A})^{-1} - I_n]\mu_y}{[1 + \alpha_1'\Sigma_y^{-1/2}(I_n - 2\Sigma_y\tilde{A})^{-1}\Sigma_y^{1/2}\alpha_1]^{1/2}} \right\}, \tag{10.12}
$$

*for all* $t = (t_1, \cdots, t_\ell)'$ *in the neighborhood of* $0 \in \Re^\ell$, *where* $\mu_y = X\beta$, $\Sigma_y = \sigma_0^2 I_n + \sigma_1^2 ZZ'$, $\tilde{A} = \sum_{i=1}^{\ell} t_i A_i/\sigma_{*i}^2$, *and* $\alpha_1 = \dfrac{\sigma_1 \Sigma_y^{-1/2} Z\alpha}{[1 + \alpha'(I_k - \sigma_1^2 Z'\Sigma_y^{-1} Z)\alpha]^{1/2}}$.

*Proof.* Note that the MGF of $Q$ is

$$
M_Q(t) = E\left[ \exp\left( \sum_{i=1}^{\ell} t_i Q_i \right) \right] = E\left[ \exp\left( y'\tilde{A}y \right) \right].
$$

Thus Equation (10.12) is obtained by replacing $tA/\sigma^2$ with $\tilde{A}$ in Equation (10.6) of Theorem 10.3. $\qquad\square$

**Lemma 10.3.** *Assume* $q = (q_1, q_2, \cdots, q_\ell)' \sim GS\chi^2_{m_1,\cdots,m_\ell}(\lambda_1, \cdots, \lambda_\ell; \eta_{11}, \cdots, \eta_{1\ell};$ $\eta_{21}, \cdots, \eta_{2\ell}; \eta_2)$, *where* $q_i = U_i'U_i$, $\lambda_i = v_i'v_i$, $\eta_{1i} = \zeta_i'v_i$, $\eta_{2i} = \zeta_i'\zeta_i$, $\eta_2 = \zeta'\zeta$, $i = 1, \cdots, \ell$, *and* $U_i$, $v_i$, $\zeta_i$, $\zeta$ *is given in* (10.10). *Then the MGF of* $q$ *is*

$$
M_q(t) = \frac{2\exp\left\{ \sum_{i=1}^{l} t_i(1 - 2t_i)^{-1}\lambda_i \right\}}{\prod_{i=1}^{l}(1 - 2t_i)^{m_i/2}}
$$

$$
\times \Phi\left\{ \frac{2\sum_{i=1}^{l} t_i(1 - 2t_i)^{-1}\eta_{1i}}{[1 + \eta_2 + 2\sum_{i=1}^{l} t_i(1 - 2t_i)^{-1}\eta_{2i}]^{1/2}} \right\}, \tag{10.13}
$$

*where* $t = (t_1, t_2, \cdots, t_l)'$ *takes values near* $0 \in R^l$.

The proof of Lemma 10.3 is shown in Wang et al. (2009).

**Theorem 10.5.** *For the model $y$ given in (10.1), let $Q_i = y'A_i y/\sigma^2_{*i}$ with nonnegative definite $A_i \in M_{n \times n}$, $m_i = rk(A_i)$, and $\sigma^2_{*i} = \frac{1}{m_i}[\sigma^2_0 tr(A_i) + \sigma^2_1 tr(A_i ZZ')]$, $i = 1, \cdots, \ell$. Assume $U \sim SN_n(v, I_n, \zeta)$, given in (10.10). Then*

$$Q_i \stackrel{d}{=} U_i' U_i \sim GS\chi^2_{m_i}(\lambda_i; \eta_{1i}; \eta_{2i}; \eta_2)$$

*if and only if, for some $\eta_{1i} \in R$ including $\eta_{1i} = 0$:*
*(i) $\Omega_i A_i$ is idempotent of rank $m_i$,*
*(ii) $\lambda_i = \mu_y' A_i \mu_y / \sigma^2_{*i}$,*
*(iii) $\eta_{1i} = \alpha_1' \Omega_i^{1/2} A_i \mu_y / \sigma_{*i}$, and*
*(iv) $\eta_{2i} = \alpha_1' P_i P_i' \alpha_1$,*

*where $\mu_y = X\beta$, $\Sigma_y = \sigma^2_0 I_n + \sigma^2_1 ZZ' = \sigma^2_{*i} \Omega_i$, $\alpha_1 = \dfrac{\sigma_1 \Sigma_y^{-1/2} Z\alpha}{[1 + \alpha'(I_k - \sigma^2_1 Z'\Sigma_y^{-1}Z)\alpha]^{1/2}}$, $v_i = P_1' \Omega_i^{1/2} A_i \mu_y / \sigma_{*i}$, $\zeta = P'\alpha_1$, $\eta_2 = \alpha_1'\alpha_1$, and $P = (P_1, P_2)$ is an orthogonal matrix in $M_{n \times n}$ such that*

$$\Omega_i^{1/2} A_i \Omega_i^{1/2} = P \begin{pmatrix} I_{m_i} & 0 \\ 0 & 0 \end{pmatrix} P' = P_i P_i'. \tag{10.14}$$

*Proof.* By Theorem 10.4, it suffices to show that (iii) and (iv) of Theorem 10.4 are equivalent to (iii) and (iv) of Theorem 10.5, respectively. Note that $\zeta = P'\alpha_1$, then $\zeta_i = P_1'\alpha_1$. From Remark 10.2, we have $U_i' U_i \sim S\chi^2_{m_i}(\lambda_i, \delta_{1i}, \delta_{2i})$ with $\delta_{1i} = \zeta_*' v_i$ and $\delta_{2i} = \zeta_*' \zeta_*$, where $\zeta_* = \zeta_i / (1 + \zeta'\zeta - \zeta_i'\zeta_i)^{1/2}$. Now,

$$\zeta_* = \zeta_i / (1 + \alpha_1'\alpha_1 - \alpha_1' P_1 P_1' \alpha_1)^{1/2} = \zeta_i / d$$

and $\eta_{ji} = d\delta_{ji}$ for $j = 1, 2$, where $d = (1 + \alpha_1' P_2 P_2' \alpha_1)^{1/2}$, so the desired result follows. $\qquad\square$

**Theorem 10.6.** *For the model $y$ given in (10.1), let $Q_i = y'A_i y/\sigma^2_{*i}$ with nonnegative definite $A_i \in M_{n \times n}$, $m_i = r(A_i)$, and $\sigma^2_{*i} = \frac{1}{m_i}[\sigma^2_0 tr(A_i) + \sigma^2_1 tr(A_i ZZ')]$, $i = 1, \cdots, \ell$. Let $Q = (Q_1, \cdots, Q_\ell)'$. Then*

$$Q \sim GS\chi^2_{m_1, \cdots, m_\ell}(\lambda_1, \cdots, \lambda_\ell; \eta_{11}, \cdots, \eta_{1\ell}; \eta_{21}, \cdots, \eta_{2\ell}; \eta_2)$$

*if and only if, for any distinct $i, j \in \{1, \cdots, \ell\}$ and some $\eta_{1i} \in \Re$ including $\eta_{1i} = 0$:*
*(i) $\Omega_i A_i$ is idempotent of rank $m_i$,*
*(ii) $\lambda_i = \mu_y' A_i \mu_y / \sigma^2_{*i}$,*
*(iii) $A_i A_j = 0$,*
*(iv) $\eta_{1i} = \alpha_1' \Omega_i^{1/2} A_i \mu_y / \sigma_{*i}$, and*
*(v) $\eta_{2i} = \alpha_1' P_i P_i' \alpha_1$,*

*where* $\mu_y = X\beta$, $\Sigma_y = \sigma_0^2 I_n + \sigma_1^2 ZZ' = \sigma_{*i}^2 \Omega_i$, $\alpha_1 = \dfrac{\sigma_1 \Sigma_y^{-1/2} Z\alpha}{[1+\alpha'(I_k - \sigma_1^2 Z'\Sigma_y^{-1} Z)\alpha]^{1/2}}$, $\eta_2 =$ $\alpha_1'\alpha_1$, *and* $P = (P_1, \cdots, P_\ell, P_{\ell+1})$ *is an orthogonal matrix in* $M_{n \times n}$ *such that*

$$\Omega_i^{1/2} A_i \Omega_i^{1/2} = P \begin{pmatrix} 0 & 0 & 0 \\ 0 & I_{m_i} & 0 \\ 0 & 0 & 0 \end{pmatrix} P' = P_i P_i' \tag{10.15}$$

*with the upper left hand* 0 *being the square matrix of order* $\sum_{j=1}^{i-1} m_j$ *(which is* 0 *for* $i = 1$), *and the lower right hand* 0 *being the square matrix of order* $\sum_{j=i+1}^{\ell+1} m_j$.

*Proof.* First, we prove the sufficiency of Theorem 10.6. Then by (i) and (iii) there exists an orthogonal matrix $P = (P_1, \cdots, P_l, P_{l+1})$ in $M_{n \times n}$ such that (10.15) holds. From (i) and (10.15), we have

$$P_i P_i' \Omega_i^{1/2} A_i = \Omega_i^{1/2} A_i. \tag{10.16}$$

Similar to Theorem 2.6, let $U = (U_1', \cdots, U_l', U_{l+1}')' = v + P'\omega$, where $U_i = v_i + P_i'\omega, v_i = P_i'\Omega_i^{1/2} A_i \mu_y / \sigma_{*i}, \omega \sim \mathrm{SN}_n(0, I_n, \alpha_1)$. It is easy to prove $\lambda = v_i'v_i, U \sim \mathrm{SN}_n(v, I_n, \zeta), \zeta = P'\alpha_1$. Then, $\zeta_i = P_i'\alpha_1$. Notice that $\eta_{1i} = \zeta_i'v_i$ and $\eta_{2i} = \zeta_i'\zeta_i$ are equivalent to (iv) and (v), respectively. From (10.11), it suffices to verify $Q \overset{d}{=} (U_1'U_1, \cdots, U_l'U_l)'$. For any given $i \in \{1, 2, \cdots, l\}$, by (10.15) and (10.16), we can get

$$\begin{aligned} Q_i &= \left(\mu_y + \Sigma_y^{1/2}\omega\right)' A_i \left(\mu_y + \Sigma_y^{1/2}\omega\right) / \sigma_{*i}^i \\ &= \left(\mu_y + \sigma_{*i}\Omega_i^{1/2}\omega\right)' A_i \left(\mu_y + \sigma_{*i}\Omega_i^{1/2}\omega\right) / \sigma_{*i}^2 \\ &= \mu_y'A_i\mu_y / \sigma_{*i}^2 + 2\omega'\Omega_i^{1/2}A_i\mu_y / \sigma_{*i} + \omega'\Omega_i^{1/2}A_i\Omega_i^{1/2}\omega \\ &= v_i'v_i + 2\omega'P_iv_i + \omega'P_iP_i'\omega \\ &= (v_i + P_i'\omega)'(v_i + P_i'\omega) \overset{d}{=} U_i'U_i. \end{aligned}$$

Let $U_{*i} = P_i'\Omega_i^{1/2} A_i y / \sigma_{*i}, i = 1, 2, \cdots, l$. Further, we have

$$U_{*i} = P_i'\Omega_i^{1/2} A_i \left(\mu_y + \Sigma_y^{1/2}\omega\right) / \sigma_{*i} = P_i'\Omega_i^{1/2}A_i\mu_y / \sigma_{*i} + P_i'\Omega_i^{1/2}A_i\Omega_i^{1/2}\omega = v_i + P_i'\omega,$$

and it is easy to see $(U_{*1}', \cdots, U_{*l}')' \overset{d}{=} (U_1', \cdots, U_l')'$. Since Q is a Borel function of $U_{*1}', \cdots, U_{*l}'$, we have $Q \overset{d}{=} (U_1'U_1, \cdots, U_l'U_l)'$ and the desired result follows.

Next, we prove the necessity of Theorem 10.6. Let $U = \left(U_1', \cdots, U_l', U_{l+1}'\right)' \sim SN_n\left(v, I_n, \zeta\right)$ and $q = (q_1, q_2, \cdots, q_l)'$ with $q_i = U_i' U_i, i = 1, 2, \cdots, l$. By Lemmas 10.2–10.3, then $M_Q(t) = M_q(t)$. For each $i \in \{1, 2, \cdots, l\}$, $Q_i \sim GS\chi^2_{m_i}\left(\lambda_i; \eta_{1i}; \eta_{2i}; \eta_2\right)$. According to Theorem 10.5, Conditions (i) and (ii) are true. Similar to the proofs of Theorem 2.6 and Lemma 2.3, we have

$$\left|I_n - 2\Sigma_y \widetilde{A}\right| = \prod_{i=1}^{l} (1 - 2t_i)^{m_i} = \prod_{i=1}^{l} \left|I_n - 2t_i \Omega_i A_i\right|, \qquad (10.17)$$

$$\frac{\alpha_1' \Sigma_y^{-1/2} \left[\left(I_n - 2\Sigma_y \widetilde{A}\right)^{-1} - I_n\right] \mu_y}{\left[1 + \alpha_1' \Sigma_y^{-1/2} \left(I_n - 2\Sigma_y \widetilde{A}\right)^{-1} \Sigma_y^{1/2} \alpha_1\right]^{1/2}} = \frac{2\sum_{i=1}^{l} t_i (1 - 2t_i)^{-1} \eta_{1i}}{\left[1 + \eta_2 + 2\sum_{i=1}^{l} t_i (1 - 2t_i)^{-1} \eta_{2i}\right]^{1/2}}, \tag{10.18}$$

where $\widetilde{A} = \sum_{i=1}^{l} t_i A_i / \sigma_{*i}^2$ and $2|t_i| < \min\{1, \rho(\Omega_i A_i)\}$, $i = 1, 2, \cdots, l$. Note that (iii) follows from (10.17). Combining (i) and (iii), there exists an orthogonal matrix $P \in M_{n \times n}$ which satisfies (10.15). For any given $i \in \{1, 2, \cdots, l\}$, let $t_j = 0$, $j = 1, 2, \cdots, l$, $j \neq i$, so that (10.18) is reduced to

$$\frac{\alpha_1' \Omega_i^{-1/2} \left[(I_n - 2t_i \Omega_i A_i)^{-1} - I_n\right] \mu_y / \sigma_{*i}}{\left[1 + \alpha_1' \Omega_i^{-1/2} (I_n - 2t_i \Omega_i A_i)^{-1} \Omega_i^{1/2} \alpha_1\right]^{1/2}} = \frac{2t_i (1 - 2t_i)^{-1} \eta_{1i}}{\left[1 + \eta_2 + 2t_i (1 - 2t_i)^{-1} \eta_{2i}\right]^{1/2}},$$

which, by Theorem 10.5, implies (iv) and (v) with $\eta_2 = \alpha_1' \alpha_1$. Thus the proof of Theorem 10.6 is completed. $\qquad \square$

**Corollary 10.2.** *For the quadratic form given in Theorem 10.6, if* $\alpha_1' \Omega_i^{1/2} A_i \mu_y = 0$, $i = 1, \cdots, \ell$, *then* $\{Q_i\}_{i=1}^{\ell}$ *is a family of independent noncentral chi-square distributed random variables and each* $Q_i \sim \chi^2_{m_i}(\lambda_i)$, *which is free of* $\eta_2 = \alpha_1' \alpha_1$, *if and only if for any distinct* $i, j \in \{1, \cdots, \ell\}$:
*(i)* $\Omega_i A_i$ *is idempotent of rank* $m_i$,
*(ii)* $\lambda_i = \mu_y' A_i \mu_y / \sigma_{*i}^2$, *and*
*(iii)* $A_i A_j = 0$,
*where* $m_i = rk(A_i)$, $\mu_y = X\beta$, $\Sigma_y = \sigma_0^2 I_n + \sigma_1^2 ZZ' = \sigma_{*i}^2 \Omega_i$, $\sigma_{*i}^2 = \frac{1}{m_i}[\sigma_0^2 tr(A_i) + \sigma_1^2 tr(A_i ZZ')]$, *and* $\alpha_1 = \dfrac{\sigma_1 \Sigma_y^{-1/2} Z\alpha}{[1 + \alpha'(I_k - \sigma_1^2 Z' \Sigma_y^{-1} Z)\alpha]^{1/2}}$.

In particular, Corollary 10.2 holds if either $\mu_y = 0$ or $\alpha_1 = 0$.

### 10.1.2 Exact inference of unknown parameters

In this section, we illustrate the applications of our results from Theorems 10.4 and 10.6. For this purpose, we need to define a new distribution, namely the noncentral skew-F distribution, which is an extension of the noncentral F distribution.

**Definition 10.2.** *Assume that* $(Q_1, Q_2) \sim GS\chi^2_{m_1,m_2}(\lambda_1, 0; \eta_{11}, 0; \eta_{21}, \eta_{22}; \eta_2)$, *where* $Q_i = U_i' U_i$ *and* $U_i$ *is given in* (10.10). *The distribution of* $F = \frac{Q_1/m_1}{Q_2/m_2}$ *is called the noncentral skew-F distribution with degrees of freedom* $m_1$ *and* $m_2$, *noncentral parameter* $\lambda_1$, *and skewness parameters* $\delta_1 = \eta_{11}/(1 + \eta_2 - \eta_{21})^{1/2}$ *and* $\delta_2 = \eta_{21}/(1 + \eta_2 - \eta_{21})$, *denoted by* $F \sim SF_{m_1,m_2}(\lambda, \delta_1, \delta_2)$.

**Remark 10.3.** *From Definition 10.2, it is easy to show that* $Q_1 \sim S\chi^2_{m_1}(\lambda, \delta_1, \delta_2)$, $Q_2 \sim \chi^2_{m_2}$. *Furthermore, by Theorem 10.2, it can be concluded that* $Q_1$ *and* $Q_2$ *are mutually independent. Hence, it can be seen that the noncentral skew-F distribution is a direct generalization of the noncentral F distribution.*

**Example 10.2** In Example 10.1, let $X = 1_{ab}$ and $Z = I_a \otimes 1_b$. It is easy to show that $y' P_z y$ and $y'(I_{ab} - P_{(X:Z)})y$ are mutually independent, where $P_z = I_a \otimes \bar{J}_b$ and $P_{(X:Z)} = P_z$. Indeed, since

$$(I_{ab} - P_{(X:Z)})\Sigma_y^{1/2}\alpha_1 = \frac{\sigma_1(I_{ab} - P_{(X:Z)})Z\alpha}{[1 + \alpha'(I_a - \sigma_1^2 Z'\Sigma_y Z)\alpha]^{1/2}} = 0$$

and

$$P_z\Sigma_y(I_{ab} - P_{(X:Z)}) = P_z(\sigma_0^2 I_{ab} + \sigma_1^2 ZZ')(I_{ab} - P_{(X:Z)}) = 0,$$

by Theorem 10.2, $P_z y$ and $(I_{ab} - P_{(X:Z)})y$ are independent and the desired result follows. Also, by Theorem 10.6, it is easy to show that

$$(y' P_z y/\sigma^2, y'(I_{ab} - P_{(X:Z)})y/\sigma_0^2)' \sim GS\chi^2_{a,a(b-1)}(\lambda_1, 0; \eta_{11}, 0; \eta_{21}, 0; \eta_2), \quad (10.19)$$

which is reduced to the joint distribution of $y' P_z y/\sigma^2 \sim S\chi^2_a(\lambda_1, \delta_1, \delta_2)$ and $y'(I_{ab} - P_{(X:Z)})y/\sigma_0^2 \sim \chi^2_{a(b-1)}$. By Definition 10.2, we have

$$F = \frac{(b-1)y'(I_a \otimes \bar{J}_b)y/\sigma^2}{y'(I_{ab} - I_a \otimes \bar{J}_b)y/\sigma_0^2} \sim SF_{a,a(b-1)}(\lambda_1, \delta_1, \delta_2).$$

Let $a = b = 2$, $\sigma_1^2 = 1$, $\sigma_0^2 = 2$, and $\alpha = 1_2$, we obtain $F \sim SF_{2,2}(\lambda_1, \delta_1, \delta_2)$, where $\lambda_1 = \mu^2$, $\delta_1 = \frac{\sqrt{2}}{2}\mu$ and $\delta_2 = \frac{1}{2}$.

Similar to the density of noncentral skew chi-square distribution, we obtain an expression for the density of noncentral skew-F distribution as follows.

**Theorem 10.7.** *Let $F \sim SF_{n_1,n_2}(\lambda,\delta_1,\delta_2)$. Then the density function of $F$ is given by*

$$f_F(x;\lambda,\delta_1,\delta_2) = \frac{n_1 e^{-\lambda/2}}{n_2 \Gamma(\tfrac{1}{2})\Gamma(\tfrac{n_1-1}{2})\Gamma(\tfrac{n_2}{2})2^{\frac{n_1+n_2}{2}-1}} h_1(x;\lambda,\delta_1,\delta_2), \qquad x > 0,$$

$$(10.20)$$

*where $\alpha_0 = \dfrac{\lambda^{-1/2}\delta_1}{(1+\delta_2-\delta_1^2/\lambda)^{1/2}}$ and*

$$h_1(x;\lambda,\delta_1,\delta_2) = \int_0^{\infty} \int_{-\sqrt{\frac{n_1 xu}{n_2}}}^{\sqrt{\frac{n_1 xu}{n_2}}} \exp\left\{-\frac{1}{2}u\left(1+\frac{n_1}{n_2}x\right)+\lambda^{1/2}v\right\}\left(\frac{n_1}{n_2}xu-v^2\right)^{\frac{n_1-3}{2}}$$

$$\times u^{n_2/2}\Phi\left\{\alpha_0(v-\lambda^{1/2})\right\}dv\,du.$$

*For the case where $\delta_1 = 0$, the density function of $F$ is*

$$f_F(x;\lambda) = e^{-\lambda/2}\,_1F_1\left(\frac{1}{2}(n_1+n_2);\frac{1}{2}n_1;\frac{\frac{1}{2}\frac{n_1}{n_2}\lambda x}{1+\frac{n_1}{n_2}x}\right)\frac{\Gamma(\frac{n_1+n_2}{2})}{\Gamma(\frac{n_1}{2})\Gamma(\frac{n_2}{2})}\frac{x^{n_1/2-1}\left(\frac{n_1}{n_2}\right)^{n_1/2}}{(1+\frac{n_1}{n_2}x)^{(n_1+n_2)/2}},x>0,$$

$$(10.21)$$

*which is free to $\delta_2$ and is denoted by $F \sim F_{n_1,n_2}(\lambda)$, where $x > 0$, $_1F_1(\kappa_1;\kappa_2;\kappa_3)$ denotes the hypergeometric function (Muirhead, 1982).*

*Proof.* Assume that $F = \dfrac{Z_1/n_1}{Z_2/n_2}$, where $Z_1 \sim S\chi_{n_1}^2(\lambda,\delta_1,\delta_2)$, $Z_2 \sim \chi_{n_2}^2$, and $Z_1$ and $Z_2$ are independent. From Theorem 2.4, the joint density function of $Z_1$ and $Z_2$ is

$$\frac{e^{-\lambda/2}\exp\left\{-\frac{z_1+z_2}{2}\right\}z_2^{n_2/2-1}}{\Gamma(\tfrac{1}{2})\Gamma(\tfrac{n_1-1}{2})\Gamma(\tfrac{n_2}{2})2^{\frac{n_1+n_2}{2}-1}}\int_{-\sqrt{z_1}}^{\sqrt{z_1}}\exp\{\lambda^{1/2}v\}(z_1-v^2)^{\frac{n_1-3}{2}}\Phi\left\{\alpha_0(v-\lambda^{1/2})\right\}dv.$$

Now make the change of variables

$$x = \frac{n_2 z_1}{n_1 z_2}, \quad u = z_2, \qquad \text{for } x > 0,\ u > 0.$$

The Jacobian of this transformation is $n_1 u/n_2$ so that the joint density function of $F$ and $Z_2$ is

$$\int_{-\sqrt{\frac{n_1 xu}{n_2}}}^{\sqrt{\frac{n_1 xu}{n_2}}} \exp\left\{-\frac{1}{2}u\left(1+\frac{n_1}{n_2}x\right)+\lambda^{1/2}v\right\}\left(\frac{n_1}{n_2}xu-v^2\right)^{\frac{n_1-3}{2}}u^{n_2/2}\Phi\left\{\alpha_0(v-\lambda^{1/2})\right\}dv$$

$$\times \frac{n_1 e^{-\lambda/2}}{n_2 \Gamma(\tfrac{1}{2})\Gamma(\tfrac{n_1-1}{2})\Gamma(\tfrac{n_2}{2})2^{\frac{n_1+n_2}{2}-1}}.$$

Now integrating with respect to $u$ over $0 < u < \infty$ gives the desired marginal density function of $F$ in (10.20). Note that when $\delta_1 = 0$, by Theorem 2.4 we have $Z_1 \sim \chi^2_{n_1}(\lambda)$. Further, we obtain $F \sim F_{n_1,n_2}(\lambda)$. By Theorem 1.3.6 of Muirhead (1982), the desired result is obtained. $\qquad\square$

Density curves of noncentral skew-F distribution are given in Figures 10.1–10.3, respectively.

In Figure 10.1, the solid curve corresponds to the density of $SF_{5,8}(5,0,10) = F_{5,8}(5)$, the noncentral F distribution with 5 and 8 degrees of freedom and non-centrality parameter 5. We can see from Figure 10.1 that the skewness parameter $\delta_1$ plays an important role between noncentral F distribution and non-central skew-F distribution. In Figure 10.2, the solid curve corresponds to the density of $SF_{10,15}(5,10,25)$ and the dashed curve corresponds to the density of $SF_{10,15}(5,-10,25)$. We know from Figure 10.2 that the signs of $\delta_1$ can change the shapes of the densities. In Figure 10.3, the solid curve corresponds to the density of $SF_{5,8}(5,2,1)$ and the dashed curve corresponds to the density of $SF_{5,8}(5,2,25)$. We know from Figure 10.3 that the values of $\delta_2$ also determine the skewness of the density curves.

**Theorem 10.8.** *Let* $F \sim \mathrm{SF}_{n_1,n_2}(\lambda,\delta_1,\delta_2)$, *then the MGF of $F$ is*

$$M_F(t) = \frac{n_1 \mathrm{e}^{-\lambda/2}}{n_2 \Gamma\left(\frac{1}{2}\right)\Gamma\left(\frac{n_1-1}{2}\right)\Gamma\left(\frac{n_2}{2}\right) 2^{\frac{n_1+n_2}{2}-1}} h_2(t;\lambda,\delta_1,\delta_2) \qquad (10.22)$$

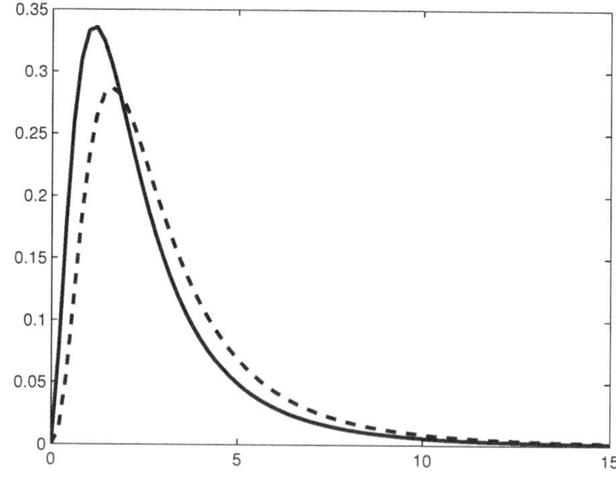

**Figure 10.1:** Density curves of $SF_{5,8}(5,0,10)$ (solid curve) and $SF_{5,8}(5,5,10)$ (dashed curve).

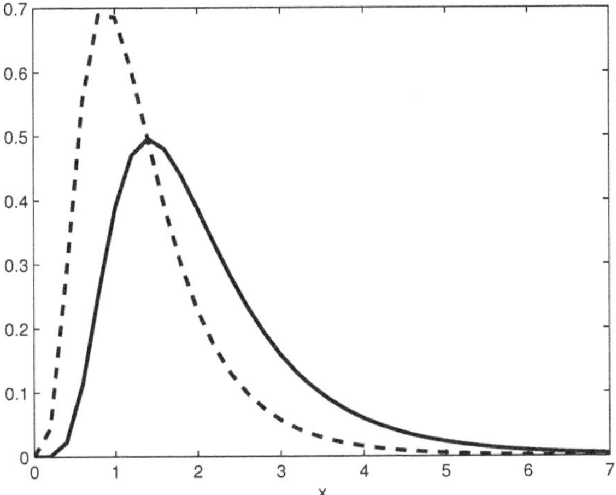

**Figure 10.2:** Density curves of $SF_{10,15}(5,10,25)$ (solid curve) and $SF_{10,15}(5,-10,25)$ (dashed curve).

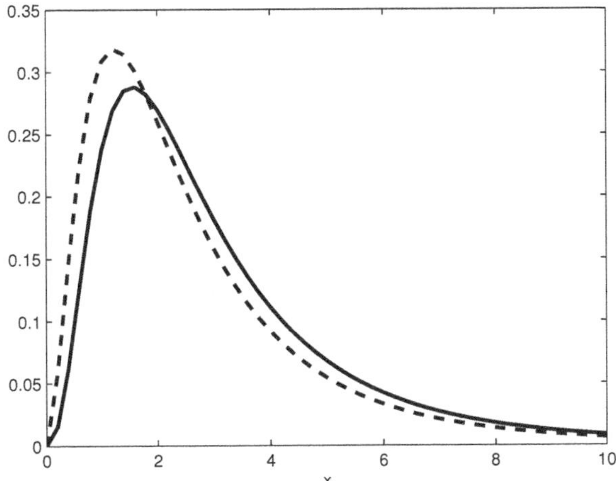

**Figure 10.3:** Density curves of $SF_{5,8}(5,2,1)$ (solid curve) and $SF_{5,8}(5,2,25)$ (dashed curve).

*where* $t \in R, \alpha_0 = \dfrac{\lambda^{-1/2}\delta_1}{\left(1+\delta_2-\delta_1^2/\lambda\right)^{1/2}}, h_2\left(x,\lambda,\delta_1,\delta_2\right) = \int_0^\infty \int_0^\infty \int_{-\sqrt{n_1 x u/n_2}}^{\sqrt{n_1 x u/n_2}} \exp$

$\left\{-\frac{1}{2}u\left(1+\frac{n_1}{n_2}x\right)+tx+\lambda^{1/2}v\right\}\left(\frac{n_1}{n_2}xu-v^2\right)^{\frac{n_1-3}{2}} \times u^{\frac{n_2}{2}}\Phi\left\{\alpha_0\left(v-\lambda^{1/2}\right)\right\}dvdudx.$

The proof of Theorem 10.8 is relatively simple, so the proof process is omitted.

Now we establish exact tests for the regression coefficient and the variance component. First, we consider the hypothesis for the variance component of the random effects

$$H_0 : \sigma_1^2 = 0 \qquad versus \qquad H_1 : \sigma_1^2 > 0. \tag{10.23}$$

A hypothesis of this form is especially important in research on longitudinal data and panel data, since model (10.1) is reduced to a usual normal linear model under $H_0$ in (10.23).

Considering the model given in (10.1), we define the test statistic

$$F_1(y) = \frac{y'(P_{(X:Z)} - P_X)y/n_1}{y'(I_n - P_{(X:Z)})y/n_2}, \tag{10.24}$$

where $n_1 = rk(X:Z) - rk(X)$ and $n_2 = n - rk(X:Z)$.

**Theorem 10.9.** *For the model $y$ given in (10.1), if $P_X ZZ' = ZZ' P_X$ and $ZZ' = cP_Z$ with a constant $c$, then*

*(i) $y'(P_{(X:Z)} - P_X)y/\sigma^2 \sim \chi_{n_1}^2$,*

*(ii) $y'(I_n - P_{(X:Z)})y/\sigma_0^2 \sim \chi_{n_2}^2$, and*

*(iii) $y'(P_{(X:Z)} - P_X)y$ and $y'(I_n - P_{(X:Z)})y$ are mutually independent,*

*where $\sigma^2 = \sigma_0^2 + c\sigma_1^2$.*

*Proof.* For (i), it suffices to show that $\lambda = 0$ and $(P_{(X:Z)} - P_X)\Omega(P_{(X:Z)} - P_X) = P_{(X:Z)} - P_X$, where $\Omega = c_1 I_n + c_2 ZZ'$, $c_1 = \sigma_0^2/\sigma^2$, $c_2 = \sigma_1^2/\sigma^2$, and $\sigma^2 = \sigma_0^2 + c\sigma_1^2$. From Theorem 10.4, we get

$$\lambda = \mu_y'(P_{(X:Z)} - P_X)\mu_y/\sigma^2 = \beta'X'(P_{(X:Z)} - P_X)X\beta/\sigma^2 = 0.$$

Further, by the conditions of Theorem 10.9, we have

$$\begin{aligned}
(P_{(X:Z)} - P_X)\Omega(P_{(X:Z)} - P_X) &= N_X P_Z(c_1 I_n + c_2 ZZ')N_X P_Z \\
&= N_X P_Z(c_1 I_n + c_2 cP_Z)N_X P_Z = (c_1 + c_2 c)N_X P_Z = P_{(X:Z)} - P_X,
\end{aligned}$$

where $N_X = I_n - P_X$. The conclusion (i) is proven.

For (ii), note that

$$y'(I_n - P_{(X:Z)})y = \varepsilon_0'(I_n - P_{(X:Z)})\varepsilon_0, \qquad \varepsilon_0 \sim N_n(0, \sigma_0^2 I_n),$$

so (ii) holds.

For (iii), it suffices to show that $(P_{(X:Z)} - P_X)y$ and $(I_n - P_{(X:Z)})y$ are independent. Since

$$(I_n - P_{(X:Z)})\Sigma_y^{1/2}\alpha_1 = \frac{\sigma_1(I_n - P_{(X:Z)})Z\alpha}{[1 + \alpha'(I_k - \sigma_1^2 Z'\Sigma_y Z)\alpha]^{1/2}} = 0$$

and

$$(P_{(X:Z)} - P_X)\Sigma_y(I_n - P_{(X:Z)}) = (P_{(X:Z)} - P_X)(\sigma_0^2 I_n + \sigma_1^2 ZZ')(I_n - P_{(X:Z)}) = 0,$$

(iii) is obtained from Theorem 10.2. Alternatively, the independence of two quadratic forms of $y$ can be obtained using Theorem 10.6. Indeed,

$$(y'(P_{(X:Z)} - P_X)y/\sigma^2, y'(I_n - P_{(X:Z)})y/\sigma_0^2)' \sim GS\chi_{n_1,n_2}^2(0,0;0,0;0,0;0),$$

which is reduced to the joint distribution of independent random variables $Z_1 \sim \chi_{n_1}^2$ and $Z_2 \sim \chi_{n_2}^2$.  $\square$

From Theorem 10.9, we know that $F_1(y)/(1+c\theta) \sim F_{n_1,n_2}$, where $\theta = \sigma_1^2/\sigma_0^2$. Note that the hypothesis given in (10.23) is equivalent to

$$H_0 : \theta = 0 \qquad versus \qquad H_1 : \theta \neq 0. \tag{10.25}$$

Let $F_{n_1,n_2}(\gamma)$ denotes the critical value of F distribution for significance level $\gamma$. By Theorem 10.9, the test for hypothesis in (10.25) is given by

$$\phi_1(F_1(y)) = \begin{cases} 1, & \text{if } F_1(y) \geq F_{n_1,n_2}(1-\gamma), \\ 0, & \text{otherwise.} \end{cases}$$

with power

$$g_1(\theta) = P(F_1(y) \geq F_{n_1,n_2}(1-\gamma)) = P\left(F_{n_1,n_2} \geq \frac{1}{1+c\theta}F_{n_1,n_2}(1-\gamma)\right).$$

For many linear mixed models, the conditions in Theorem 10.9 can be satisfied. Now we give two classic examples to illustrate it. For example, in Example 10.1, it is easy to see that $ZZ' = bP_Z = b(I_a \otimes \bar{J}_b)$ and $P_X ZZ' = ZZ' P_X = b\bar{J}_{ab}$.

**Example 10.3** Consider the two-way classification model with skew-normal random effects given by

$$y = X\beta + Z\varepsilon + \varepsilon_0,$$

where $\beta = (\mu, \beta_1, \cdots, \beta_a)'$, $X = (1_{ab} : I_a \otimes 1_b)$, $Z = 1_a \otimes I_b$, $\beta$ is the vector of fixed effects, $\varepsilon \sim SN_b(0, \sigma_1^2 I_b, \alpha)$, $\varepsilon_0 \sim N_{ab}(0, \sigma_0^2 I_{ab})$, and $\varepsilon$ and $\varepsilon_0$ are independent. It is easy to check that $ZZ' = aP_Z = a(\bar{J}_a \otimes I_b)$ and $P_X ZZ' = ZZ' P_X = a\bar{J}_{ab}$. Also, conditions of Theorem 10.9 still hold if $\beta_i$'s in this model are random effects and $\varepsilon_1$ is the vector of fixed effects.

Second, we consider a linear hypothesis of fixed effects in model (10.1) as

$$H_0 : H\beta = h \qquad versus \qquad H_1 : H\beta \neq h, \tag{10.26}$$

where $H \in M_{m_2 \times p}$ is of rank $m_2$ and $\mathcal{M}(H') \subset \mathcal{M}(X')$. This hypothesis is equivalent to

$$H_0 : H\vartheta = 0 \qquad versus \qquad H_1 : H\vartheta \neq 0, \tag{10.27}$$

where $\vartheta = \beta - \beta_0$ and $\beta_0$ is a solution of $H\beta = h$. Therefore, without loss of generality, we assume that $h = 0$.

Consider the test statistic

$$F_2(y) = \frac{(H\hat{\beta})'(H(X'X)^- H')^{-1}(H\hat{\beta})/m_2}{y'(I_n - P_{(X:Z)})y/n_2}, \tag{10.28}$$

where $\hat{\beta} = (X'X)^- X'y$ and $n_2 = n - rk(X : Z)$.

**Theorem 10.10.** *For the model given in (10.1), assume that*
*(i) $X'Z = 0$,*
*(ii) $\lambda = (H\beta)'(H(X'X)^- H')^{-1}(H\beta)/\sigma_0^2$,*
*(iii) $\delta_1 = \alpha_1' \Omega^{1/2} A\mu_y/(d\sigma_0)$, and*
*(iv) $\delta_2 = \alpha_1' P_1 P_1' \alpha_1/d^2$,*
*then*
*(a) $(H\hat{\beta})'(H(X'X)^- H')^{-1}(H\hat{\beta})/\sigma_0^2 \sim S\chi_{m_2}^2(\lambda, \delta_1, \delta_2)$, and*
*(b) $(H\hat{\beta})'(H(X'X)^- H')^{-1}(H\hat{\beta})$ and $y'(I_n - P_{(X:Z)})y$ are mutually independent,*
*where* $A = X(X'X)^- H'(H(X'X)^- H')^{-1}H(X'X)^- X'$, $\mu_y = X\beta$, $\Sigma_y = \sigma_0^2 I_n +$
$\sigma_1^2 ZZ' = \sigma_0^2 \Omega$, $\alpha_1 = \dfrac{\sigma_1 \Sigma_y^{-1/2} Z\alpha}{[1+\alpha'(I_k - \sigma_1^2 Z'\Sigma_y^{-1}Z)\alpha]^{1/2}}$, $d = (1 + \alpha_1' P_2 P_2' \alpha_1)^{1/2}$, *and* $P = (P_1, P_2)$ *is an orthogonal matrix in* $M_{n \times n}$ *such that*

$$\Omega^{1/2} A\Omega^{1/2} = P \begin{pmatrix} I_{m_2} & 0 \\ 0 & 0 \end{pmatrix} P' = P_1 P_1'. \tag{10.29}$$

*Proof.* For (a), it suffices to show that $\sigma^2 = \sigma_0^2$, $\lambda = \mu_y' A\mu_y/\sigma_0^2$ and $A\Omega A = A$, where $\Omega = c_1 I_n + c_2 ZZ'$, $c_1 = 1$, $c_2 = \sigma_1^2/\sigma_0^2$, and $A = X(X'X)^- H'(H(X'X)^- H')^{-1} H(X'X)^- X'$.

Note that $A^2 = A$, so $tr(A) = rk(A) = m_2$. By (i), we obtain

$$\sigma^2 = \frac{1}{m_2}[\sigma_0^2 tr(A) + \sigma_1^2 tr(AZZ')] = \sigma_0^2.$$

By (ii), we know

$$\begin{aligned} \lambda &= (H\beta)'(H(X'X)^- H')^{-1}(H\beta)/\sigma_0^2 \\ &= (X\beta)'(X(X'X)^- H'(H(X'X)^- H')^{-1}H(X'X)^- X')(X\beta)/\sigma_0^2 = \mu_y' A\mu_y/\sigma_0^2. \end{aligned}$$

Further, it is readily verified that

$$A\Omega A = A(c_1 I_n + c_2 ZZ')A = A^2 = A,$$

so that (a) holds. For (b), it suffices to show that $(H(X'X)^- H')^{-1/2}(H\hat{\beta})$ and $(I_n - P_{(X:Z)})y$ are mutually independent. Note that

$$(H(X'X)^- H')^{-1/2} H(X'X)^- X'\Sigma_y (I_n - P_{(X:Z)})$$
$$= (H(X'X)^- H')^{-1/2} H(X'X)^- X'(\sigma_0^2 I_n + \sigma_1^2 ZZ')(I_n - P_{(X:Z)}) = 0.$$

The desired result follows by Theorem 10.2. $\qquad\square$

**Remark 10.4.** *With the conditions given in Theorem 10.10, $F_2(y) \sim SF_{m_2,n_2}$ $(\lambda, \delta_1, \delta_2)$. Under $H_0$ in (10.26), $\lambda = 0$, $\delta_1 = 0$, and $F_2(y) \sim F_{m_2,n_2}$. Therefore, the test for hypothesis given in (10.26) is*

$$\phi_2(F_2(y)) = \begin{cases} 1, & \text{if } F_2(y) \geq F_{m_2,n_2}(1-\gamma), \\ 0, & \text{otherwise.} \end{cases}$$

*with power*

$$g_2(\lambda, \delta_1, \delta_2) = P(F_2(y) \geq F_{m_2,n_2}(1-\gamma)) = P(SF_{m_2,n_2}(\lambda, \delta_1, \delta_2) \geq F_{m_2,n_2}(1-\gamma)).$$

Finally, we consider a special case of skew-normal mixed effects model, namely, the skew-normal multivariate linear regression model, given by

$$y = X\beta + \varepsilon, \qquad \varepsilon \sim SN_n(0, \sigma_1^2 I_n, \alpha). \tag{10.30}$$

For the hypothesis given in (10.26), define the test statistic

$$F_3(y) = \frac{(H\hat{\beta})'(H(X'X)^- H')^{-1}(H\hat{\beta})/m_2}{y'(I_n - P_X)y/n_3}, \tag{10.31}$$

where $\hat{\beta} = (X'X)^- X'y$ and $n_3 = n - rk(X)$.

For $(H\hat{\beta})'(H(X'X)^- H')^{-1}(H\hat{\beta})$ in (10.31), it is easy to show that the conditions given in Theorem 10.4 are satisfied, so that

$$(H\hat{\beta})'(H(X'X)^- H')^{-1}(H\hat{\beta})/\sigma_1^2 \sim S\chi_{m_2}^2(\lambda, \delta_1, \delta_2),$$

where $\lambda = (H\beta)'(H(X'X)^- H')^{-1}(H\beta)/\sigma_1^2$, $\delta_1 = \alpha'AX\beta/(d\sigma_1)$, $\delta_2 = \alpha'A\alpha/d^2$, $d = (1 + \alpha'P_2 P_2'\alpha)^{1/2}$, and $A$ and $P_2$ are given in Theorem 10.10. Further, it is easy to show that

$$((H\hat{\beta})'(H(X'X)^- H')^{-1}(H\hat{\beta})/\sigma_1^2, y'(I_n - P_X)y/\sigma_1^2)' \sim GS\chi_{m_2,n_3}^2(\lambda, 0; \eta_{11}, 0; \eta_{21}, 0; \eta_2),$$

which is reduced to the joint distribution of independent random variables $Z_1 \sim S\chi_{m_2}^2(\lambda, \delta_1, \delta_2)$ and $Z_2 \sim \chi_{n_3}^2$. Thus, $F_3(y) \sim SF_{m_2,n_3}(\lambda, \delta_1, \delta_2)$, and $H_0 : H\beta = 0$ is rejected if $F_3(y) \geq F_{m_2,n_3}(1-\gamma)$.

### 10.1.3 Monte Carlo simulation

This section examines the Type I error probability and power of the proposed method in this book through a Monte Carlo simulation, especially whether the simulated Type I error probability can maintain the nominal significance level.

For convenience, consider the following hypothesis testing problem

$$H_0 : \beta_1 = 0 \qquad versus \qquad H_1 : \beta_1 \neq 0. \tag{10.32}$$

Let $H = (1, 0, \ldots, 0) \in M_{1 \times p}$, then the hypothesis testing problem (10.26) degenerates into (10.32). Therefore, at different significance levels, the Type I error probability and power of $F_2(y)$ for hypothesis testing problem (10.32) are discussed. In the model, take the sample size n=15, 30 and 60, regression coefficient $\beta_1$=0.1, 0.5, 1 and 2, standard deviation component $\sigma_0$=1, 1.5 and 3, $\sigma_1$=1.5, 2 and 4. Let $\alpha = \alpha^* 1_n$, where $\alpha^*$=0, 1 and 2. Let $X = I_a \otimes I_b$, $n = ab$, and $Z$ satisfies $X'Z = 0$. The specific simulation results are shown in Tables 10.1 and 10.2.

**Table 10.1:** Simulated Type I error probabilities for $F_2(y)$.

| $n$ | $\alpha^*$ | $\sigma_0$ | $\sigma_1$ | $\gamma$ | | | |
|---|---|---|---|---|---|---|---|
| | | | | 0.025 | 0.05 | 0.075 | 0.1 |
| 15 | 0 | 1 | 1.5 | 0.0224 | 0.0494 | 0.0722 | 0.0942 |
| | | | 2 | 0.0230 | 0.0460 | 0.0720 | 0.0972 |
| | | | 4 | 0.0238 | 0.0530 | 0.0734 | 0.1012 |
| 15 | 1 | 1.5 | 1.5 | 0.0264 | 0.0504 | 0.0704 | 0.1042 |
| | | | 2 | 0.0242 | 0.0496 | 0.0744 | 0.1024 |
| | | | 4 | 0.0232 | 0.0468 | 0.0724 | 0.0990 |
| 30 | 1 | 1.5 | 1.5 | 0.0256 | 0.0498 | 0.0716 | 0.0954 |
| | | | 2 | 0.0248 | 0.0506 | 0.0750 | 0.0996 |
| | | | 4 | 0.0262 | 0.0482 | 0.0742 | 0.0968 |
| 30 | 2 | 3 | 1.5 | 0.0258 | 0.0518 | 0.0748 | 0.1008 |
| | | | 2 | 0.0252 | 0.0504 | 0.0736 | 0.0964 |
| | | | 4 | 0.0230 | 0.0506 | 0.0734 | 0.0982 |
| 60 | 2 | 3 | 1.5 | 0.0252 | 0.0532 | 0.0742 | 0.1032 |
| | | | 2 | 0.0248 | 0.0482 | 0.0726 | 0.0998 |
| | | | 4 | 0.0260 | 0.0504 | 0.0738 | 0.1004 |

**Table 10.2:** Simulated powers for $F_2(Y)$ ($\sigma_0 = 1$).

| $n$ | $\alpha^*$ | $\sigma_1$ | $\beta_1$ | $\gamma$ | | | |
|---|---|---|---|---|---|---|---|
| | | | | 0.025 | 0.05 | 0.075 | 0.1 |
| 15 | 0 | 1.5 | 0.1 | 0.0310 | 0.0658 | 0.0920 | 0.1186 |
| | | | 0.5 | 0.1032 | 0.1728 | 0.2284 | 0.2758 |
| | | | 1 | 0.3462 | 0.4886 | 0.5720 | 0.6306 |
| | | | 2 | 0.9018 | 0.9558 | 0.9754 | 0.9840 |
| 15 | 1 | 1.5 | 0.1 | 0.0308 | 0.0562 | 0.0854 | 0.1132 |
| | | | 0.5 | 0.1042 | 0.1730 | 0.2262 | 0.2782 |
| | | | 1 | 0.3340 | 0.4724 | 0.5556 | 0.6226 |
| | | | 2 | 0.8992 | 0.9546 | 0.9724 | 0.9822 |
| 30 | 1 | 2 | 0.1 | 0.0348 | 0.0710 | 0.0988 | 0.1280 |
| | | | 0.5 | 0.2322 | 0.3326 | 0.4078 | 0.4584 |
| | | | 1 | 0.7394 | 0.8340 | 0.8798 | 0.9062 |
| | | | 2 | 0.9998 | 0.9999 | 0.9999 | 0.9999 |
| 30 | 2 | 2 | 0.1 | 0.0292 | 0.0564 | 0.0882 | 0.1098 |
| | | | 0.5 | 0.0736 | 0.1220 | 0.1658 | 0.2050 |
| | | | 1 | 0.2088 | 0.3036 | 0.3748 | 0.4288 |
| | | | 2 | 0.7096 | 0.8102 | 0.8580 | 0.8898 |
| 60 | 2 | 4 | 0.1 | 0.0504 | 0.0916 | 0.1294 | 0.1664 |
| | | | 0.5 | 0.4738 | 0.5858 | 0.6630 | 0.7084 |
| | | | 1 | 0.9774 | 0.9900 | 0.9942 | 0.9958 |
| | | | 2 | 0.9999 | 0.9999 | 0.9999 | 0.9999 |

From Table 10.1, with different sample sizes and parameters, the Type I error probabilities of noncentral skew-F statistic $F_2(y)$ are close to the corresponding nominal significance levels. This shows that the Type I error probability of $F_2(y)$ is free of the sample size $n$ and parameters $\sigma_0$, $\sigma_1$ and $\alpha^*$. In addition, from Table 10.2, when $\beta_1$ deviates from the null hypothesis $H_0$ in (10.32), the powers of $F_2(y)$ increased significantly with the increase in sample size. Therefore, from the simulated results of Tables 10.1–10.2, the noncenter skew-F statistic can effectively control the Type I error probability, and has a higher testing power.

### 10.1.4 Illustrative example

In this section, we will analyze a data set to illustrate the proposed approaches.

**Example 10.4** The data set was obtained from a study of leaf area indices (LAI) of robinnia pseudoscacia in the Huaiping forest farm of Shannxi Province from June to October in 2010 (with permission of the authors). The stand age (in years), slope aspect (in degrees) and LAI are given in Table 10.3. The frequency histogram of LAI is given in Figure 10.4. For testing the normality of the data,

**Table 10.3:** The observed values of stand age (in year), slope aspect (in degree) and LAI.

| Batch | Stand age ($X_1$) | Slope aspect ($X_2$) | LAI ($y$) | | | |
|---|---|---|---|---|---|---|
| | | | June ($y_1$) | July ($y_2$) | September ($y_3$) | October ($y_4$) |
| 1 | 9 | 140 | 4.87 | 3.32 | 2.05 | 1.5 |
| 2 | 9 | 120 | 5 | 3.02 | 2.12 | 1.46 |
| 3 | 10 | 180 | 4.72 | 3.28 | 2.24 | 1.55 |
| 4 | 8 | 70 | 5.16 | 3.63 | 2.56 | 1.27 |
| 5 | 9 | 70 | 5.11 | 3.68 | 2.67 | 1.26 |
| 6 | 8 | 50 | 5.03 | 3.79 | 2.61 | 1.37 |
| 7 | 13 | 76 | 5.36 | 3.68 | 2.42 | 1.87 |
| 8 | 13 | 80 | 5.17 | 4.06 | 2.58 | 1.75 |
| 9 | 14 | 76 | 5.56 | 4.13 | 2.56 | 1.81 |
| 10 | 13 | 122 | 4.48 | 2.92 | 1.84 | 1.98 |
| 11 | 14 | 130 | 4.55 | 3.05 | 1.94 | 1.89 |
| 12 | 15 | 150 | 4.69 | 3.02 | 1.95 | 1.71 |
| 13 | 19 | 120 | 2.54 | 2.78 | 2.29 | 1.29 |
| 14 | 19 | 120 | 3.09 | 2.35 | 1.94 | 1.34 |
| 15 | 19 | 130 | 2.79 | 2.4 | 2.2 | 1.29 |
| 16 | 18 | 50 | 3.8 | 3.28 | 1.56 | 1.1 |
| 17 | 18 | 70 | 3.61 | 3.45 | 1.4 | 1.04 |
| 18 | 18 | 70 | 3.53 | 2.85 | 1.36 | 1.08 |
| 19 | 24 | 70 | 2.51 | 3.05 | 1.6 | 0.86 |
| 20 | 25 | 50 | 2.41 | 2.78 | 1.5 | 0.7 |
| 21 | 25 | 70 | 2.8 | 2.72 | 1.88 | 0.82 |
| 22 | 24 | 140 | 3.23 | 2.64 | 1.63 | 1.19 |
| 23 | 24 | 100 | 3.46 | 2.88 | 1.66 | 1.24 |
| 24 | 25 | 156 | 3.12 | 3 | 1.62 | 1.14 |

the p-values from SAS output for the Shapiro-Wilk test, Kolmogorov-Smirnov test and Cramer-von Mises test are 0.0007, 0.0463 and 0.0098, respectively. We can conclude that the LAI is not normally distributed at a 5% significance level. Also the chi-square goodness-of-fit test is used to test the null hypothesis that the LAI is skew-normally distributed. By Table 10.3, the value of the test statistic $\chi^2 = 5.4523 < \chi_3^2(0.95) = 7.8147$, so the null hypothesis is not rejected at the 5% significance level. Hence, the distribution of LAI can be considered approximately skew-normal. Based on the method of moment estimation, the LAI is approximately distributed as $SN(1.2585, 1.8332^2, 2.7966)$ and its density curve is given in Figure 10.4.

Obviously, the LAI data belongs to the longitudinal data. Additionally, one of the most popular models for fitting longitudinal data is the linear mixed model (See Diggle et al., 2002; Wu, 2013; Wu, 2009), which introduces the random effects to account for the between-individual variation and within-individual correlation

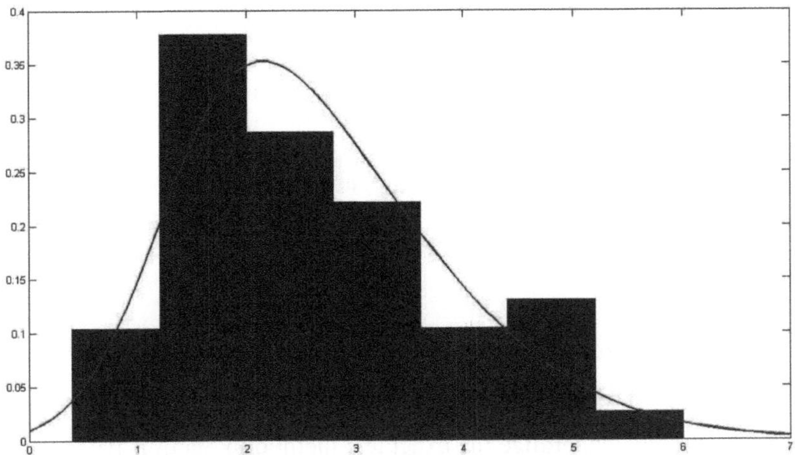

**Figure 10.4:** Frequency histogram of the LAI with superimposed skew-normal density curve.

in the LAI data. Therefore, we define LAI as the response variable (Denoted by $y$) and define stand age and slope aspect as the covariate variables (Denoted by $X_1$ and $X_2$, respectively). Then the model of LAI is written as

$$y = X\beta + Z\varepsilon + \varepsilon_0, \tag{10.33}$$

where $y = (y_1', y_2', y_3', y_4')'$ with $y_i$ being $24 \times 1$ observed values given in Table 10.3, $X = (1_{96} : I_4 \otimes (X_1 : X_2))$ with $X_i$ given in Table 10.3, $Z = I_4 \otimes 1_{24}$, $\beta = (\beta_0, \beta_1, \cdots, \beta_8)'$ is a $9 \times 1$ regression coefficients, $\varepsilon \sim SN_4(0, \sigma_1^2 I_4, \alpha)$, $\varepsilon_0 \sim N_{96}(0, \sigma_0^2 I_{96})$, and $\varepsilon$ and $\varepsilon_0$ are independent.

Consider the hypothesis of the form

$$H_0 : \sigma_1^2 = 0 \qquad versus \qquad H_1 : \sigma_1^2 > 0. \tag{10.34}$$

We define the test statistic as

$$F_1(y) = \frac{y'(P_{(X:Z)} - P_X)y/3}{y'(I_{96} - P_{(X:Z)})y/84} = 47.9703. \tag{10.35}$$

Since $F_1(y) > F_{3,84}(0.95) = 2.7132$, the null hypothesis $H_0$ in (10.34) is rejected at the 5% nominal significance level, namely, the skew-normal random effects are significant.

In order to consider the hypothesis of regression coefficients of interest as

$$H_0 : \beta_1 = \beta_2 \qquad versus \qquad H_1 : \beta_1 \neq \beta_2, \tag{10.36}$$

we simplify the model (10.33) as

$$y_1 = 1_{24}\beta_0 + X_1\beta_1 + X_2\beta_2 + \varepsilon, \tag{10.37}$$

where $\varepsilon \sim SN_{24}(0, \sigma_*^2 I_{24}, \alpha_*)$. By (10.31), we have

$$F_3(y_1) = \frac{(H\hat{\beta}_*)^2 / (H(X_*'X_*)^- H')}{y_1'(I_{24} - P_{X_*})y_1 / 21} = 64.8690,$$

where $H = (0, 1, -1)$, $X_* = (1_{24} : X_1 : X_2)$, and $\hat{\beta}_* = (X_*'X_*)^- X_*'y_1$. Since $F_3(y_1) > F_{1,21}(0.95) = 4.3248$, the null hypothesis $H_0$ in (10.36) is rejected at the 5% nominal significance level.

## 10.2   Skew-normal mixed effect model with k+1 random effects

In this section, we generalize the exact test method in Section 10.1 from a skew-normal mixed-effects model with two random effects to a skew-normal mixed-effects model with a k+1 random effect. Therefore, we consider the following model

$$y = X\beta + \sum_{i=1}^{k} Z_i \varepsilon_i + \varepsilon_0, \tag{10.38}$$

where $y$ is a $n \times 1$ random vector, $X$ and $Z_i$ are $n \times p$ and $n \times q_i$ design matrices, respectively, $\beta$ is a $p \times 1$ vector of regression coefficients, $\varepsilon_i$ is a $q_i \times 1$ vector of random effects, and $\varepsilon_0$ is a $n \times 1$ vector of random errors. We assume that $\varepsilon_0$, $\varepsilon_1$, $\cdots$, $\varepsilon_k$ are mutually independent and

$$\varepsilon_0 \sim SN_n(0, \sigma_0^2 I_n, \alpha), \qquad \varepsilon_i \sim N_{q_i}(0, \sigma_i^2 I_{q_i}), \; i = 1, \cdots, k,$$

The model (10.38) is the normal variance components model when $\alpha = 0$ and skew-normal multivariate linear regression model when $\sigma_i^2 = 0 \; (i = 1, \cdots, k)$. For convenience, expressions with similar meanings to those in Section 10.1 appear in this section and will use the same symbols.

### 10.2.1   Quadratic form and its Cochran's theorem

The following conclusions are similar to subsections 10.1.1 and 10.1.2, so the proof process is omitted.

**Theorem 10.11.** *For the model given in (10.38), we conclude the following. (i) The MGF of $y$ is*

$$M_y(t) = 2\exp\left(t'\mu_y + \frac{t'\Sigma_y t}{2}\right)\Phi\left\{\frac{\sigma_0 \alpha' t}{(1 + \alpha'\alpha)^{1/2}}\right\} \qquad t \in \Re^n, \tag{10.39}$$

*where $\mu_y = X\beta$ and $\Sigma_y = \sum_{i=1}^{k} \sigma_i^2 Z_i Z_i' + \sigma_0^2 I_n$.*

*(ii) The density function of y is*

$$f_y(x; \mu_y, \Sigma_y, \alpha_1) = 2\phi_n(x; \mu_y, \Sigma_y)\Phi(\alpha_1'\Sigma_y^{-1/2}(x - \mu_y)) \qquad x \in \Re^n, \qquad (10.40)$$

*where* $\alpha_1 = \dfrac{\sigma_0 \Sigma_y^{-1/2}\alpha}{[1 + \alpha'(I_n - \sigma_0^2\Sigma_y^{-1})\alpha]^{1/2}}$. *We denote* $y \sim SN_n(\mu_y, \Sigma_y, \alpha_1)$.

*(iii) The mean vector and covariance matrix of y are*

$$E(y) = \mu_y + \sqrt{\frac{2}{\pi}}\frac{\Sigma_y^{1/2}\alpha_1}{(1 + \alpha_1'\alpha_1)^{1/2}}, Cov(y) = \Sigma_y^{1/2}\left(I_n - \frac{2\alpha_1\alpha_1'}{\pi(1 + \alpha_1'\alpha_1)}\right)\Sigma_y^{1/2}. \quad (10.41)$$

**Theorem 10.12.** *For the model given in (10.38), suppose* $B_i \in M_{k_i \times n}$ $(i = 1, 2)$, *then* $B_1 y$ *and* $B_2 y$ *are mutually independent if and only if*

*(i)* $B_1\Sigma_y B_2' = 0$ *and*

*(ii) either* $B_1\Sigma_y^{1/2}\alpha_1 = 0$ *or* $B_2\Sigma_y^{1/2}\alpha_1 = 0$,

*where* $\Sigma_y = \sum_{i=1}^k \sigma_i^2 Z_i Z_i' + \sigma_0^2 I_n$ *and* $\alpha_1 = \dfrac{\sigma_0\Sigma_y^{-1/2}\alpha}{[1 + \alpha'(I_n - \sigma_0^2\Sigma_y^{-1})\alpha]^{1/2}}$.

**Theorem 10.13.** *For the model* $y$ *given in (10.38), let* $Q_i = y'A_i y/\sigma_{*i}^2$ *with non-negative definite* $A_i \in M_{n \times n}$, $m_i = rk(A_i)$, *and* $\sigma_{*i}^2 = \frac{1}{m_i}[\sigma_0^2 tr(A_i) + \sum_{j=1}^k \sigma_j^2 tr(A_i Z_j Z_j')]$, $i = 1, \cdots, \ell$. *Let* $Q = (Q_1, \cdots, Q_\ell)'$. *Then*

$$Q \sim GS\chi^2_{m_1, \cdots, m_\ell}(\lambda_1, \cdots, \lambda_\ell; \eta_{11}, \cdots, \eta_{1\ell}; \eta_{21}, \cdots, \eta_{2\ell}; \eta_2)$$

*if and only if, for any distinct* $i, j \in \{1, \cdots, l\}$ *and some* $\eta_{1i} \in R$ *including* $\eta_{1i} = 0$:

*(i)* $\Omega_i A_i$ *is idempotent of rank* $m_i$,

*(ii)* $\lambda_i = \mu_y'A_i\mu_y/\sigma_{*i}^2$,

*(iii)* $A_i A_j = 0$,

*(iv)* $\eta_{1i} = \alpha_1'\Omega_i^{1/2}A_i\mu_y/\sigma_{*i}$, *and*

*(v)* $\eta_{2i} = \alpha_1'P_iP_i'\alpha_1$,

*where* $\mu_y = X\beta$, $\Sigma_y = \sum_{j=1}^k \sigma_j^2 Z_j Z_j' + \sigma_0^2 I_n = \sigma_{*i}^2\Omega_i$, $\alpha_1 = \dfrac{\sigma_0\Sigma_y^{-1/2}\alpha}{[1 + \alpha'(I_n - \sigma_0^2\Sigma_y^{-1})\alpha]^{1/2}}$, $\eta_2 = \alpha_1'\alpha_1$, *and* $P = (P_1, \cdots, P_\ell, P_{\ell+1})$ *is an orthogonal matrix in* $M_{n \times n}$ *such that*

$$\Omega_i^{1/2}A_i\Omega_i^{1/2} = P\begin{pmatrix} 0 & 0 & 0 \\ 0 & I_{m_i} & 0 \\ 0 & 0 & 0 \end{pmatrix}P' = P_iP_i' \qquad (10.42)$$

*with the upper left hand 0 being the square matrix of order $\sum_{j=1}^{i-1} m_j$ (which is 0 for $i = 1$), and the lower right hand 0 being the square matrix of order $\sum_{j=i+1}^{\ell+1} m_j$.*

**Corollary 10.3.** *In Theorem 10.13, if $\alpha_1' \Omega_i^{1/2} A_i \mu_y = 0$, $i = 1, \cdots, \ell$, then $\{Q_i\}_{i=1}^{\ell}$ is a family of independent noncentral chi-square distributed random variables and each $Q_i \sim \chi_{m_i}^2(\lambda_i)$, which is free of $\eta_2 = \alpha_1' \alpha_1$, if and only if for any distinct $i, j \in \{1, \cdots, \ell\}$:*

*(i) $\Omega_i A_i$ is idempotent of rank $m_i$,*

*(ii) $\lambda_i = \mu_y' A_i \mu_y / \sigma_{*i}^2$, and*

*(iii) $A_i A_j = 0$,*

*where $m_i = rk(A_i)$, $\mu_y = X\beta$, $\Sigma_y = \sum_{j=1}^{k} \sigma_j^2 Z_j Z_j' + \sigma_0^2 I_n = \sigma_{*i}^2 \Omega_i$, $\sigma_{*i}^2 = \frac{1}{m_i}[\sigma_0^2 tr(A_i) + \sum_{j=1}^{k} \sigma_j^2 tr(A_i Z_j Z_j')]$, and $\alpha_1 = \frac{\sigma_0 \Sigma_y^{-1/2} \alpha}{[1 + \alpha'(I_n - \sigma_0^2 \Sigma_y^{-1})\alpha]^{1/2}}.*

In particular, Corollary 10.3 holds if either $\mu_y = 0$ or $\alpha_1 = 0$.

### 10.2.2   Exact inference of unknown parameters

In this section, we will obtain exact tests for fixed effects and variance components based on the Theorem 10.13. First, we consider the significance testing of all the random effects

$$H_0 : \sigma_1^2 = \cdots = \sigma_k^2 = 0 \qquad versus \qquad H_1 : \text{not all } \sigma_i^2 \text{ are equal to 0.} \quad (10.43)$$

It is clear that model (10.38) is reduced to a skew-normal multivariate linear regression model under $H_0$.

Denote $I_n - P_n = N_B$, $B \in M_{n \times k}$. Define test statistics

$$F_4(y) = \frac{y'\left(P_{(X:Z_1:\cdots:Z_k)} - P_X\right)y/n_1}{y'N_{(X:Z_1:\cdots:Z_k)}y/n_2}, \qquad (10.44)$$

where $n_1 = rk(X : Z_1 : \cdots : Z_k) - rk(X)$, $n_2 = n - rk(X : Z_1 : \cdots : Z_k)$.

Note that

$$y'N_{(X:Z_1:\cdots:Z_k)}y = \varepsilon_0' N_{(X:Z_1:\cdots:Z_k)}\varepsilon_0,$$

and

$$y'\left(P_{(X:Z_1:\cdots:Z_k)} - P_X\right)y = \varepsilon_0'(P_{(X:Z_1:\cdots:Z_k)} - P_X)\varepsilon_0 \qquad \text{under } H_0.$$

By Theorem 10.13, it is easy to show that under $H_0$ in (10.43)

$$(y'(P_{(X:Z_1:\cdots:Z_k)} - P_X)y/\sigma_0^2, y'N_{(X:Z_1:\cdots:Z_k)}y/\sigma_0^2)' \sim GS\chi_{n_1,n_2}^2(0,0;0,0;\eta_{21},\eta_{22};\eta_2).$$

Since $(P_{(X:Z_1:\cdots:Z_k)} - P_X)N_{(X:Z_1:\cdots:Z_k)} = 0$, $y'(P_{(X:Z_1:\cdots:Z_k)} - P_X)y$ and $y'N_{(X:Z_1:\cdots:Z_k)}y$ are mutually independent under $H_0$. By Definition 10.2, $F_4(y) \sim F_{n_1,n_2}$ under $H_0$ in (10.43). Hence, $H_0$ is rejected if $F_4(y) \geq F_{n_1,n_2}(1-\gamma)$, where $F_{n_1,n_2}(1-\gamma)$ denotes the critical value of $F$ distribution for significance level $\gamma$.

When the significance testing of all the random effects is rejected, we need to test the existence of every random effect one by one. Hence, we consider the significance testing of some random effect

$$H_0 : \sigma_i^2 = 0 \qquad versus \qquad H_1 : \sigma_i^2 > 0. \tag{10.45}$$

Define the test statistic

$$F_5(y) = \frac{y'A^*y/n_3}{y'N_{(z^*:z_i)}y/n_2}, \tag{10.46}$$

where $A^* = P_{(z^*:z_i)} - P_{Z^*}$, $n_3 = rk(P_{(z^*:z_i)}) - rk(P_{Z^*})$, and $Z^* = (X : Z_1 : \cdots : Z_{i-1} : Z_{i+1} : \cdots : Z_k)$.

**Theorem 10.14.** *Let* $t_i = tr(A^*Z_iZ_i')/n_3$. *For the model $y$ given in* (10.38), *if* $P_{Z^*}Z_iZ_i' = Z_iZ_i'P_{Z^*}$ *and* $Z_iZ_i' = t_iP_{Z_i}$, *then*

*(i)* $(y'A^*y/\sigma^2, y'N_{(z^*:z_i)}y/\sigma_0^2)' \sim GS\chi^2_{n_3,n_2}(0,0;0,0;\eta_{21},\eta_{22};\eta_2)$, *and*

*(ii)* $F_5(y) \sim (1+t_i\theta_i)F_{n_3,n_2}$,
*where* $\sigma^2 = \sigma_0^2 + t_i\sigma_i^2$ *and* $\theta_i = \sigma_i^2/\sigma_0^2$.

*Proof.* For (i), it suffices to show that $\lambda_1 = \lambda_2 = 0$, $A^*N_{(z^*:z_i)} = 0$, $A^* = A^*\Omega_1 A^*$, and $N_{(z^*:z_i)} = N_{(z^*:z_i)}\Omega_2 N_{(z^*:z_i)}$, where $\Omega_1 = \sigma^{-2}\Sigma_y$ and $\Omega_2 = \sigma_0^{-2}\Sigma_y$.

By Theorem 10.13, we have

$$\lambda_1 = \mu_y'A^*\mu_y = \beta'X'(P_{(z^*:z_i)} - P_{Z^*})X\beta = 0,$$
$$\lambda_2 = \mu_y'N_{(z^*:z_i)}\mu_y = \beta'X'N_{(z^*:z_i)}X\beta = 0,$$
$$A^*N_{(z^*:z_i)} = (P_{(z^*:z_i)} - P_{Z^*})N_{(z^*:z_i)} = 0.$$

Further, by conditions of Theorem 10.14, we obtain

$$A^*\Omega_1 A^* = (P_{(z^*:z_i)} - P_{Z^*})\left(\sum_{j=1}^{k}\sigma_j^2 Z_jZ_j' + \sigma_0^2 I_n\right)(P_{(z^*:z_i)} - P_{Z^*})/\sigma^2$$

$$= N_{Z^*}P_{Z_i}(t_i\sigma_i^2 P_{Z_i} + \sigma_0^2 I_n)N_{Z^*}P_{Z_i}/\sigma^2 = \frac{\sigma_0^2 + t_i\sigma_i^2}{\sigma^2}N_{Z^*}P_{Z_i} = A^*,$$

and

$$N_{(Z^*:Z_i)}\Omega_2 N_{(Z^*:Z_i)} = N_{(Z^*:Z_i)}\Big(\sum_{j=1}^{k}\sigma_j^2 Z_j Z_j' + \sigma_0^2 I_n\Big)N_{(Z^*:Z_i)}/\sigma_0^2 = N_{(Z^*:Z_i)}.$$

The desired result is obtained.

For (ii), it suffices to show that $y'A^*y$ and $y'N_{(Z^*:Z_i)}y$ are mutually independent. Since

$$A^*\Sigma_y N_{(Z^*:Z_i)} = (P_{(Z^*:Z_i)} - P_{Z^*})\Big(\sum_{j=1}^{k}\sigma_j^2 Z_j Z_j' + \sigma_0^2 I_n\Big)N_{(Z^*:Z_i)} = 0,$$

(ii) is obtained from Theorem 10.12. □

Note that the hypothesis given in (10.45) is equivalent to

$$H_0 : \theta_i = 0 \qquad versus \qquad H_1 : \theta_i > 0, \tag{10.47}$$

where $\theta_i = \sigma_i^2/\sigma_0^2$. By Theorem 10.14, the test for hypothesis in (10.47) is given by

$$\phi_3(F_s(Y)) = \begin{cases} 1, & \text{if } F_s(Y) \geq F_{n_3,n_2}(1-\gamma), \\ 0, & \text{otherwise.} \end{cases}$$

with power

$$g_3(\theta_i) = P(F_s(Y) \geq F_{n_3,n_2}(1-\gamma)) = P\Big(F_{n_3,n_2} \geq \frac{1}{1+t_i\theta_i}F_{n_3,n_2}(1-\gamma)\Big).$$

Finally, we consider a linear hypothesis of fixed effects of interest in model (10.38) as

$$H_0 : c_i'\beta_i = d_i \qquad versus \qquad H_1 : c_i'\beta_i \neq d_i, \tag{10.48}$$

where $X = (X_1,\cdots,X_q)$, $\beta = (\beta_1',\cdots,\beta_q')'$, $\beta_i$ is the subvector of fixed effects $\beta$, $X_i$ is the corresponding design matrix of $\beta_i$, $c_i \in \mathcal{M}(X_i')$, and $X_i'X_j = 0$ for any $i \neq j$. This hypothesis is equivalent to

$$H_0 : c_i'\vartheta_i = 0 \qquad versus \qquad H_1 : c_i'\vartheta_i \neq 0, \tag{10.49}$$

where $\vartheta_i = \beta_i - \beta_{i0}$ and $\beta_{i0}$ is a solution of $c_i'\beta_i = d_i$. Therefore, without loss of generality, we assume that $d_i = 0$.

Next, we give the test statistic for hypothesis (10.48). Denote $N_x = I_n - P_x$ and $\sigma_*^2 = (\sigma_0^2,\cdots,\sigma_k^2)'$.

**Theorem 10.15.** *For the model Y given in* (10.38), *assume that*

*(i) $N_X \Sigma_y = \Sigma_y N_X = \sum_{i=0}^{k} \rho_i V_i$,*

*(ii) there exists an eigenvalue $\rho_l$ such that $P_{X_i} \Sigma_y = \rho_l P_{X_i}$,*

*(iii) $\lambda_1 = (c_i' \beta_i)^2 / (\rho_l c_i' (X_i' X_i)^- c_i)$,*

*(iv) $\eta_{11} = \alpha_1' \Omega^{1/2} A_1 \mu_y / \rho_l^{1/2}$, and*

*(v) $\eta_{2t} = \alpha_1' P_t P_t' \alpha_1, t = 1, 2,$*
*then*

*(a) $(y' A_1 y / \rho_l, y' A_2 y / \rho_l)' \sim GS\chi^2_{1,n_l}(\lambda_1, 0; \eta_{11}, 0; \eta_{21}, \eta_{22}; \eta_2)$, and*

*(b) $F_6(y) = \dfrac{y' A_1 y}{y' A_2 y / n_l} \sim SF_{1,n_l}(\lambda_1, \delta_1, \delta_2)$,*
*where $\rho_i$'s are $k+1$ non-zero distinct eigenvalues of $N_X \Sigma_y$ and are $k+1$ non-zero distinct linearly independent combinations of $\sigma_*^2$, $V_i$'s are orthogonal projectors such that $V_i V_j = 0 \ (i \neq j)$ and $\sum_{i=0}^{k} V_i = N_X$, $A_1 = X_i (X_i' X_i)^- c_i (c_i' (X_i' X_i)^- c_i)^{-1} c_i' (X_i' X_i)^- X_i'$, $A_2 = V_l$, $n_l = rk(V_l)$, $\delta_1 = \eta_{11}/(1 + \eta_2 - \eta_{21})^{1/2}$, $\delta_2 = \eta_{21}/(1 + \eta_2 - \eta_{21})$, $\mu_y = X\beta$, $\Sigma_y = \sum_{j=1}^{k} \sigma_j^2 Z_j Z_j' + \sigma_0^2 I_n = \rho_l \Omega$, $\alpha_1 = \dfrac{\sigma_0 \Sigma_y^{-1/2} \alpha}{[1 + \alpha' (I_n - \sigma_0^2 \Sigma_y^{-1}) \alpha]^{1/2}}$, $\eta_2 = \alpha_1' \alpha_1$, and $P = (P_1, P_2, P_3)$ is an orthogonal matrix in $M_{n \times n}$ such that*

$$\Omega^{1/2} A_t \Omega^{1/2} = P \begin{pmatrix} 0 & 0 & 0 \\ 0 & I_{m_t} & 0 \\ 0 & 0 & 0 \end{pmatrix} P' = P_t P_t' \tag{10.50}$$

*with the upper left hand 0 being the square matrix of order $\sum_{j=1}^{t-1} m_j$ (which is 0 for $t = 1$), and the lower right hand 0 being the square matrix of order $\sum_{j=t+1}^{3} m_j$.*

*Proof.* For (a), it suffices to show that $A_1 A_2 = 0$, $\sigma_{*1}^2 = \sigma_{*2}^2 = \rho_l$, $\lambda_1 = \mu_y' A_1 \mu_y / \rho_l$, $\lambda_2 = 0$, and $A_t \Omega A_t = A_t, t = 1, 2$.

By (i), we obtain $A_1 A_2 = 0$ and

$$\Sigma_y = N_X \Sigma_y N_X + P_X \Sigma_y P_X = \sum_{i=0}^{k} \rho_i V_i + P_X \Sigma_y P_X,$$

so that $\sigma_{*2}^2 = n_l^{-1} tr(A_2 \Sigma_y) = tr\left(A_2 \left(\sum_{i=0}^{k} \rho_i V_i + P_X \Sigma_y P_X\right)\right) = \rho_l$. Note that $A_1^2 = A_1$, so $tr(A_1) = rk(A_1) = 1$. By (ii), $\sigma_{*1}^2 = tr(A_1 \Sigma_y) = \rho_l$. By (iii), we know

$$\begin{aligned}
\lambda_1 &= (c_i' \beta_i)^2 / (\rho_l c_i' (X_i' X_i)^- c_i) \\
&= (X\beta)' (X_i (X_i' X_i)^- c_i (c_i' (X_i' X_i)^- c_i)^{-1} c_i' (X_i' X_i)^- X_i')(X\beta)/\rho_l = \mu_y' A_1 \mu_y / \rho_l.
\end{aligned}$$

Similarly, we can prove that $\lambda_2 = 0$. Further, it is easy to show that

$$A_t \Omega A_t = A_t \Sigma_y A_t / \rho_t = A_t^2 = A_t, \quad t = 1, 2,$$

so that (a) holds. (b) is obtained from (a) and Definition 10.2. $\qquad\square$

By Theorem 10.15, we have $\lambda_1 = \eta_{11} = 0$ and $F_6(y) \sim F_{1,n_l}$ under $H_0$. Therefore, the test for the hypothesis given in (10.48) is

$$\phi_4(F_6(y)) = \begin{cases} 1, & \text{if } F_6(y) \geq F_{1,n_l}(1-\gamma), \\ 0, & \text{otherwise.} \end{cases}$$

with power

$$g_4(\lambda_1, \delta_1, \delta_2) = P(F_6(Y) \geq F_{1,n_l}(1-\gamma)) = P(SF_{1,n_l}(\lambda_1, \delta_1, \delta_2) \geq F_{1,n_l}(1-\gamma)).$$

**Remark 10.5.** *For hypothesis $H_0 : c_*'\beta = 0$, it is easy to establish the corresponding test statistics as long as the notations $c_i$, $\beta_i$ and $X_i$ are replaced by $c_*$, $\beta$ and $X$ in Theorem 10.15.*

## 10.2.3 Monte Carlo simulation

In this section, we intend to study the behavior of Type I error probability and power of the proposed test. In particular, we would like to see if the simulated Type I error probabilities of the proposed test can maintain the nominal significance level.

For simplicity and convenience, we consider the hypothesis (10.52) in the two-way classification model with skew-normal random errors. For the test statistic $F_4(y)$ given in (10.53), simulation studies on the Type I error probability and power have been carried out at the various values of nominal level $\gamma$. In the simulation, it is assigned that $\alpha = \tilde{\alpha} 1_n$ with $\tilde{\alpha} = 0, 0.5$ and 2. We use a variety of unknown parameter configurations and three different settings of sample size: (i) $(a,b) = (5,5)$, (ii) $(a,b) = (10,8)$, and $(a,b) = (20,10)$. These settings are selected to investigate the performance of the proposed test under different nominal levels and different sample sizes. For each parameter setting, 5000 skew-normal random vectors are generated from (10.51) based on the method proposed by Arellano-Valle et al. (2005).

Table 10.4 presents the simulated Type I error probabilities of the test statistic $F_4(y)$ for various combinations of $a, b, \tilde{\alpha}$, and $\sigma_0^2$. The Type I error probabilities of $F_4(y)$ are very close to the various nominal levels across the wide array of scenarios, which have nothing to do with $\sigma_0^2$ for the fixed values of $a, b$ and $\tilde{\alpha}$. Table 10.5 reports the simulated powers of the test statistic $F_4(y)$ for various

**Table 10.4:** Simulated sizes of $F_4(Y)(\sigma_1^2 = \sigma_2^2 = 0)$.

| $a$ | $b$ | $\alpha_*$ | $\sigma_0^2$ | $\gamma$ | | | |
|---|---|---|---|---|---|---|---|
| | | | | 0.025 | 0.05 | 0.075 | 0.1 |
| 5 | 5 | 0 | 1 | 0.0232 | 0.0496 | 0.0772 | 0.1002 |
| | | | 2 | 0.0232 | 0.0496 | 0.0772 | 0.1002 |
| | | | 4 | 0.0232 | 0.0496 | 0.0772 | 0.1002 |
| 10 | 8 | 0.5 | 1 | 0.0242 | 0.0488 | 0.0730 | 0.0974 |
| | | | 2 | 0.0242 | 0.0488 | 0.0730 | 0.0974 |
| | | | 4 | 0.0242 | 0.0488 | 0.0730 | 0.0974 |
| 20 | 10 | 2 | 1 | 0.0254 | 0.0494 | 0.0744 | 0.1006 |
| | | | 2 | 0.0254 | 0.0494 | 0.0744 | 0.1006 |
| | | | 4 | 0.0254 | 0.0494 | 0.0744 | 0.1006 |

combinations of $a, b, \widetilde{\alpha}$, and $\sigma_2^2$. In cases where $\sigma_1^2$ and $\sigma_2^2$ depart from the null hypothesis $H_0$ in (10.52), the power increases significantly with the sample size enlarging. In short, the overall picture that emerges from the simulation results is that the proposed test is extremely satisfactory, and it is applicable regardless of sample size.

**Table 10.5:** Simulated powers of $F_4(Y)(\sigma_0^2 = 1, \sigma_1^2 = 0)$.

| $a$ | $b$ | $\alpha_*$ | $\sigma_2^2$ | $\gamma$ | | | |
|---|---|---|---|---|---|---|---|
| | | | | 0.025 | 0.05 | 0.075 | 0.1 |
| 5 | 5 | 0 | 0.1 | 0.0572 | 0.0992 | 0.1412 | 0.1806 |
| | | | 0.2 | 0.1012 | 0.1668 | 0.2234 | 0.2672 |
| | | | 0.3 | 0.1566 | 0.2362 | 0.2982 | 0.3498 |
| | | | 0.5 | 0.2704 | 0.3692 | 0.4412 | 0.4930 |
| | | | 1.0 | 0.5110 | 0.6102 | 0.6708 | 0.7172 |
| 10 | 8 | 0.5 | 0.1 | 0.1738 | 0.2630 | 0.3228 | 0.3690 |
| | | | 0.2 | 0.3970 | 0.5022 | 0.5730 | 0.6242 |
| | | | 0.3 | 0.5906 | 0.6850 | 0.7386 | 0.7790 |
| | | | 0.5 | 0.8134 | 0.8644 | 0.8958 | 0.9160 |
| | | | 1.0 | 0.9616 | 0.9746 | 0.9826 | 0.9878 |
| 20 | 10 | 2 | 0.1 | 0.4834 | 0.5934 | 0.6652 | 0.7126 |
| | | | 0.2 | 0.8442 | 0.9002 | 0.9272 | 0.9402 |
| | | | 0.3 | 0.9572 | 0.9738 | 0.9816 | 0.9870 |
| | | | 0.5 | 0.9966 | 0.9980 | 0.9984 | 0.9988 |
| | | | 1.0 | 1.0000 | 1.0000 | 1.0000 | 1.0000 |

### 10.2.4 Illustrative examples

In this section, we will analyze two examples to demonstrate the effectiveness of the above-mentioned method.

**Example 10.5** Consider the two-way classification model with skew-normal random errors given by

$$y = 1_{ab}\mu + (I_a \otimes 1_b)\varepsilon_2 + (1_a \otimes I_b)\varepsilon_1 + \varepsilon_0, \tag{10.51}$$

where $1_m = (1, \cdots, 1)' \in \Re^m$, $\mu \in \Re$ is a fixed effect, $\varepsilon_2$ and $\varepsilon_1$ are random effects, and $\varepsilon_0$ is a error term. Suppose that $\varepsilon_2 \sim N_a(0, \sigma_2^2 I_a)$, $\varepsilon_1 \sim N_b(0, \sigma_1^2 I_b)$, $\varepsilon_0 \sim SN_{ab}(0, \sigma_0^2 I_{ab}, \alpha)$, and $\varepsilon_2$, $\varepsilon_1$ and $\varepsilon_0$ are mutually independent. Denote $X = 1_{ab}$, $Z_2 = I_a \otimes 1_b$, $Z_1 = 1_a \otimes I_b$.

Consider the hypothesis of the form

$$H_0 : \sigma_1^2 = \sigma_2^2 = 0 \qquad versus \qquad H_1 : \text{not all } \sigma_i^2 \text{ are equal to 0.} \tag{10.52}$$

We define the test statistic as

$$\begin{aligned}
F_4(y) &= \frac{y'(P_{(X:Z_2:Z_1)} - P_X)y/(a+b-2)}{y'(I_{ab} - P_{(X:Z_2:Z_1)})y/((a-1)(b-1))} \\
&= \frac{y'[(I_a - \bar{J}_a) \otimes \bar{J}_b + \bar{J}_a \otimes (I_b - \bar{J}_b)]y/(a+b-2)}{y'[(I_a - \bar{J}_a) \otimes (I_b - \bar{J}_b)]y/((a-1)(b-1))}.
\end{aligned} \tag{10.53}$$

It is clear that $F_4(y) \sim F_{(a+b-2),(a-1)(b-1)}$ under $H_0$ in (10.52). Hence, $H_0$ is rejected if $F_4(y) > F_{(a+b-2),(a-1)(b-1)}(1-\gamma)$.

Next, we consider the hypothesis of the form

$$H_0 : \sigma_1^2 = 0 \qquad versus \qquad H_1 : \sigma_1^2 > 0. \tag{10.54}$$

Note that $Z_1 Z_1' = a\bar{J}_a \otimes I_b = aP_{Z_1}$ and $P_{(X:Z_2)}Z_1 Z_1' = a\bar{J}_a \otimes \bar{J}_b = Z_1 Z_1' P_{(X:Z_2)}$. By Theorem 10.14, we have

$$\begin{aligned}
F_5(y) &= \frac{y'(P_{(X:Z_2:Z_1)} - P_{(X:Z_2)})y/(b-1)}{y'(I_{ab} - P_{(X:Z_2:Z_1)})y/((a-1)(b-1))} \\
&= \frac{y'[\bar{J}_a \otimes (I_b - \bar{J}_b)]y/(b-1)}{y'[(I_a - \bar{J}_a) \otimes (I_b - \bar{J}_b)]y/((a-1)(b-1))} \\
&\sim (1 + a\sigma_1^2/\sigma_0^2)F_{(b-1),(a-1)(b-1)}.
\end{aligned} \tag{10.55}$$

Therefore, $H_0$ in (10.54) is rejected if $F_5(y) \geq F_{(b-1),(a-1)(b-1)}(1-\gamma)$.

**Remark 10.6.** *Suppose that $\sigma_1^2 = 0$ and $\alpha = 0$, then model (10.51) is reduced to a one-way classification model with normal random effects, namely*

$$y = 1_{ab}\mu + (I_a \otimes 1_b)\varepsilon_2 + \varepsilon_0, \tag{10.56}$$

*where $\varepsilon_2 \sim N_a(0, \sigma_2^2 I_a)$ and $\varepsilon_0 \sim N_{ab}(0, \sigma_0^2 I_{ab})$. Consider the hypothesis of the form*

$$H_0 : \sigma_2^2 = 0 \qquad versus \qquad H_1 : \sigma_2^2 > 0. \tag{10.57}$$

*It is well known that the ANOVA test for hypothesis in (10.57) may be undefined, because the ANOVA estimate for $\sigma_2^2$ can turn out to be negative with positive probability (See Scheffe (1956)). However, we can construct a uniformly most powerful unbiased test (UMPUT) for hypothesis in (10.57) based on Theorem 10.14.*

Clearly, $Z_2 Z_2' = b(I_a \otimes \bar{J}_b) = bP_{Z_2}$ and $P_X Z_2 Z_2' = b\bar{J}_{ab} = Z_2 Z_2' P_X$. By Theorem 10.14, we get

$$F_5(y) = \frac{y'[(I_a - \bar{J}_a) \otimes \bar{J}_b]y/(a-1)}{y'[I_a \otimes (I_b - \bar{J}_b)]y/(a(b-1))} \sim (1 + b\sigma_2^2/\sigma_0^2)F_{(a-1),a(b-1)},$$

and $H_0$ is rejected if $F_5(y) > F_{(a-1),a(b-1)}(1-\gamma)$, which is a UMPUT for hypothesis in (10.57) (See Theorem 3.3 given by Wu and Wang (2004)).

**Example 10.6** Consider the random regression coefficient model with skew-normal random errors given by

$$y = (I_k \otimes 1_n)u_* + (I_k \otimes X)v_* + \varepsilon, \tag{10.58}$$

where $y = (y_1', \cdots, y_k')'$, $y_i = (y_{i1}, \cdots, y_{in})'$, and $y_i$ is the random vector of the $i$th subclass, $X$ is a $n \times p$ design matrix with full column rank, $u_*$ is a $k \times 1$ random intercept vector with distribution $N_k(1_k\mu, \sigma_{u_*}^2 I_k)$, $v_*$ is a $kp \times 1$ random regression coefficient with distribution $N_{kp}(1_k \otimes \beta, \sigma_{v_*}^2 I_{kp})$, $\varepsilon$ is a $kn \times 1$ random error vector with distribution $SN_{kn}(0, \sigma_\varepsilon^2 I_{kn}, \alpha)$, and $u_*, v_*$ and $\varepsilon$ are mutually independent.

Denote $u_* = 1_k\mu + \eta$ and $v_* = 1_k \otimes \beta + \xi$, where $\eta \sim N_k(0, \sigma_{u_*}^2 I_k)$ and $\xi \sim N_{kp}(0, \sigma_{v_*}^2 I_{kp})$. Then model (10.58) can be rewritten as

$$y = 1_{kn}\mu + (1_k \otimes X)\beta + (I_k \otimes 1_n)\eta + (I_k \otimes X)\xi + \varepsilon. \tag{10.59}$$

Consider the hypothesis of the form

$$H_0 : h'\beta = 0 \qquad versus \qquad H_1 : h'\beta \neq 0, \tag{10.60}$$

where $h \in \mathcal{M}(X')$.

Let $X^* = (1_{kn} : 1_k \otimes X)$. Suppose that $X'X = aI_p$ $(a > 0)$ and $1'_n X = 0$, then $\Sigma_y = n\sigma_{u_*}^2 (I_k \otimes \bar{J}_n) + a\sigma_{v_*}^2 (I_k \otimes P_X) + \sigma_\varepsilon^2 I_{kn}$. Further, we obtain

$$
\begin{aligned}
N_{X^*}\Sigma_y &= (n\sigma_{u_*}^2 + \sigma_\varepsilon^2)(I_k - \bar{J}_k) \otimes \bar{J}_n + (a\sigma_{v_*}^2 + \sigma_\varepsilon^2)(I_k - \bar{J}_k) \otimes P_X + \sigma_\varepsilon^2 I_k \otimes (I_n - \bar{J}_n - P_X) \\
&= \Sigma_y N_{X^*} = \sum_{i=0}^{2} \rho_i V_i,
\end{aligned}
$$

where $\rho_0 = \sigma_\varepsilon^2$, $\rho_1 = a\sigma_{v_*}^2 + \sigma_\varepsilon^2$, $\rho_2 = n\sigma_{u_*}^2 + \sigma_\varepsilon^2$, $V_0 = I_k \otimes (I_n - \bar{J}_n - P_X)$, $V_1 = (I_k - \bar{J}_k) \otimes P_X$, and $V_2 = (I_k - \bar{J}_k) \otimes \bar{J}_n$. Thus it is easy to show that

$$
P_{1_k \otimes X}\Sigma_y = (a\sigma_{v_*}^2 + \sigma_\varepsilon^2)(\bar{J}_k \otimes P_X) = \rho_1 P_{1_k \otimes X}.
$$

By Theorem 10.15, we have

$$
\begin{aligned}
F_6(y) &= \frac{ak(h'\hat{\beta})^2/(h'h)}{y'V_1 y/(p(k-1))} \\
&= \frac{ak(h'\hat{\beta})^2/(h'h)}{y'[(I_k - \bar{J}_k) \otimes P_X]y/(p(k-1))} \sim SF_{1,p(k-1)}(\lambda_1, \delta_1, \delta_2), \quad (10.61)
\end{aligned}
$$

where $\hat{\beta} = (1'_k \otimes X')y/(ak)$, $\lambda_1 = ak(h'\beta)^2/(\rho_1 h'h)$, $\delta_1 = \eta_{11}/(1 + \eta_2 - \eta_{21})^{1/2}$, $\delta_2 = \eta_{21}/(1 + \eta_2 - \eta_{21})$, $\eta_{11} = \dfrac{\sigma_\varepsilon \alpha'(1_k \otimes X)P_h \beta}{\rho_1[1 + \alpha'(I_{kn} - \sigma_\varepsilon^2 \Sigma_y^{-1})\alpha]^{1/2}}$, $\eta_{21} = \dfrac{\sigma_\varepsilon^2 \alpha'(1_k \otimes X)P_h(1_k \otimes X)'\alpha}{ak\rho_l[1 + \alpha'(I_{kn} - \sigma_\varepsilon^2 \Sigma_y^{-1})\alpha]}$, and $\eta_2 = \dfrac{\sigma_\varepsilon^2 \alpha'\Sigma_y^{-1}\alpha}{1 + \alpha'(I_{kn} - \sigma_\varepsilon^2 \Sigma_y^{-1})\alpha}$.

# References


Abdel-Karim A H. Application of generalized inference. The Dissertation for the Degree of Doctor of Philosophy, Colorado State University, 2005.

Adhikari S. Matrix variate distribution for probabilistic structural dynamics. AIAA Journal, 2007, 45: 1748–1762.

Arellano-Valle R B and Azzalini A. The centred parametrization for the multivariate skew-normal distribution. Journal of Multivariate Analysis, 2008, 99: 1362–1382.

Arellano-Valle R B, Bolfarine H and Lachos V H. Skew-normal linear mixed models. Journal of Data Science, 2005, 3(4): 415–438.

Arellano-Valle R B, Contreras-Reyes J E and Quintero F O L. A skew-normal dynamic linear model and Bayesian forecasting. Computational Statistics, 2019, 34(3): 1055–1085.

Arendacka B. Generalized confidence intervals on the variance component in mixed linear models with two variance components. Statistics, 2005, 39(4): 275–286.

Arnold B C and Lin G D. Characterizations of the skew-normal and generalized chi distributions. Sankhya, 2004, 66: 593–606.

Azzalini A and Arellano-Valle R B. Maximum penalized likelihood estimation for skew-normal and skew-t distributions. Journal of Statistical Planning and Inference, 2013, 143(2): 419–433.

Azzalini A and Capitanio A. The Skew-normal and Related Families. New York: Cambridge University Press, 2014.

Azzalini A and Dalla Valle A. The multivariate skew-normal distribution. Biometrika, 1996, 83(4): 715–726.

Azzalini A. A class of distributions which includes the normal ones. Scandinavian Journal of Statistics, 1985, 12(2): 171–178.

Azzalini A. The skew-normal distribution and related multivariate families. Scandinavian Journal of Statistics, 2005, 32(2): 159–188.

Balakrishnan N and Scarpa B. Multivariate measures of skewness for the skew-normal distribution. Journal of Multivariate Analysis, 2012, 104: 73–87.

Bartoletti S and Loperfido N. Modelling air pollution data by the skew-normal distribution. Stochastic Environmental Research and Risk Assessment, 2010, 24: 513–517.

Basso R M, Lachos V H and Cabral C R B. Robust mixture modeling based on scale mixtures of skew-normal distributions. Computational Statistics & Data Analysis, 2010, 54(12): 2926–2941.

Burch B D. Confidence intervals for variance components in unbalanced one-way random effects model using non-normal distributions. Journal of Statistical Planning and Inference, 2011, 141(12): 3793–3807.

Carmichael B and Coen A. Asset pricing with skewed-normal return. Finance Research Letters, 2013, 10: 50–57.

Chi E M and Weerahandi S. Comparing treatments under growth curve models: Exact tests using generalized p-values. Journal of Statistical Planning and Inference, 1998, 71(1-2): 179–189.

Contreras-Reyes J E and Arellano-Valle R B. Growth estimates of cardinalfish (Epigonus crassicaudus) based on scale mixtures of skew-normal distributions. Fisheries Research, 2013, 147: 137–144.

Contreras-Reyes J E and Arellano-Valle R B. Kullback-leibler divergence measure for multivariate skew-normal distributions. Entropy, 2012, 14: 1606–1626.

Counsell N, Cortina-Borja M and Lehtonen A. Modelling psychiatric measures using skew-normal distributions. European Psychiatry, 2011, 26: 112–114.

Diggle P. Analysis of Longitudinal Data. New York: Oxford University Press, 2002.

Driscoll M F and Gundberg Jr W R. A history of the development of Craig's Theorem. The American Statistician, 1986, 40(1): 65–70.

Efron B. Bootstrap methods: Another look at the jackknife. The Annals of Statistics, 1979, 7(1): 1–26.

Eling M. Fitting insurance claims to skewed distributions: Are the skew-normal and skew-student good models. Insurance Mathematics & Economics, 2012, 51: 239–248.

Fan Y H and Wang S G. Nonnegative estimates of variance components in two way classification models with random effects. Chinese Journal of Engineering Mathematics, 2007, 24(2): 303–310.

Figueiredo F and Gomes M I. The skew-normal distribution in SPC. Revstat-Statistical Journal, 2013, 11: 83–104.

Fruhwirth-Schnatter S and Pyne S. Bayesian inference for finite mixtures of univariate and multivariate skew normal and skew-t distributions. Biostatistics, 2020, 11(2): 317–336.

Gamage J, Mathew T and Weerahandi S. Generalized p-values and generalized confidence regions for the multivariate Behrens-Fisher problem and MANOVA. Journal of Multivariate Analysis, 2004, 88(1): 177–189.

Genton M G, He L and Liu X. Moments of skew-normal random vectors and their quadratic forms. Statistics & Probability Letters, 2001, 51(4): 319–325.

Genton M G. Discussion of "The Skew-Normal". Scandinavian Journal of Statistics, 2005, 32(2): 189–198.

Ghidey W, Lesaffre E and Eilers P. Smooth random effects distribution in a linear mixed model. Biometrics, 2004, 60: 945–953.

Gilder K, Ting N and Tian L. Confidence intervals on intraclass correlation coefficients in a balanced two-factor random design. Journal of Statistical Planning and Inference, 2007, 137(4): 1199–1212.

Graybill F A and Deal R B. Combining unbiased estimators. Biometrics, 1959, 15(4): 543–550.

Gui W H and Guo L. Statistical inference for the location and scale parameters of the skew normal distribution. Indian Journal of Pure & Applied Mathematics, 2018, 49: 633–650.

Gupta A K and Huang W J. Quadratic forms in skew normal variates. Journal of Mathematical Analysis and Applications, 2002, 273: 558–564.

Gupta A K and Nagar D K. Matrix Variate Distributions. Boca Raton: Chapman and Hall/CRC, 2000.

Gupta A K, Nguyen T T and Sanqui J A T. Characterization of the skew-normal distribution. Annals of the Institute of Statistical Mathematics, 2004, 56: 351–360.

Gupta A K, Varga T and Bodnar T. Elliptically Contoured Models in Statistics and Portfolio Theory (2nd ed.). New York: Springer, 2013.

Gupta R C and Brown N. Reliability studies of the skew-normal distribution and its application to a strength-stress model. Communications in Statistics-theory and Methods, 2001, 30: 2427–2445.

Hannig J, Iyer H and Patterson P. Fiducial generalized confidence intervals. Journal of the American Statistical Association, 2006, 101(473): 254–269.

Hossain A and Beyene J. Application of skew-normal distribution for detecting differential expression to microRNA data. Journal of Applied Statistics, 2015, 42: 477–491.

Hsu B M, Wu C W and Shu M H. Generalized confidence intervals for the process capability index Cpm. Metrika, 2008, 68(1): 65–82.

Hu X Y. Advanced Theory of Probability. Beijing: Science Press, 2009.

Hu Y P, Xue L G and Zhao J. Skew-normal partial functional linear model and homogeneity test. Journal of Statistical Planning and Inference, 2020, 204: 116–127.

Hutton J L and Stanghellini E. Modelling bounded health scores with censored skew-normal distributions. Statistics in Medicine, 2011, 30: 368–376.

Jin L B, Xu W L and Zhu L P. Penalized maximum likelihood estimation for skew normal mixtures (in Chinese). Scientia Sinica Mathematica, 2019, 49: 1225–1250.

Jose K K and Luke J A. Confidence intervals for process capability indices for the unbalanced one way random effect ANOVA model. Quality and Reliability Engineering International, 2012, 28(4): 371–375.

Karlsson S and Skoglund J. Maximum-likelihood based inference in the two-way random effects model with serially correlated time effects. Empirical Economics, 2004, 29: 79–88.

Khatri C G. 14 Quadratic forms in normal variables. Handbook of Statistics, 1980, 1: 443–469.

Kim H M and Genton M G. Characteristic functions of scale mixtures of multivariate skew-normal distributions. Journal of Multivariate Analysis, 2011, 102: 1105–1117.

Krishnamoorthy K and Guo H Z. Assessing occupational exposure via the one-way random effectsmodel with unbalanced data. Journal of Statistical Planning and Inference, 2005, 128(1): 219–229.

Krishnamoorthy K and Lin Y. Confidence limits for stress-strength reliability involving Weibull models. Journal of Statistical Planning and Inference, 2010, 140(7): 1754–1764.

Krishnamoorthy K and Lu Y. Inferences on the common mean of several normal populations based on the generalized variable method. Biometrics, 2003, 59(2): 237–247.

Krishnamoorthy K and Mathew T. Inferences on the means of log-normal distributions using generalized p-values and generalized confidence intervals. Journal of Statistical Planning and Inference, 2003, 115(1): 103–121.

Krishnamoorthy K, Lu F and Mathew T. A parametric bootstrap approach for ANOVA with unequal variances: fixed and random models. Computational Statistics & Data Analysis, 2007, 51(12): 5731–5742.

Krishnamoorthy K, Mallick A and Mathew T. Inference for the log-normal mean and quantiles based on samples with left and right type I censoring. Technometrics, 2011, 53(1): 72–83.

Kundu D and Gupta R D. Estimation of $P[Y<X]$ for Weibull distributions. IEEE Transactions on Reliability, 2006, 55(2): 270–280.

Lachos V H, Dey D K and Cancho V G. Robust linear mixed models with skew-normal independent distributions from a Bayesian perspective. Journal of Statistical Planning and Inference, 2009, 139: 4098–4110.

Laha R G. On the stochastic independence of two second degree polynomial statistics in normally distributed variates. Annals of Mathematical Statistics, 1956, 27: 790–796.

Li X M and Li G Y. Confidence intervals on sum of variance components with unbalanced designs. Communications in Statistics-Theory and Methods, 2005, 34(4): 833–845.

Li X M, Xu X Z and Li G Y. Fiducial inference of Generalized p-value. Science in China, Series A, 2007, 37(6): 733–741.

Li X M. Comparison of confidence intervals on between group variance in unbalanced heteroscedastic one-way random models. Communications in Statistics-Simulation and Computation, 2007, 36(2): 381–390.

Liao X, Peng Z X and Nadarajah S. Asymptotic expansions for moments of skew-normal extremes. Statistics & Probability Letters, 2013, 83: 1321–1329.

Liao X, Peng Z X and Nadarajah S. Rates of convergence of extremes from skew-normal samples. Statistics & Probability Letters, 2014, 84: 40–47.

Lin S H and Lee J C. Exact tests in simple growth curve models and one-way ANOVA with equicorrelation error structure. Journal of Multivariate Analysis, 2003, 84(2): 351–368.

Lin S H and Lee J C. Generalized inferences on the common mean of several normal populations. Journal of Statistical Planning and Inference, 2005, 134(2): 568–582.

Lin T I and Lee J C. Estimation and prediction in linear mixed models with skew-normal random effects for longitudinal data. Statistics in Medicine, 2008, 27: 1490–1507.

Lin T I, Lee J C and Yen S Y. Finite mixture modelling using the skew normal distribution. Statistica Sinica, 2007, 17: 909–927.

Ma C X and Tian L L. A parametric bootstrap approach for testing equality of inverse gaussian means under heterogeneity. Communications in Statistics-Simulation and Computation, 2009, 38(6): 1153–1160.

Ma T F and Wang S G. Test of variance components of linear mixed model. Applied Mathematics—A Journal of Chinese Universities, Series A, 2007, 22(4): 433–440.

Ma Z W, Chen Y J and Wang T H. The inference on the location parameters under multivariate skew normal settings. In Proceedings of the International Econometric Conference of Vietnam, Ho-Chi-Minh City, Vietnam, 14–16 January 2019, pp. 146–162.

Maleki M and Wraith D. Mixtures of multivariate restricted skew-normal factor analyzer models in a Bayesian framework. Computational Statistics, 2019, 34(3): 1039–1053.

Mathew T and Nordstrom K. Wishart and Chi-square distributions associated with matrix quadratic forms. Journal of Multivariate Analysis, 1997, 61: 129–143.

Mathew T and Webb D W. Generalized p values and confidence intervals for variance components: Applications to army test and evaluation. Technometrics, 2005, 47(3): 312–322.

Mathew T, Sebastian G and Kurian K M. Generalized confidence intervals for process capability indices. Quality and Reliability Engineering International, 2007, 23(4): 471–481.

Mazzuco S and Scarpa B. Fitting age-specific fertility rates by a flexible generalized skew normal probability density function. Journal of the Royal Statistical Society, 2015, 178: 187–203.

Montanari A and Viroli C. A skew-normal factor model for the analysis of student satisfaction towards university courses. Journal of Applied Statistics, 2010, 37: 473–487.

Muirhead R J. Aspects of Multivariate Statistical Theory. New York: Wiley, 1982.

Nadarajah S and Li R. The exact density of the sum of independent skew normal random variables. Journal of Computational and Applied Mathematics, 2017, 311: 1–10.

Otiniano C E G, Rathie P N and Ozelim L. On the identifiability of finite mixture of skew-normal and skew-t distributions. Statistics & Probability Letters, 2015, 106: 103–108.

Pan, J J. The joint distribution and asymptotic independence of the quadratic form and linear form of normal variable. Advances in Mathematics, 1966, 9(2): 183–189.

Park J. The generalized p-value in one-sided testing in two sample multivariate normal populations. Journal of Statistical Planning and Inference, 2010, 140(4): 1044–1055.

Pewsey A. Modelling asymmetrically distributed circular data using the wrapped skew-normal distribution. Environmental and Ecological Statistics, 2006, 13: 257–269.

Pewsey A. Problems of inference for Azzalini's skew-normal distribution. Journal of Applied Statistics, 2000a, 27: 859–870.

Pewsey A. The wrapped skew-normal distribution on the circle. Communications in Statistics-theory and Methods, 2000b, 29: 2459–2472.

Pigeon M, Antonio K and Denuit M. Individual loss reserving with the multivariate skew normal framework. Astin Bulletin, 2013, 43: 399–428.

Pinheiro J C, Liu C H and Wu Y N. Efficient algorithms for robust estimation in linear mixed-effects models using a multivariate t-distribution. Journal of Computational and Graphical Statistics, 2001, 10: 249–276.

Roy A and Mathew T. A generalized confidence limit for the reliability function of a two-parameter exponential distribution. Journal of Statistical Planning and Inference, 2005, 128(2): 509–517.

Said K K, Ning W and Tian Y. Likelihood procedure for testing changes in skew normal model with applications to stock returns. Communications in Statistics-Simulation and Computation, 2017, 46(9): 6790–6802.

Scheffe H. Alternative models for the analysis of variance. The Annals of Mathematical Statistics, 1956, 27(2): 251–271.

Sinha S K. Bootstrap tests for variance components in generalized linear mixed models. Canadian Journal of Statistics, 2009, 37(2): 219–234.

Su N C and Gupta A K. On some sampling distributions for skew-normal population. Journal of Statistical Computation and Simulation, 2015, 85: 3549–3559.

Taniguchi M, Petkovic A and Kase T. Robust portfolio estimation under skew-normal return processes. European Journal of Finance, 2015, 21: 1091–1112.

Thiuthad P and Pal N. Hypothesis testing on the location parameter of a skew-normal distribution (SND) with application. In Proceedings of the ITM Web of Conferences, International Conference on Mathematics (ICM 2018) Recent Advances in Algebra, Numerical Analysis, Applied Analysis and Statistics, Tokyo, Japan, 21–22 November 2018, pp. 03003.

Tian L. Interval estimation and hypothesis testing of intraclass correlation coefficients: The generalized variable approach. Statistics in Medicine, 2005, 24(11): 1745–1753.

Tian L. Testing equality of inverse Gaussian means under heterogeneity, based on generalized test variable. Computational Statistics and Data Analysis, 2006, 51(2): 1156–1162.

Tsui K W and Weerahandi S. Generalized p-values in significance testing for hypotheses in the presence of nuisance parameters. Journal of the American Statistical Association, 1989, 84(406): 602–607.

Verbeke G and Lesaffre E. The effect of misspecifying the random effects distribution in linear mixed models for longitudinal data. Computational Statistics & Data Analysis, 1997, 23: 541–556.

Wang S G, Shi J H and Yin S J. Introduction to Linear Models. Beijing: Science Press, 2004.

Wang T H, Li B K and Gupta A K. Distribution of quadratic forms under skew normal settings. Journal of Multivariate Analysis, 2009, 100: 533–545.

Wang T. Versions of Cochran's theorem for general quadratic expressions in normal matrices. Journal of Statistical Planning and Inference, 1997, 58: 283–297.

Wang Z J and Zou C L. Mathematical Statistics Course. Beijing: Higher Education Press, 2014.

Wang Z Y, Wang C and Wang T H. Estimation of location parameter in the skew normal setting with known coefficient of variation and skewness. International Journal of Intelligent Technologies & Applied Statistics, 2016, 9: 191–208.

Weerahandi S and Berger V W. Exact inference for growth curves with intraclass correlation structure. Biometrics, 1999, 55(3): 921–924.

Weerahandi S and Johnson R A. Testing reliability in a stress-strength model when X and Y are normally distributed. Technometrics, 1992, 34(1): 83–91.

Weerahandi S. Exact Statistical Methods for Data Analysis. New York: Springer-Verlag, 1995.

Weerahandi S. Generalized confidence intervals. Journal of the American Statistical Association, 1993, 88(423): 899–905.

Weerahandi S. Generalized Inference in Repeated Measures. New York: John Wiley & Sons, 2004.

Weerahandi S. Testing variance components in mixed models with generalized p-values. Journal of the American Statistical Association, 1991, 86(413): 151–153.

Wimmer G and Witkovský V. Between group variance component interval estimation for the unbalanced heteroscedastic one-way random effects model. Journal of Statistical Computation and Simulation, 2003, 73(5): 333–345.

Wong C S, Masaro J and Wang T. Multivariate versions of Cochran's theorems. Journal of Multivariate Analysis, 1991, 39: 154–174.

Wu J P, Jiang G Y and Wong A C M. Likelihood analysis for the ratio of means of two independent log-normal distributions. Biometrics, 2002, 58(2): 463–469.

Wu L D, Li X P and Bian G R. Probability Theory. Beijing: Higher Education Press, 1979.

Wu L. Mixed Effects Models for Complex Data. Boca Raton: CRC Press, 2009.

Wu M X, Tian Y and Liu A. Robust inference in linear mixed model with skew normal-symmetric error. Frontiers of Mathematics in China, 2017a, 12: 1483–1500.

Wu M X, Yu K F and Liu A. Simultaneous optimal estimation in linear mixed models. Metrika, 2012, 75: 471–489.

Wu M X, Zhao J and Wang T H. The ANOVA-type inference in linear mixed model with skew normal error. Journal of Systems Science and Complexity, 2017b, 30(3): 710–720.

Wu M X. Introduction to the Linear Mixed-Effect Model. Beijing: Science Press, 2013.

Xiong S F, Mu W Y and Xu X Z. Generalized inference for a class of linear models under heteroscedasticity. Communications in Statistics-theory and Methods, 2008, 37(8): 1225–1236.

Xu L W, Mei B and Chen R R. Parametric bootstrap tests for unbalanced nested designs under heteroscedasticity. Journal of Statistical Computation and Simulation, 2014, 84(9): 2059–2070.

Xu L W, Qu K Y and Wu M X. Parametric bootstrap tests for unbalanced three-factor nested designs under heteroscedasticity. Communications in Statistics-Simulation and Computation, 2016, 45(1): 322–338.

Xu L W, Yang F, Chen R R and Yu S H. A parametric bootstrap test for two-way ANOVA model without interaction under heteroscedasticity. Communications in Statistics-Simulation and Computation, 2015, 44(5): 1264–1272.

Xu L W. The Bootstrap Statistical Inference of Complex Data and its Applications. Beijing: Science Press, 2016.

Xu X Z and Liu F. Statistical inference of mixed ration. Science in China, Series A, 2008, 38(1): 106–120.

Yang F Q, Xu L W and Abula A. Parameter bootstrap test of variance component in one-way random effects model. Proceedings of Statistical Education and Applied Statistics Symposium, Beijing, 2012, 234–237.

Ye R D and Jiang L. A parameter bootstrap inference for panel data model. Applied Mathematics—A Journal of Chinese Universities, Series A, 2018, 33(4): 379–386.

Ye R D and Luo K. Statistical Inference Research on Several Mixed Effects Models. Beijing: Science Press, 2016.

Ye R D and Qi J. Bootstrap inference of variance component function in skew-normal one-way classification random effect model. Journal of Applied Statistics and Management, 2022, 41(2): 311–21.

Ye R D and Wang S G. Inferences on the intraclass correlation coefficients in the unbalanced two-way random effects model with interaction. Journal of Statistical Planning and Inference, 2009, 139(2): 396–410.

Ye R D and Wang T H. Inferences in linear mixed models with skew-normal random effects. Acta Mathematica Sinica, English Series, 2015, 31(4): 576–594.

Ye R D, Fang B N and Du W X. Bootstrap tests for the location parameter under the skew-normal population with unknown scale parameter and skewness parameter. Mathematics, 2022, 10: 921.

Ye R D, Ge W T and Luo K. Bootstrap inference on the variance component functions in the two-way random effects model with interaction. Journal of Systems Science and Complexity, 2021, 34: 774–791.

Ye R D, Ge W T and Luo K. Bootstrap inference on variance component functions in the unbalanced two-way random effects model. Communications in Statistics-Simulation and Computation, 2022, 51(9): 5373–5386.

Ye R D, Ma T F and Luo K. Inferences on the reliability in balanced and unbalanced one-way random models. Journal of Statistical Computation and Simulation, 2014, 84(5): 1136–1153.

Ye R D, Ma T F and Wang S G. Inferences on the common mean of several inverse Gaussian populations. Computational Statistics and Data Analysis, 2010, 54(4): 906–915.

Ye R D, Wang T H and Gupta A K. Distribution of matrix quadratic forms under skew-normal settings. Journal of Multivariate Analysis, 2014, 131: 229–239.

Ye R D, Wang T H and Sukparungsee S. Tests in variance components models under skew-normal settings. Metrika, 2015, 78: 885–904.

Ye R D, Xu L J and Luo K. A parametric bootstrap approach for one-way classification model with skew-normal random effects. Applied Mathematics—A Journal of Chinese Universities, 2019, 34(4): 423–435.

Yue L L, Shi J H and Song W X. A parametric bootstrap approach for two-way error component regression models. Communications in Statistics-Simulation and Computation, 2015, 46(5): 3952–3961.

Zacks S. Parametric Statistical Inference. Oxford: Pergamon, 1981.

Zhang D and Davidian M. Linear mixed models with flexible distributions of random effects for longitudinal data. Biometrics, 2001, 57: 795–802.

Zhang D and Davidian M. Linear mixed models with flexible distributions of random effects for longitudinal data. Biometrics, 2001, 57(3): 795–802.

Zhang G Y, Christensen R and Pesko J. Parametric bootstrap and objective Bayesian testing for heteroscedastic one-way ANOVA. Statistics & Probability Letters, 2021, 174: 109095.

Zhao H B. Exact tests in panel data using generalized p-values. Communications in Statistics-Theory and Methods, 2008, 37(1): 18–36.

Zhao J, Cheng W H and Wu M X. Generalized p-value tests of variance components in panel data model. Applied Mathematics—A Journal of Chinese Universities, Series A, 2014, 29(2): 171–179.

Zhao J, Wang S G and Wang L. Exact tests of variance components in nested error components regression model. Chinese Journal of Applied Probability and Statistics, 2014, 30(1): 31–39.

Zhong K L. Probability Theory Course. Beijing: China Machine Press, 2010.

# Index

For Product Safety Concerns and Information please contact our
EU representative GPSR@taylorandfrancis.com Taylor & Francis
Verlag GmbH, Kaufingerstraße 24, 80331 München, Germany